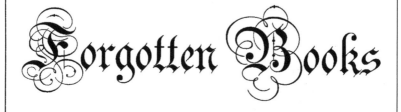

ISBN 978-1-5285-0192-7
PIBN 10109801

1 MONTH OF
FREE
READING

at

www.ForgottenBooks.com

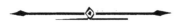

By purchasing this book you are eligible for one month membership to ForgottenBooks.com, giving you unlimited access to our entire collection of over 1,000,000 titles via our web site and mobile apps.

To claim your free month visit:

www.forgottenbooks.com/free109801

THE BRISTOL

Medico-Chirurgical Journal.

A JOURNAL OF THE MEDICAL SCIENCES FOR THE
WEST OF ENGLAND AND SOUTH WALES

PUBLISHED UNDER THE AUS ICES OF

THE BRISTOL MEDICO-CHIRURGICAL SOCIETY.

EDITOR:

R. SHINGLETON SMITH, M.D., B.Sc.,

WITH WHOM ARE ASSOCIATED

J. MICHELL CLARKE, M.A., M.D., W. H. HARSANT,
B. M. H. ROGERS, B.A., M.D., B.Ch., AND JAMES SWAIN, M.S., M.D.

ASSISTANT-EDITOR:

L. M. GRIFFITHS.

EDITORIAL SECRETARY:

JAMES TAYLOR.

———

*"Scire est nescire, nisi id me
Scire alius sciret."*

———

VOL. XVII.

BRISTOL: J. W. ARROWSMITH.
LONDON: J. & A. CHURCHILL, 7 GREAT MARLBOROUGH STREET.
1899.

CONTENTS OF VOLUME XVII.

Page.

The Surgical Treatment of Myoma of the Uterus. By W. ROGER
WILLIAMS, F.R.C.S.   4

A Case of Hysterectomy for Fibroid Tumour of Uterus, with Intra-
Abdominal Treatment of Pedicle. By W. H. C. NEWNHAM,
M.A., M.B. Cantab.   8

Symphysiotomy. By WALTER C. SWAYNE, M.D. Lond...   11

A Case of Acute Ulcerative Endocarditis. By H. L. ORMEROD,
M.D.R.U.I., M.R.C.S., L.R.C.P.   15

Achondroplasia. By CHARLES E. S. FLEMMING, M.R.C.S., L.R.C.P.   21

The Bacteriology of Some Suppurations Complicating Pulmonary
Disease. By J. O. SYMES, M.D., D.P.H.   30

On the Temperature in Cases of Apoplexy, and on the Occurrence
(1) of Œdema and (2) of Loss of the Knee-Jerk in the Paralysed
Limbs in Hemiplegia. By J. MICHELL CLARKE, M.A., M.D.
Cantab., F.R.C.P.   97

Fracture of the Patella. By A. W. PRICHARD, M.R.C.S.   104

Idiopathic Thrombosis of the Portal and Contributory Veins. By
BERTRAM M. H. ROGERS, B.A., M.D., B.Ch. Oxon.   107

A Case of Extreme Bradycardia. By R. GEORGE FENDICK, M.R.C.S.,
and GEORGE PARKER, M.D. Cantab. With Notes on the Eye-
Symptoms by F. RICHARDSON CROSS, M.B. Lond., F.R.C.S. ...   113

A Case of Dislocation of the Hand and Carpus Backwards. By
TRAFFORD MITCHELL, M.D. Glasg.   121

The Antiseptic and Disinfectant Properties of Soap. By J. O. SYMES,
M.D. Lond., D.P.H.   193

CONTENTS.

Page.

On the Treatment of Subacute Bronchitis. By F. H. EDGEWORTH, M.B., B.Sc., B.A. Cantab. 197

Some Groups of Interesting Cases of Abdominal Surgery. By CHARLES A. MORTON, F.R.C.S. Eng. 203

Some Unusual Operations on Lunatics and their Results. By J. PAUL BUSH, M.R.C.S. Eng. 219

A Simple Form of Influence Machine for X-Ray Work. By WILLIAM COTTON, M.A., M.D. Ed. 222

Medical Bristol in the Eighteenth Century. By W. H. HARSANT, F.R.C.S. Eng. 297

The Varieties of Uterine Neoplasms and their Relative Frequency. By W. ROGER WILLIAMS, F.R.C.S. Eng. 314

A Case of Neuritic Muscular Atrophy ("Peroneal" Type). By J. E. SHAW, M.B. Ed. 319

Irreducible Intussusception: with Notes on a Fatal Case. By G. L. KERR PRINGLE, M.D. Ed. 322

PROGRESS OF THE MEDICAL SCIENCES 36, 121, 236, 326

REVIEWS OF BOOKS 50, 138, 254, 342

NOTES ON PREPARATIONS FOR THE SICK 77, 160, 280, 366

MEETINGS OF SOCIETIES 79, 161, 367

THE LIBRARY OF THE BRISTOL MEDICO-CHIRURGICAL SOCIETY 89, 177, 282, 370

LOCAL MEDICAL NOTES 92, 181, 287, 374

SCRAPS 93, 190, 295, 381

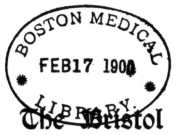
The Bristol
Medico=Chirurgical Journal.

MARCH, 1899.

THE SURGICAL TREATMENT OF MYOMA OF THE UTERUS.

BY

W. Roger Williams, F.R.C.S.

Uterine myomata are of such common occurrence, and they so frequently give rise to serious symptoms, that every practitioner ought to be well acquainted with the chief features of the disease, and with the appropriate therapeutic indications. Modern principles of treatment differ so widely from those hitherto prevalent, that I deem no apology necessary for formulating my views on the subject.

I am not one of those who believe that the mere presence of these tumours is *ipso facto* an indication for operation; for in most cases myomata cause no dangerous symptoms, and in many others such symptoms as do occur may be relieved by palliative treatment. Uterine myomata are less dangerous to life than ovarian cystomata, and their removal is more hazardous; hence radical treatment is only exceptionally required. To justify removal there must be some urgent indication. Probably not more than one-fifth of all cases ever need active surgical intervention, but in about half of these—the patient's life being directly endangered—surgical treatment is urgently called for.

Severe and oft-repeated hemorrhage, undermining the

2

patient's health, is an indication for operative interference, when other treatment has failed. Pressure-symptoms, indicative of dangerous complications (intestinal obstruction, peritonitis, urinary complications, etc.), whether associated with incarceration or not, may also require it. Myomata that have become inflamed, through septic infection, torsion of pedicle or otherwise, must be promptly removed. Tumours complicated with pregnancy may require surgical intervention, when they cause dystocia, and under some other circumstances. It is generally desirable to remove tumours that project into the vagina, and all very large tumours incompatible with comfortable existence. In persons near the climacteric, it is no use putting off operation, in the expectation that the tumour will subside when the catamenia cease; for this is an event that rarely happens, as is evident by noting the large proportion of patients of post-climacteric ages in any statistical list of operations.[1]

In operating for non-malignant uterine tumours, it is well to bear in mind the old surgical maxim, "*Non nocere.*" Healthy organs should not be sacrificed unnecessarily; and it is of great importance to preserve the ovaries, wholly or in part. Two contingencies must be specially provided against; viz., *sepsis* and *hemorrhage.* Strict aseptic precautions are a *sine quâ non;* for it is only by this means that successful results can be attained. For the arrest of hemorrhage, it is necessary to have accurate knowledge of the course and relations of the ovarian and uterine blood-vessels, and of the seats of election for their ligation, compression, etc.

Removal per vaginam.—The removal of myomata that have descended into the vagina is an ancient procedure. It was practically the only form of surgical treatment in vogue, until Amussat,[2] in 1840, opened up the cervix and removed a myoma from within the corpus uteri.

It must be borne in mind that septic infection of myomata

---

[1] Of 250 operated cases tabulated by Péan, 100 were between fifty and sixty years of age, and 70 between forty and fifty. (*Semaine méd.*, Avril 5, 1893.)

[2] *Mém. sur l'anat. path. des tumeurs fibreuses de l'utérus et sur la possibilité d'extirper ces tumeurs, etc.*, 1842.

projecting into the uterus and vagina is a most dangerous complication, which is apt to be caused by any form of traumatism. Consequently vaginal removal should only be attempted when complete extirpation of the tumour seems feasible.   It is a mistake to attempt to imitate the natural process of expulsion by partial operation, by incision into the capsule, by decortication, by gouging or burning the tumour-substance, etc., for in nineteen out of twenty cases the natural efforts at elimination end fatally, and the results of the artificial imitation thereof are hardly less disastrous.   For similar reasons, ligation and torsion of the pedicle are also to be condemned, as well as the use of the *écraseur*, the galvano-cautery snare, and the curette, for all these proceedings favour inflammation and septic infection, of which many fatal instances might be adduced.   In a less degree, the same objection applies also to dilatation of the cervix by sponge tents, laminaria, etc.

The removal of myomata growing into the vagina from the inferior segment of the uterus, and of tumours that have descended from the uterus into the vagina, or that have become engaged in the cervical canal, may generally be best effected by enucleation *per vaginam*.

Pedunculated tumours of no great size are best removed by cutting through the pedicle close to the tumour with scissors curved on the flat.   If feasible, the pedicle may be previously ligatured or seized with pressure-forceps.   A tampon of iodoform gauze is afterwards introduced into the vagina.

As a rule, however, the class of tumours to which I am now referring do not have a distinct pedicle.   Moreover, they are generally solitary, or at any rate only one has attained considerable size.   They are also softer than is usual with most myomata, even when they are not of the " œdematous " variety, to which many of them belong.

Such local conditions as salpingitis, hydro-pyo- and hæmato-salpinx, pelvic and ovarian abscess, generally contra-indicate vaginal extirpation.   The operation is easier in parous women than in nulliparæ.   Care must be taken not to perforate the uterus, and so wound the peritoneum.

The *modus operandi* is as follows :—The field of operation

having been thoroughly disinfected, and the bowels evacuated, the patient is anæsthetised and placed in lithotomy position, with Clover's crutch between the knees. The bladder is then emptied, and the vagina irrigated with antiseptic solution.[1] Simons's specula and retractors will be found invaluable for ensuring a good view of the parts.

An assistant, pressing on the hypogastric region, pushes the uterus downwards ; and the surgeon, seizing the tumour with a powerful volsella, brings it down as far as possible, and with a strong blunt-pointed scissors, a crucial incision is made into its most accessible part. The severed capsule is now peeled off, a blunt enucleator being used to aid the fingers if necessary. The bared part of the tumour is next seized with the volsella, and as it is depressed the capsule is gradually separated right up to its base, when the tumour is shelled out. It may be necessary to remove large tumours piecemeal (*morcellement*), cutting them up with scissors, aided by powerful forceps, such as those introduced by Péan. Bleeding points are seized with pressure forceps, which may generally be removed before the completion of the operation. All but the stump of the capsule is cut away.

In drawing down the tumour, the uterus may be more or less inverted. Provided this is duly recognised, and care is taken to avoid wounding the displaced organ (as also the bladder, which is often displaced as well), such an occurrence facilitates the operation, and there is no difficulty in afterwards correcting the displacement. When the tumour is embedded in the substance of the inferior segment of the uterus, the overlying uterine tissues must be incised, until the capsule is exposed. The tumour is then enucleated as above described. The wound is afterwards tamponed with a long strip of iodoform gauze, which is removed a few days later.

In properly selected cases the dangers of this proceeding are slight : Leopold [2] has had a run of forty-six operations without a single fatality, and Chrobak [3] forty-three operations with but

---

[1] If corrosive sublimate or similar mercurial solutions be employed, they must be weak and used with caution, for many fatal cases of mercurial poisoning have resulted from the intra-uterine injection of such solutions.

[2] *Centralbl. f. Gynäk.*, 1894, xviii. 617.

[3] *Samml. klin. Vortr.*, n.F., 1892, No. 43 (*Gynäk.*, No. 17, 369)

one death. This mode of treatment has the great advantage of removing the disease without mutilating the patient.

For the removal of tumours contained wholly within the uterine cavity, it is best to resort either to some modification of Amussat's proceeding, or to laparotomy—the intra-uterine tumour being removed by modified Cæsarean section. The former procedure is well adapted for dealing with tumours that fall short of the largest dimensions, and for inflamed and suppurating tumours ; the latter is reserved for tumours too large for removal *per vaginam*.

In vaginal extirpation, the first step is to render the tumour accessible. To effect this, the vaginal fornix is divided—anteriorly, or all round if necessary—and the bladder, having been detached from the cervix, is drawn up with a retractor, as in vaginal hysterectomy. The anterior wall of the cervix is then divided by a median longitudinal incision, and the cervical canal is laid open, until the tumour is exposed. The latter is seized with the volsella, drawn down, and deep incision is made into it. One lip of this incision is grasped with morcellation forceps, and all that it holds is cut away. By repetition of this process the whole tumour is removed piecemeal. The gravity of the operation depends much upon the size and condition of the tumour to be removed. Péan has extirpated very large tumours, such as are usually dealt with by laparotomy, in this way, with three deaths in forty operations. Vaginal hysterectomy for myomata, large enough to require removal, is an operation that is hardly ever really called for.

Removal by Abdominal Section.—Abdominal section ought to be regarded as a means for dealing with certain exceptional cases, rather than as the routine operative treatment. Most tumours of the largest size may be included in this category ; as well as subperitoneal tumours, especially such as are stalked and cystic ; interstitial tumours of abdominal evolution, especially when multiple and of considerable size ; intra-ligamentous myomata, and submucous intra-uterine tumours, too large for removal *per vaginam*.

A median incision is made through the abdominal wall below the umbilicus. As the bladder is often unduly elevated, its lower end should be well above the pubes; and the peritoneal sac should be first opened at its upper end. Should there be adhesions between the tumour and the great omentum, intestines, etc., these must be cautiously separated. If the union is too firm for this, omental adhesions are best overcome by excising the adherent portion of the omentum; and intestinal adhesions by excising the peritoneum covering the adherent part of the tumour. If a stalked tumour is found it may be removed, just as if it were an ovarian tumour, by transfixing the pedicle near to the uterus with a blunt needle carrying a double silk thread, each half being tied separately, and the threads cut short. The pedicle is then cut through on the distal side of the ligature, and dropped. The mortality ought not to exceed three or four per cent. As the desirability of sparing the reproductive organs whenever possible, becomes more generally recognised, the superiority of a conservative proceeding, like abdominal enucleation, over any form of hysterectomy will become apparent, especially for comparatively young women, who may bear children after this operation.

Abdominal enucleation is the best means for removing sessile subperitoneal tumours; intra-parietal tumours of abdominal evolution, especially such as grow from the fundus and anterior surface of the uterus; and intra-ligamentous myomata. When the appendages are extensively diseased, hysterectomy may be preferable.

Schröder and Martin have especially identified themselves with the improvement of this operation. The tumour, having been explored and freed from adhesions, is brought up into the wound. To prevent hemorrhage during the operation, a constricting india-rubber cord is temporarily fixed round the uterus below the tumour. To effect this, in some few cases, it may be necessary first of all to divide each broad ligament, after having ligatured the utero-ovarian blood-vessels on both sides (i.) at the pelvic margin near the infundibular pelvic ligament; (ii.) near the uterine insertion of the round ligament. The field of operation is shut off from the rest of the abdomen by packing aseptic sponges or gauze compresses—wrung out in hot sterilised water—round the uterus.

Enucleation is commenced by making a longitudinal incision into the projecting part of the tumour, so as to divide its capsule. The tumour is then seized and shelled out with the fingers, aided by a blunt enucleator. If necessary, it may be cut up and removed piecemeal. Redundant tissue about its bed is cut away, and the cavity is uniformly closed throughout by one or more rows of super-imposed buried catgut sutures. Over these the divided peritoneum is drawn, and its infolded serous margins are united by a row of Lembert's sutures. The elastic constrictor is removed, and any bleeding points are secured. The toilet of the peritoneum is performed. Lastly, the stump is examined, and when satisfactory hæmostasis has been secured, it is dropped into the abdomen, and the operation is completed as in ovariotomy.

Should the uterine cavity be opened, as frequently happens in dealing with large tumours, it may be closed with a continuous catgut suture, over which other rows of buried sutures are placed. Zweifel's[1] results show that there is no scientific basis for the prejudice against opening the uterine cavity, on account of the supposed risk of septic infection; and his experience agrees with the results of bacteriological research, which have repeatedly demonstrated the absence of pathogenic microbes from the healthy uterus. In the highly exceptional event of intractable hemorrhage taking place from the sutured pedicle, the bed of the tumour may be opened up, and plugged with a long strip of iodoform gauze. The margins of the uterine wound are then sutured to the parietal peritoneum at the lower part of the abdominal incision, on each side, the free end of the gauze tampon being brought out at its lower angle. The rest of the abdominal wound is then closed in the usual way. To make assurance doubly sure, Alexander[2] anchors the fundus uteri to the abdominal wound with silkworm-gut sutures, passed through the entire thickness of the latter, and tied externally. When the cavity of the uterus has been opened, some surgeons pack the bed of the tumour with a strip of iodoform gauze, the free end of which is passed into the vagina. Of 141 such

[1] *Centrabl. f. Gynäk.*, 1894, xviii. 321.
[2] *Brit. M. J.*, 1898, i. 1318.

operations by Martin,[1] 26 died, or 18.4 per cent., but th
includes all his early operations before the *technique* was per-
fected ; of the 20 cases reported, only 1 was lost. Engström [2]
has done 100 operations, with only 5 deaths ; but in more than
half his cases the tumours removed were not very large. With
regard to the remaining operations practised for the removal
of myomata, partial hysterectomy (hystero-myomectomy) is
preferable to abdominal panhysterectomy, and the latter is
preferable to panhysterectomy by the "combined method";
but the truth is, the more the field of these mutilating
proceedings is contracted the better.

A CASE OF HYSTERECTOMY FOR FIBROID TUMOUR OF UTERUS, WITH INTRA-ABDOMINAL TREATMENT OF PEDICLE.[3]

BY

W. H. C. NEWNHAM, M.A., M.B. Cantab.,

Physician-Accoucheur, Bristol General Hospital.

I HAVE put together the notes of this case thinking it would be
of interest to the Society, inasmuch as it is the first operation
of this description that has been done in Bristol.

It is a far more satisfactory operation than the old one of
treating the pedicle with some kind of mechanical clamp outside
the abdominal wall, for the following reasons :—

(1) It is absolutely aseptic, while in the old operation there
was always danger of suppuration of the pedicle.

(2) No mechanical means are required for arresting hemorrhage, as all vessels are tied at the time of division.

(3) There is no drag on the pedicle and practically no risk
of peritonitis.

[1] *Deutsche med. Wchnschr.*, 1893, xix. 709.

[2] *Mitth. a. d. gynaek. Klin. d. O. Engström in Helsingfors*, 1897, i. 1.

[3] Paper read before the Bristol Medico-Chirurgical Society,
January 11th, 1899.

(4) Bland Sutton asserts (and certainly has proved it in his own operations) that this method possesses no more risk than an ordinary ovariotomy. The latest statistics shew that the mortality is less than it was with the old fashioned operation, which the late Mr. Greig Smith clung to even to the end of his life.

The patient, M. H., aged 35, was sent to me by Dr. Freeman on November 1st, 1898. She had had two children, the last ten years ago. Menstruation commenced at the age of 13, always lasted five to six days, and was always excessive.

About a year before admission patient had noticed some swelling of the abdomen; at the same time she had great pain in this region, which varied in intensity. Four months ago she noticed the swelling had increased considerably in size and was causing still more pain: her periods also now became more excessive.

On examination there was a large, soft, semi-fluctuating tumour to be felt in the median line of the abdomen, rising out of the pelvis. It was extremely painful if handled at all; the sound passed three inches, and the tumour was apparently in front of the uterus itself. By some of my colleagues it was thought it might be the bladder or some diverticulum of that organ.

On November 10th, the patient being placed under ether, I made a long incision into the abdominal cavity, and at once brought out a large fibroid tumour (produced) growing from the fundus of the uterus. A pedicle needle threaded with stout silk was passed through the broad ligament, and the ovarian arteries and veins were ligatured on each side and cut away from the uterus. The ovaries were left untouched, this being considered a very important part of the operation. It is not at all necessary to remove the ovaries, and it is considered much better for the patient to retain them if possible.

The pedicle needle was now pushed through the broad ligament on each side below the uterine arteries, and these were ligatured after some slight difficulty. This appears to be the most difficult step of the operation.

A semi-circular incision was now made with the convexity upwards on the anterior aspect of the uterus, below the point where the tumour joined the body of the uterus: a similar flap was made posteriorly in the same manner, and then the tumour and upper part of the uterus were cut away, carrying the knife down deeply below the flaps and taking away as much as possible. A few bleeding points in the flaps were tied, and then they were brought into exact apposition by means of silk sutures sewn deeply through the flaps. Then, there being no hemorrhage, the pedicle was dropped into the pelvis and the abdominal wall sutured in the ordinary manner.

The patient was put to bed, and from that time had not a bad symptom. She was able to get up on November 28th, or eighteen days after the operation.

Now, is not this a contrast to the old hysterectomy, with a sloughing pedicle hanging out from the abdominal wall with foul pus discharging from the stump, the chance of peritonitis from dragging on the pedicle, the risk of hemorrhage which may easily be fatal from slipping or loosening of the clamp, the danger of some drop or so of foul pus getting into the peritoneal cavity, the separation and final healing of the stump not taking place for many weary weeks? Whereas this patient runs no risk, but is well and walking about on the eighteenth day after the operation.

———

In the discussion on Dr. Newnham's case, Dr. AUST LAWRENCE stated that this mode of operation would in the future in a good many cases be preferred to the old plan of fixing the stump outside the abdomen, and he looked forward to the mortality being very much reduced in this class of operation. Dr. Aust Lawrence, however, spoke against any operation being done in a large number of cases of myoma uteri, as the symptoms did not warrant interference in at least 80 per cent. of the cases.—Mr. ROGER WILLIAMS suggested that the operation done in this case might more appropriately be called " Abdominal myomectomy," since nothing but the tumour was removed. He was glad to see that the importance of preserving as much as possible of the reproductive organs was now beginning to be recognised. For the treatment of a non-malignant disease like myoma of the uterus, he thought myomectomy was a much superior operation to hysterectomy, which should be reserved for a few exceptional cases not otherwise operable. After myomectomy, women might bear healthy children; and with Zweifel's *technique*, the mortality of myomectomy was only about 5 per cent.—Dr. WALTER SWAYNE, recalled to the recollection of those present a paper by Stuart Nairne, of Glasgow *(Prov. Med. Journ.*, 1889*)*, in which he not only dealt in this manner with the stump after hysterectomy, but related a long series of cases of myomectomy with most successful results. The retaining of the ovaries, if healthy, apart from the quicker convalescence, was a great advantage of the more modern method of operating. In considering the relations between the success of the intraperitoneal and extraperitoneal methods of treatment, it should be remembered that many of the former cases were operated on for small tumours, and the results were likely to be superior to those in cases where large tumours with dense adhesions existed; apart from this, however, the more modern method was undoubtedly superior to the old, and no doubt would become generally adopted in the future.— Mr. CARWARDINE spoke in favour of hysterectomy by retroperitoneal treatment of the stump when possible.—Mr. MORTON thought that though the treatment of the pedicle by constriction with a wire in the extraperitoneal method seemed a barbarous and unsurgical proceeding, yet it was well to remember that it had a smaller mortality than the intraperitoneal method, and that was the main consideration. We could not, of course, judge of the respective merits of the two methods unless we had a series of cases treated by each ; one case was of no value for such a purpose. He thought the best plan was to begin the operation with everything prepared for either method, and then to be guided by the condition of the growth. He thought, from an examination of the specimen, that Dr. Newnham's case was one particularly suited for the intraperitoneal method.— In reply, Dr. NEWNHAM said : It is evident that Mr. Morton has not seen the latest statistics on the subject of mortality, for in the hands of

Bland Sutton and some German surgeons the mortality is reduced to the same level as the rate for ordinary ovariotomy. It is manifestly very easy to open the abdomen and remove a fibroid with an ordinary thin pedicle; but the difficulty arises when it is necessary to remove the tumour and the greater part of the uterus itself, the one not being capable of being distinguished from the other.

SYMPHYSIOTOMY.

BY

WALTER C. SWAYNE, M.D. Lond.,

Obstetric Physician to the Bristol Royal Infirmary.

THIS operation was originally proposed by Sigault, a French medical student, in 1768, as a substitute for Cæsarean section, and he performed the first successful operation in 1778, as a result of which it was warmly advocated and often performed for a few years; the first operation in England being performed by Welchman, a Warwickshire surgeon, in 1782. As, however, the results proved disappointing, the maternal mortality being very high and not much inferior to that after Cæsarean section, being about 33 per cent. in the former to 42 per cent.[2] in the latter case, it fell into disuse in a comparatively short time. Being revived by Morisani, of Naples, in 1866, it was practised with greater success, and, the mortality falling greatly on the introduction of antiseptic methods, rose again into favour; and at the present time a large number of cases of recent date are on record.

Originally introduced as a substitute for Cæsarean section, it has now come to be regarded as the proper substitute for craniotomy, since, although the maternal mortality is rather larger, the child, instead of certain destruction awaiting it, has a very good chance of survival. It has also been performed deliberately at term in cases of contracted pelvis instead of the induction of premature labour, and here the results as

---

[1] Read before the Bristol Medico-Chirurgical Society, December 14th, 1898.

[2] Churchill's *Midwifery.*

regards the life of the fœtus are also very much better, but the maternal mortality is higher. The combined mortality rate in the hands of Pinard and Tarnier[1] respectively is 18.36 for the former in symphysiotomy, and 20.29 for the latter in induced labour. As a substitute for craniotomy it is always performed as an operation of emergency, and it is under this head that the operation described in this paper was performed.

The general indications for its use may be briefly stated as follows:—(1) Absolute contraction of the pelvis when the conjugate diameter is above 2¾ inches; (2) relative contraction when the fœtal head, not being enlarged by hydrocephalus, is too large to pass through a normal sized or only slightly contracted pelvis. It is not suitable for cases in which a tumour impacted in the pelvis or bony outgrowth prevents the descent of the head. An essential condition for its performance is, that the child should be alive. The time for operating is when the first stage of labour is complete or almost complete, and the cervix so dilated as to allow of the easy application of the forceps and the passage of the head through it. It should not be performed for rigidity of the soft parts, or when great rigidity is present. Most careful attention to antiseptic measures is necessary, and the patient should as far as possible be prepared as if for an abdominal section, the pubes being shaved and the skin cleansed as perfectly as circumstances will admit. The operation itself is performed by two methods—the subcutaneous and the open methods. The former is the preferable, as the longer the incision in this region the greater the difficulty in preventing contamination of the wound. All that is necessary is, that the incision should be of sufficient length to allow of the free passage of the finger behind the pelvic articulation.

Two assistants are necessary in addition to the anæsthetist, as after section of the joint care must be taken to avoid the too wide separation of the bones during the passage of the head through the pelvis. The dangers to the patient are from hemorrhage and sepsis : the first, however, is easily controlled, and the second should not be likely nowadays. The open method by long incision is said to cause less hemorrhage, since

---

[1] *Presse méd.*, 1895, 265.

this is usually produced by laceration of the soft parts and vessels around the joint on its separation, but the increased risk of contamination rightly seems to render the subcutaneous method preferable. The most experienced operators do not consider that wiring or suturing the bones together is of any material advantage, and in several cases partial necrosis of the bones and troublesome fistulæ have resulted where this method of treatment has been adopted. The gain in space which is the result of the operation is as follows :—As much as 1¼ inches may be gained as a maximum : that is, when the maximum divergence consistent with the integrity of the sacro-iliac joints is caused, the divergence is just about three inches, and beyond this it should never be allowed to pass. Since the transverse diameter increases very nearly to the same extent as does the distance between the separated ends of the bone, it is obvious what an increase in the sectional area of the pelvic canal can be gained. In the case described the true conjugate was estimated at 2¾ inches; and as the separation of the bones during the extraction was about 2¼ inches, nearly an inch was gained in the antero-posterior and about 2¼ inches in the transvere diameters bringing the available space up to that required for an ordinary forceps extraction, namely, to 3¾ inches antero-posterior, and to considerably more than the normal in the transverse, which, although not measured, was obviously contracted, though not to so great an extent as the antero-posterior. The following is the history of the case:—

Mrs. S., aged 25, primipara, at the full term of pregnancy. Labour pains commenced at 3 a.m. on the 22nd of October, 1898. A midwife attended her, and finding that no progress had been made by the evening of that day, administered a grain of opium in pill. Twenty-four hours later, as the head did not advance, she called in a medical man, who, finding on examination that the pelvis was very contracted, advised her removal to the Bristol Royal Infirmary, to which she was admitted on the evening of the 23rd of October. On admission her condition was as follows :—

The patient is a small woman, showing marked signs of rickets. The abdomen, distended by the enlarged uterus, is more than usually prominent, and the fundus uteri reaches to the ensiform cartilage; the pains strong, and recurring every five minutes. Abdominal palpation shows that the fœtus is lying in the third position, the head presenting; the fœtal movements vigorous, and the uterine contractions strong and regular. On auscultation the fœtal heart is heard to the right of the middle line and below the umbilicus, rate about 140 to the minute. The head was felt to be above the brim, and could not be pressed down into the pelvis. On vaginal examination the promontory of the sacrum was easily reached, and the diagonal conjugate was found to be 3¼ inches, the os nearly fully dilated, and the soft parts soft and dilatable. The transverse diameter was also found to be lessened, and the ilio-pectineal line within easy reach throughout its whole length. After an attempt to effect delivery with axis-traction forceps—which, as expected, was unsuccessful,—it was decided to attempt delivery by symphysiotomy. After careful cleansing of the external parts and skin, an incision about 1¼ inches long was made just above the upper edge of the pubes in the middle line, and carried down for a short distance through the soft parts below the upper level of the symphysis, but not extending more than half an inch below. The incision was carried above through the interval of the tendons of the recti, and a short transverse incision was made to the left side to allow of the introduction of the finger, when the posterior surface of the symphysis was cleared and a sickle-shaped Galbiati's knife introduced, and the separation of the fibro-cartilage commenced above in order to obtain a groove to guide the blade, as the joint was found to be to the left of the middle line. The knife was then carried down the back of the joint and its probe-pointed end made to project against the anterior vaginal wall, the urethra being pressed to one side by means of a sound. The knife was then worked through the joint from below upwards and behind forwards, and the joint divided. The two halves of the pelvis at once sprang apart, separating about an inch, and rather free hemorrhage occurred. This was controlled by iodoform gauze pushed into the wound. The wound was now covered with a sponge-cloth wrung out of hydrarg. perchlor. solution 1—1000. The head immediately descended to a certain extent, and the axis traction forceps were applied. Under steady, but not too strong, traction the head descended, the patient's thighs being supported by two assistants, and delivery effected in about twenty-five minutes. The placenta was expressed twenty minutes later, and a slight laceration of the perineum repaired and the uterus washed out with hot perchloride of mercury solution (1—3000). The superficial wound was sewn up with silkworm-gut sutures, two stitches taking up the fibrous structures on the front of the bone, the packing pressed backwards from between the bones, the bones pressed together, and the sutures tied, the pelvis being brought together by strong traction on the ends of a long piece of unbleached calico bandage passed around the pelvis, the wound dressed with iodoform gauze, and a strong bandage fixed firmly around the pelvis.

The further progress of the case was uneventful. The wound united by first intention, except a small portion at the lower end where the skin adaptation was not quite accurate. The temperature on two occasions reached 100° F. The sutures were removed on the sixth day. The calico support to the pelvis was replaced on the third day by a strong webbing belt tightly buckled around the ilia, while a second belt encircled the trochanters. The catheter was used for the first four days. The patient was allowed out of bed on the twentieth day, and went home on the twenty-eighth day. She has had no disturbance of locomotion, and walked over two miles to be shown at a medical meeting in the seventh week after operation. The child, a male, was born alive, and at birth its condition was as follows: Weight, 8 lbs.; length, 21 ins. Measurements of the head: Maximum vertico-mental diameter, 5¼ ins.; sub-occipito bregmatic diameter, 3¾; occipito-frontal, 4¼; fronto-mental, 3½; biparietal, 3⅜; bitemporal, 3¼; bimastoid, 3. The child, now three months old, weighs 12 lbs., and seems perfectly healthy. The mother was able to nurse it; she did so for six weeks entirely, and still does so partially.

I examined the mother on January 14th, as she complained of some prolapse of the anterior vaginal wall. I found the symphysis with a separation of about ⅜ inch, apparently perfectly firm, and the conjugate diameter not appreciably altered; otherwise she appeared to be in perfect health.

The conditions under which the operation was performed were extremely favourable. Labour was not so far advanced as to prejudice the mother's chance of recovery; in fact, the os was only fully dilated just before the application of the forceps; plenty of assistants were at hand, a good light and all appliances for carrying out antiseptic and aseptic methods; but at the same time the difficulties which would arise in less favourable circumstances are not insuperable, and the operation itself is not in reality much more difficult than a severe craniotomy, which latter, if a living child is to be operated on, is a most loathsome proceeding. For the very careful notes of the case I am indebted to Mr. A. L. Flemming, resident obstetric officer, and Mr. P. G. Stock.

After the reading of Dr. W. C. Swayne's paper, Dr. J. G. SWAYNE said that about 1777, when the operation was first introduced, his grandfather, Dr. Griffiths, was beginning his medical education, and afterwards practised in this city more than fifty years. Mr. J. C. Swayne, Dr. J. G. Swayne's father, was Dr. Griffiths's apprentice; he passed the College of Surgeons in 1808, and practised for forty years in Bristol, until he retired in 1848. If symphysiotomy had ever been performed here, he would have heard of it from his grandfather, father, or Mr. Richard Smith, the senior surgeon to the Bristol Infirmary. This was almost certainly the first case in which the operation had been performed in this city.

A CASE OF ACUTE ULCERATIVE ENDOCARDITIS.[1]

BY

H. L. ORMEROD, M.D.R.U.I., M.R.C.S., L.R.C.P.

CASES of ulcerative or malignant endocarditis are always interesting, but my special reasons for bringing this one before the Society are:

(1) Its unusual acuteness.

(2) The persistent pyrexia, without any rigor or marked remission in temperature.

(3) It is another example of the value of Widal's test in cases of, or resembling, enteric fever.

[1] Read before the Bristol Medico-Chirurgical Society, November 9th, 1898.

The patient was a farmer, aged twenty-nine years, of some-what slight build, who, with the exception of occasional mild rheumatic attacks, none of which were sufficiently severe to induce him to consult a medical man, had always enjoyed good health.   There is nothing of interest in the family history.

first saw him on Monday, October 17th, 1898.   He then told me that for the past week or ten days he had felt tired, and suffered a good deal from headache and pains in the back and limbs, but had continued his work until the previous day; the bowels had acted regularly each day, and he had not observed anything unusual about the motions.   For some days he had been suffering from a small sore on the outer side of the left heel, caused by his boot, but had had no tenderness or enlarge-ment of the lymphatic glands, nor could I get any history of lymphangitis.

When I first saw him he was up and dressed, complaining of general malaise, frontal headache, pain in lower part of the back and limbs, chiefly in the larger joints, and of some slight cough, with rusty-coloured tenacious expectoration. There was no history of shivering.   Temperature was 103°, skin just moist, no redness of joints and no effusion into them, but slight tenderness over them and some pain on movement. Respirations about twenty per minute, and no abnormal sounds to be heard in the lungs.   There was, however, a loud diastolic aortic murmur, with, so far as I could ascertain, very little if any displacement of the apex-beat.   Pulse about 100.   Tongue clean and moist, and abdomen apparently normal.   I suspected that he was suffering from a small patch of deep-seated pneumonia, and possibly influenza.   I ordered him to bed, and treated him with salicylate of sodium, with liquor ammoniæ acetatis and sal volatile.

For the first five days of my attending him he appeared to be progressing satisfactorily; the temperature ranged from 103°—104°, cough and expectoration diminished, the cardiac bruit did not alter in character.   The bowels continued to act once each day, the motions being dark-coloured and formed; tongue remained moist and was very little furred; there was still, however, some headache and pains in the joints, especially shoulders, elbows, hips and knees, with tenderness over them, but no effusion; and although I could not detect any abnormal physical signs in the lungs, I saw no reason to change my diagnosis. On the evening of the fifth day patient was a little delirious, and when I saw him on the sixth day (Saturday) was certainly worse. Temperature was 104°, but the pulse and respiration had risen to 120 and 24 respectively; still, there was no alteration in the physical signs of the chest. The tongue was becoming dry; abdomen a little flatulent, with some tenderness over region of the bladder, but no gurgling over cæcum, and no typhoid spots; the spleen extended to edge of the ribs; there was still a little delirium; no deafness, but some slight tinnitus, probably due to the salicylate of sodium, I thought, and the patient answered questions sharply. Pupils equal and of about the normal size, reacted readily to light; skin much more moist; trace of albumen, but no blood in urine, and some tremor of muscles. The patient was lying on his back, but he had done so all through the illness, on account of the pain in the shoulders. The next day (Sunday) pulse had risen to over 140, and respiration to 36; delirium continued, tongue was dryer; three light-coloured loose motions had been passed in the previous twenty-four hours; spleen could be distinctly felt just below edge of ribs; there was no increase of abdominal distension, but slight gurgling over the cæcum; no typhoid spots, but two small patches of petechiæ—one just over the left anterior superior iliac spine, and the other in right hypochondrium; tremor much more marked and subsultus present. Towards night, delirium increased, temperature rose to 105°, and urine was passed unconsciously. At midday next day patient would still answer questions rationally, pulse and respiration 144 and 48 respectively; the aortic diastolic bruit was still the only murmur present; there was some impaired resonance and bronchial breathing at the base of left lung, but no crepitation or sign of any general bronchial catarrh. Dozens of petechiæ over chest, abdomen, back, and especially the extremities, those on the hands and feet being the largest. There was no evidence of any affection of the cranial nerves. Abdomen a little more distended, but no tenderness, and no action of the bowels since the previous

3

morning. The blood did not give the typhoid reaction to
Widal's test. The patient gradually became more and more
drowsy, general diffuse râles became audible over both lungs;
temperature rose steadily to 106.2°, and in spite of 30 grs.
of quinine and frequently-repeated doses of phenacetin, together with cold sponging, only fell to 104.6° before death,
which took place early next morning, or on the ninth day of
my attendance.

At the *post-mortem* examination, made thirty-two hours after
death, in which Dr. J. O. Symes kindly assisted me, the heart
was found to be a little enlarged, the left ventricle being hypertrophied. The aortic valves, which were incompetent and also
considerably thickened and puckered, had several small vegetations upon them and also some ulceration ; there were also
two small patches of lymph upon, and slight ulceration of, the
endocardium of the left ventricle, otherwise the heart appeared
normal. There were petechial patches over the visceral pleura ;
but the lungs, with the exception of considerable engorgement
and *post-mortem* changes, were normal. Spleen was about twice
the natural size, studded with small infarcts ; the kidneys
also were dotted with petechiæ and a few infarcts ; the intestines normal ; liver normal. We could not obtain leave
to examine the brain. Cultures were subsequently made
from the infarcts by Dr. Symes, and found to consist of pure
streptococci ; and in sections of the aortic valves, kindly made
for me by Mr. A. L. Flemming, are to be seen streptococci and
staphylococci.

The complete absence of any rigor or of marked remissions
in the temperature, which are so characteristic of ulcerative
endocarditis, made the nature of the case somewhat uncertain ;
indeed, until after the fifth day, I saw no reason to doubt the
original diagnosis of a small deep-seated pneumonia. At about
this date, however, the enlarged spleen and typhoidal condition of
the patient led me to strongly suspect enteric fever, especially with
the history of an indefinite onset of about ten days, followed by
the continued pyrexia ; still the rapid downward progress of the
case, with the absence of deafness, bronchial catarrh, or definite
intestinal symptoms, with the exception of the loose motions on

one day, combined with the clean tongue and mental acuteness of the patient, seemed strongly against this view, and pointed rather to a form of septicæmia, and my opinion was subsequently strengthened by the absence of the Widal reaction. With the exception of the small sore on the foot previously referred to, and which did not appear to have caused any constitutional symptoms, I could discover no external source, and was thus led to a diagnosis of ulcerative endocarditis of the acute typhoidal type.   I regret, however, that no cultures were made from the blood before death.

These cases are quite different in their clinical symptoms from the more common forms of ulcerative endocarditis, namely, the subacute and chronic cases, and are especially severe and fatal, the patient usually being seized with a rigor when apparently in good health, or convalescent from an acute illness, especially rheumatism, and are said by Mitchell Bruce to always result in death within fourteen days ; in fact, a case has been known to terminate fatally in two days. The failure of every means of cure hitherto employed in these acute cases serves to impress on us the importance of preventive treatment ; to protect subjects with chronic valvular disease against zymotic diseases, and also attend with special care to the treatment of suppuration. When ulceration has occurred, the case must be managed on the general principles applicable to all acute specific fevers.   Drugs in great variety have been tried with little benefit, including mercurials, quinine, and other antipyretics, eucalyptus, turpentine, salicylates, and sulphocarbolates. The two latter have, however, been attended with success in a few instances in the chronic form of the disease. During the past few months some cases have been treated with injections of the anti-streptococcus serum, and although some good may very possibly be done in the subacute or chronic cases, so far as I can find, no acute case has been successfully treated by this means, and, indeed, from the rapidly fatal issue of these cases, so powerful a dose of the serum would be required that the percentage of recoveries by this means of treatment would be extremely small.

In conclusion, in addition to Dr. Symes and Mr. Flemming

for pathological help, I must thank Dr. Shingleton Smith for clinical assistance in the case.

In the discussion which followed the reading of Dr. Ormerod's case, Dr. SHINGLETON SMITH commented on the rarity of these cases of acute fulminating septic endocarditis. He alluded to the difficulty of differentiating them from enteric fever, and to the utility of the Widal test for this purpose. In allusion to the streptococcic serum, he stated that his experience of it in a fatal case of pemphigus foliaceus had not been favourable.—Dr. WALDO said this case bears out the view that when pneumonia is associated with ulcerative endocarditis the latter is of an unusually malignant type. There are present in this condition all the signs of septic infection, and, as Wilks has well said, this disease should be regarded as one of arterial pyæmia. The treatment, in his experience, was always unfavourable. He had administered intestinal antiseptics of various kinds, and had given perchloride of mercury hypodermically, but, he must confess, with very little good result.—Dr. B. M. H. ROGERS showed a heart with large vegetations on two of the aortic valves, which was taken from the body of a gipsy girl, aged 11, who died in the Children's Hospital, after only three days' illness. She was taken ill on a Thursday, and when admitted to the Hospital was practically moribund. A loud murmur was heard over the base of the heart, its loudest spot being over the pulmonary artery. At the necropsy the left ventricle wall was found to be much hypertrophied, and two vegetations were present on the aortic valves. There were no infarcts found anywhere. For some months previous to her fatal illness, her parents had noticed that her abdomen was much enlarged, and at the necropsy this was ascertained to be due to a much enlarged spleen. The substance of this organ was very hard, not friable as is usually met with in cases of malignant endocarditis. He mentioned this case to illustrate the exceedingly rapidly fatal issue that may follow infection of this sort, death resulting after only three days' illness.—Dr. G. PARKER said that in a case of ulcerative endocarditis recently under his care the patient's blood showed the presence of staphylococcus albus, but no serum at present existed which had any effect upon this organism. He had used the streptococcal serum as well as quinine, and injections of corrosive sublimate, without influencing the course of the disease.—Dr. J. O. SYMES said that the organism in Dr. Ormerod's case proved on cultivation to be the streptococcus longus, and colonies of the same were found in sections of the valves. The blood did not give Widal's reaction. In another case, with well-marked vegetations on the valves, no organisms could be found in the tissues after death. He did not regard this as a true infective endocarditis. For purposes of diagnosis, two or three cubic centimetres of blood should be taken from a vein and cultures made. Treatment by anti-streptococcus serum was a specific treatment, and useless against other infections.—Dr. WALTER SWAYNE said it was important to know if those who had used the anti-streptococcic serum largely had noticed any ill effects to follow ; it was generally stated that ill effects were not experienced, and, that being so, it would appear that the empirical use of the serum was not only justifiable, but to be recommended, since the difficulty of identifying scientifically a true case of streptococcic infection was not only great but required time which might be of the greatest value. He would feel inclined to use the serum in suspected cases without waiting for bacteriological verification of the true source of the poisoning, although such a course might be said to be scientifically incorrect. —Dr. F. H. EDGEWORTH said that though a definite diagnosis during life of infective endocarditis could only be made in the presence of three phenomena—a heart-murmur, fever, and infective emboli—and this endocarditis could only be held to be definitely due to streptococci when examination of the blood proved their presence; yet insomuch as this form of endocarditis was in the majority of cases due to these particular micro-organisms and there was no evidence that the injection of anti-streptococcic serum ever did harm, it was permissible for one to use this method of treatment in cases where the evidence was incomplete. He had found in several cases of rheumatic fever with endocarditis, where the fever continued after the arthritis had subsided and there was no lesion other than the cardiac one to account for the fever, that an injection of anti-streptococcic serum had caused a rapid disappearance of the fever, whilst apparently the cardiac mischief did not subsequently further advance.—Mr. ROGER WILLIAMS mentioned that in certain cases of acute mastitis with septic complications the latter had been found to be due to the presence of staphylococci, which some pathologists thought were harmless, and he asked whether any analogous condition was found in ulcerative endocarditis.

ACHONDROPLASIA.[1]

BY

CHARLES E. S. FLEMMING, M.R.C.S., L.R.C.P.

ACHONDROPLASIA, more pleasantly but less properly called fœtal rickets, though not common, is of sufficient importance in its after-effects to be of more interest than a mere pathological curiosity. It is a disease of intra-uterine life, characterised by great shortness of the limbs, which are bent and markedly out of proportion to a fully developed trunk, and an enlarged abdomen. The head is rather large, and there is considerable thickening of the skin of the whole body.

Mrs. H., an anæmic, but otherwise healthy woman, mother of one healthy child, was in the eighth month of her pregnancy confined of a stillborn male child; the second stage was prolonged, and owing to the soft state of the head there was some

---

[1] A Paper read before the Bath and Bristol Branch of the British Medical Association, November 30th, 1898.

difficulty in diagnosing the presentation, which was first vertex. The child died, apparently during labour. The placenta was normal in appearance. The child had a remarkable appearance.

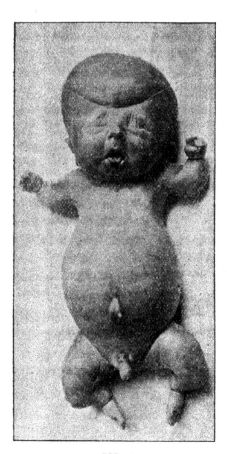

FIG. I.

Photograph of Stillborn Child affected with Achondroplasia. Reduced one-fourth.

(Fig. I.) Except for the enlarged belly, there was little to note in the trunk; the head was rather large, but so soft and shapeless that the nurse's description of it as " real pudden-headed " was not hyperbolical; its condition is well shown by the mark of the string which had to be used to hold it in position for photographing. Only towards the base of the skull could any resisting bone be felt. The face was expressionless and heavy, the nose wide and flat, and the skin about the face and neck appeared very thick, so much so that in the neck it was in a large fold. The most marked deformity was in the limbs; these were very short in proportion to the trunk, markedly curved and bent, with relatively small hands and feet. The width from shoulder to shoulder was normal, but the arms were very short and deformed; the arm and forearm both bent to nearly a right angle, the concavity being forwards and inwards; in addition the wrists were strongly pronated. For the purpose of photographing, the body was "displayed proper," as they say in heraldry, so that the pronation is less marked in the picture than it was in reality. The hands were very small, but not deformed.

The legs, like the arms, were short and bent; the curve of the thigh was a double one, and not so acute as in the arm; the most marked curve was at about the junction of the lower and middle thirds, and had its concavity forwards; above this was a slight curve backwards, and a little inwards. The legs had the most marked deformity of all, being bent backwards to less than a right angle. The feet were in a position of equino-varus, due to deformity rather of the leg than of the tarsus.

The skin was everywhere thickened, and on section it was clear that this thickening was due to an increase in the deeper areolar layer, and not merely to an increase in the subcutaneous fat; and in the penis, where there is no fat, the skin was markedly thick. The tongue appeared too large for the mouth, as it does in those cases of sporadic cretinism where there is a great increase of connective tissue at its root.

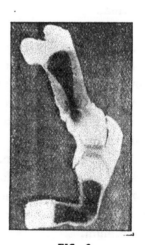

FIG. 2.

Photograph of longitudinal section of Femur and Tibia from the same case. Four-fifths actual size.

There was no gross nor microscopical change in the thyroid, and all the organs of the thorax and abdomen appeared normal. The cartilaginous epiphyses of the long bones (Fig. 2) were enlarged in every direction, and did not present the usual white line at their junction with the diaphyses.

The bones were easily cut with a knife from end to end; the shafts of the long bones had merely a thin casing of bone (owing to the obliquity of the section, this appears thicker in the femur than it really was), and the cancellous bone inside felt only gritty to the knife. The cranial bones were no stiffer than a sheet of writing paper. The clavicle and ribs, though soft, were normal in shape and size, and the pelvis presented no marked deformity.

When examining the minute anatomy of the cartilage in a section of a normal epiphysis at the same period of fœtal life, we see from above downwards the oval masses of proliferating

cartilage cells, the calcification of their capsules and the formation of the primary areolæ, then the excavation of the secondary
areolæ in this calcified cartilage by the osteoclasts, and finally
the deposition of new bone on the walls of the secondary areolæ
by the osteoblasts.   Now in a section of the same bone, tibia,
from the case of achondroplasia, we see a sparseness of the
proliferating cartilage cells, and only a few calcified capsules
with shrunken cells, *i.e.*, a deficiency of the primary areolæ,
and the proliferating cells abut immediately on a mass of
osteoblasts and osteoclasts in which are but few calcified
or ossifying trabeculæ; it is noteworthy that the process,
such as it is, is fairly regular.   Further on, in the shaft,
we find great quantities of these round cells and a few
bony trabeculæ, but the periosteal layer of bone appears fairly
normal.

In the section of a parietal bone we see greatly delayed
ossification.   The appearance of the cartilage suggests no loss
of power to grow, but an almost complete incapacity to carry
out its bone-forming duties; the cells grow, but refuse to calcify,
and the round cells crowd round and absorb them, the deficient
calcification apparently interfering with the ossifying function
of the osteoblasts.

It would seem then, that while owing to some dystrophy the
skeleton maintained for a long while its embryonic form, there
was some special affection of the epiphyseal cartilage whereby
its ossification was not only delayed but reduced almost to a
minimum.

While then the periosteum is forming bone, the cartilage on
which the length of the bone depends is inactive, the consequence being that although the bone has a normal, or nearly
normal, transverse diameter, it is at the same time greatly
reduced in length.   Bones in the growth of which the cartilage
takes but a small part, such as the clavicle and the ribs, are not
shortened, and bones developed in membrane are of natural
size.

The lesions of the long bones produced by the delay in ossification are so symmetrical and of such a nature that they cannot
be considered as due to any external accidental cause.   They

are evidently due entirely to muscular action. (Fig. 3.) The biceps has bent forwards the humerus, and the flexors and pronators of the wrist have rotated and flexed the radius and ulna.

In the lower extremity, as a longitudinal section shows, there is a forward curve of the femur due undoubtedly to the action of the quadriceps extensor; the slight curve above, backwards and inwards, is, I suppose, produced by the adductors of the thigh and flexors of the leg. The tibia is evidently doubled up by the gastrocnemius and soleus.

The following short description of this disease is gathered from published papers, the most important being one by Dr. Porak[1] of Paris. Achondroplasia is characterised by lesions of the skeleton which are symmetrical and chiefly in

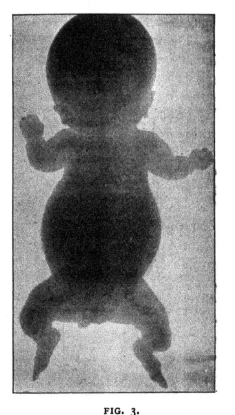

FIG. 3.

Radiogram of the same case. Reduced one-fourth.

the long bones; these are thick, short, hard, and compact, and where bent the bending is always in the diaphyses and in the same direction. It is not a question of local, or rather special lesions of the bones, for these are accompanied by profound nutritional lesions, in particular a great thickening of the skin.

The affection does not show itself in the trunk or the head, except at the base of the skull, which is contracted, and has the bones prematurely united. Some cases are, however, hydrocephalic. It is a disease which comes on and completes its evolu-

[1] *De l'Achondroplasie.*

tion in the earlier months of pregnancy, so that when the child is born the lesions are cured and the initial disorders escape observation.   However, one authority says that the disease may be active until the twenty-sixth week.

The bone when formed is very hard, and the epiphyses are greatly enlarged.   The whole appearance of a case of achondroplasia may be best described as cretinoid, and the disease is probably closely allied to, if not a phase of, sporadic cretinism. The chief, if not the only, difference between my case and those already described is the length of time during which the disease remained active.   When it has ceased early, we should expect shortening, but little bending, of the bones; but when it has lasted long and the muscles grown strong, the bending of the bones will probably be increased in proportion to the lateness of recovery.

It is necessary to distinguish these cases from inherited syphilis and from rickets.   In the former there is a great overgrowth at the diaphyso-epiphyseal junction, where later the tissues degenerate, and we may then find dislocation of the epiphyses.   There are characteristic osteophytic productions under the periosteum, and the long bones far from being shortened may actually be lengthened.   There are generally other concomitant signs of syphilis.   Rickets as a rule does not occur until about the second year of life.   Kassowitz, however, says that it is a frequent occurrence in stillborn or early dying children, but passes unnoticed, as it is not perceived until a child begins to walk, but it does not seem to be obvious why the lesions of the ribs and arms should not be observed.

In rickets the lesions are not so symmetrical, the ribs are nearly always affected; the curves in the long bones may be merely exaggerations of the natural curves, and most often are due to pressure, and they are accompanied by actual, not merely relative, thickening of the bone; as a rule the curves that occur early are near the epiphyses, and the lesions are often isolated. The microscopic appearance of a rickety epiphysis is characteristic; there is an increased proliferation of cartilage cells, the line of junction with the diaphysis is markedly irregular, the secondary areolæ are large, vascular, and irregularly disposed, islets of cartilage are seen in the osteoid trabeculæ and in the medullary cavities, and medullary cavities occur in the epiphyseal cartilage.

In the discussion which followed, Dr. F. H. EDGEWORTH said: Achondroplasia is probably not such a very rare disease, though cases do not come under observation for treatment. I know by sight at least four persons in Bristol who are affected with it, in addition to the one whose photographs are here reproduced (Figs. 4 and 5), and who was admitted to the Bristol Royal Infirmary eighteen months ago for

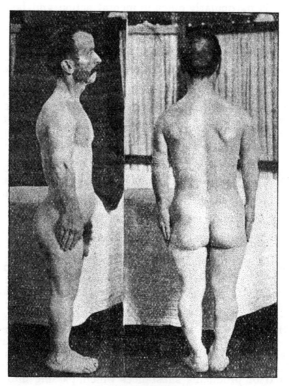

FIGS. 4 & 5.

Case of Achondroplasia.

gastro-intestinal catarrh by the house physician, Dr. Stack, who recognised the skeletal condition.

The patient, now 59 years of age, is one of a numerous family, the other members of which are of normal stature. He has no children. His height is 4 feet 8 inches, and the pictures show that this shortness of stature is due to deficiency in the length of the long bones of the legs. The long bones of the arms are similarly very short. The trunk shows no abnormality. The muscles are very well developed, through having short bellies and tendons. Skiagrams of the limbs show that the bones. are of normal transverse diameters, and the only defects observable are a shortness of the diaphyses and a slight exaggeration of the ordinary curves. The shape of the head is peculiar. There is a short basicranial axis associated with a globular vault, great vertical height and prominent forehead, producing, as it has been said, a pouter-pigeon aspect. (This conformation of head has been shown by Thomson and Symington[1] to be a direct result of the early synostosis of the basicranial axis, and the consequent expansion of the growing brain in other directions.) There are no myxœdematous features : the skin is not thickened and is of healthy tint, the thyroid is of normal size, the tongue is normal, there are no supra-clavicular masses of fat, the abdomen is normal, and there is not the least trace of mental hebetude—in fact the man is particularly quick in mental action and bodily movement.

The etiology of achondroplasia is obscure. It was shown by Thomson and Symington that the essential skeletal abnormalities of the disease are of two kinds—premature synostosis of the basicranial axis, and defective endochondral ossification, so that the diaphyses of long bones are shorter than usual.

It was also pointed out by these observers that the only condition to which achondroplasia has any resemblance is sporadic cretinism, in which precisely the same osseous abnormalities are present.

Figs. 6 and 7 of a case of sporadic cretinism, which was under my care a year or two ago, clearly show the similar changes in the shape of the head and in the length of the limbs.

Achondroplasia differs however from sporadic cretinism in that the thyroid body is normal, and in the majority of cases there is an absence of cretinoid features, e.g. enlarged tongue, supra-clavicular masses of fat, enlarged abdomen, myxœdematous condition of the skin, defective intellect. Mr. Flemming's case is exceptional in that these cretinoid features were present ; indeed, were it not that the thyroid body was normal, one would be fully justified in calling it one of sporadic cretinism.

These facts lead to the following suggestion. It is well known that the thyroid body is originally a gland pouring a secretion into the alimentary canal. This function ceases early in the vertebrate family history and in the individual life-history of the higher vertebrates; and the only trace in adult life of this part played in the past is the foramen cæcum at the base of the tongue and an atrophied duct passing up in front of the hyoid bone, portions of which, persisting, may form troublesome mucus-secreting cysts. But another function is superimposed on the gland, by reason of which it continues in existence and develops—that of producing substances which, passing into the lymphatics and thence into the blood, keep the body in good health, and the failure of which from disease brings about a myxœdematous condition.

Now, in the usual cases of achondroplasia, e.g. the man above described, there can be but little doubt that the thyroid body ultimately performs its function of producing an internal secretion. The skeletal changes, however, indicate that probably during early fœtal life this function was absent or deficient. Achondroplasia, then, is possibly due to a retardation in the development of this function. The cases. may thus be cretins in early intra-uterine life; and whilst, on the development of the secondary function of the thyroid, the tissue

[1] *Rep. Lab. Roy. Coll. Phys., Edinb.*, 1892, iv. 237.

changes other than the osseous rapidly improve, the latter from their very nature persist and leave indelible traces of the events of the past.

Mr. Flemming suggests that in his case the disease had remained active much longer than usual. This suggestion, it may be remarked, is in harmony with the cretinoid condition of the child, and probably the "internal" secretion of the thyroid had not yet begun to be formed.

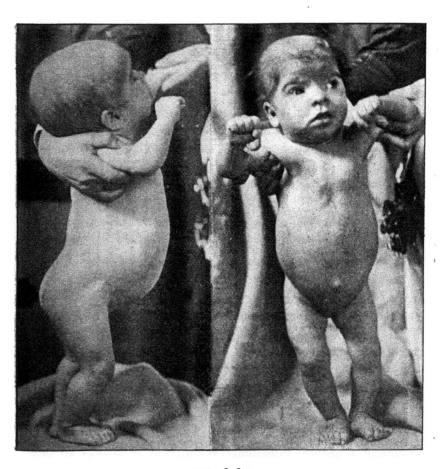

FIGS. 6 & 7.

Case of Sporadic Cretinism.

THE BACTERIOLOGY OF SOME SUPPURATIONS COMPLICATING PULMONARY DISEASE.[1]

BY

J. O. SYMES, M.D., D.P.H.,

Bacteriologist to the Bristol Royal Infirmary.

Pneumonia.—The first series of cases to which I wish to draw attention is that in which, together with either lobar or catarrhal pneumonia, there existed one or more foci of suppuration in other parts. I have examined seven such cases. In four of these the lung was apparently the starting point of the infection.

Case 1.—Aged 3 years. Was admitted suffering from lobar pneumonia, during which cerebral symptoms developed. At the necropsy there was well-marked croupous pneumonia and pleurisy, together with suppurative infiltration of the lateral ventricles of the brain, without general meningitis. Friedländer's pneumo-bacillus was isolated from the lung and from the pus on the ependyma.

Case 2.—Aged 21 years. Admitted with broncho-pneumonia, which terminated fatally. The necropsy showed suppurative peritonitis, and pus in the right middle ear, in addition to broncho-pneumonia. The suppurative lesions were not recognised during life. Pneumococci were present in the pus from all three situations.

Case 3.—Aged 6 years. Clinically there were signs of broncho-pneumonia and meningitis, and the *post-mortem* examination showed catarrhal patches in both lungs and pus in both tympanic cavities. There was no meningitis. Pneumococci were detected in the pus from the ears, in the consolidated areas of lung-tissue, and in the spleen.

Case 4.—Admitted with lobar pneumonia of left lung, and died soon after admission. In addition to pleuro-pneumonia, suppurative pericarditis was found at the *post-mortem* examination, and bacteriological examination showed the existence of pneumococci in lung, in pericardium, and in spleen.

These cases, especially those in which the organism was cultivated from the spleen, illustrate the fact that pneumonia is frequently a general infection. Whether it is always so one cannot say with certainty. It is interesting in this connection to note that in severe cases the pneumococcus cannot infrequently be demonstrated during life in the blood. Thus Kohn isolated the pneumococcus from the blood in nine out of thirty-two

---

[1] Read before the Bristol Medico-Chirurgical Society, February 8th, 1899.

cases of pneumonia. Of these nine positive cases seven died, and the other two were complicated respectively by empyema and pneumococcus suppuration. Of the twenty-three negative cases only five died, so that one may conclude that the presence of the pneumococcus in the blood of a patient suffering from pneumonia is to be regarded as a bad prognostic indication.

There is evidently scope for *ante-mortem* as well as *post-mortem* blood examination in cases of pneumococcus infection.

A point of practical importance suggested by the cases just quoted is the necessity for examining the ears in all cases of pneumonia with cerebral symptoms, and if signs of pus be detected of evacuating it by incising the membrana tympani.

The following case might perhaps have been fairly classed with the four preceding :—

A child of 15 years was admitted in a typhoidal state, with delirium, and other well-marked cerebral symptoms. There was no optic neuritis, and Widal's test was negative. Later there were signs of broncho-pneumonia, and death ensued. The *post-mortem* examination showed a general pneumococcus infection, there being broncho-pneumonia, suppurative cerebral and spinal meningitis, and pus in tympanic cavities. The right membrana tympani was perforated. The history showed that when eight years old there had been suppuration of the right middle-ear and perforation of the membrane. The question then arises: Was the right tympanic cavity the starting point of the infection ?

In three out of the first four cases in which otitis media existed there seems little doubt but that this was secondary to the lung condition.

Personally, I do not know whether the pneumococcus is found in *chronic* middle-ear discharges; but as it is normally present in the mouth and pharynx, it is not unlikely that it should reach the ear and, exciting a suppuration, be the starting point of a general infection. On the other hand, it is equally possible that the old ear-mischief was again lit up by a pneumococcal infection from the lung. Again, the case may have been one of simple cerebro-spinal meningitis, a disease of which the pneumococcus is frequently the exciting cause.

The danger to life of **middle-ear suppuration**, although no symptoms of mastoid implication can be clinically detected, is well illustrated by the following cases :—

Case 1.—Admitted with membranous stomatitis and tonsillitis. Died of broncho-pneumonia. Bacteriological examination of the membrane before and after death showed staphylococcus albus and aureus only. Cultures taken at the *post-mortem* examination from consolidated areas of the lung and from pus in the right tympanic cavity showed streptococci. There had been discharge from the right ear for six months previously, and one may assume that this was the exciting cause of the streptococcic pneumonia.

Case 2.—Aged 5 years. Was admitted with discharge from right ear of many months' duration. No mastoid tenderness, but broncho-pneumonia and signs of meningitis. The necropsy showed pus in right tympanic cavity, extra-dural abscess, sinus thrombosis and multiple suppurative centres in the lung, all of which gave rise' on culture to abundant growth of streptococcus longus. There was no meningitis.

In acute cases of middle-ear disease with **mastoid implication** calling for operative interference, I have on several occasions found the streptococcus to be either the predominant organism, or to be present in pure culture. It apparently is the most common causative agent, whilst second comes the pneumo-coccus, staphylococcus being a secondary infection. It would be of great interest to determine whether the streptococcus is constantly present in chronic ear discharges. In the throat the streptococcus appears to be normally present, at times attaining to a high state of virulence, and exciting tonsillitis and stoma-titis. It may be that it undergoes similar changes of virulence in the ear, or possibly when introduced from without it finds in the chronically inflamed tympanic cavity a suitable nidus, and excites a suppuration of more than ordinary intensity.

The last case of pneumonia with suppuration which I purpose mentioning occurred in a case of enteric fever.

During life, in addition to the regular symptoms of the disease, there was marked deafness and retraction of the head, together with signs of pneumonic consolidation. At the necropsy the right tympanic cavity was full of pus, there was a septic thrombus in the kidney, and broncho - pneumonia. Bacillus coli was isolated from kidney, ear, and lung. As the necropsy was made thirty-six hours after death, it is doubtful whether this result has any true value. In abdominal diseases, and especially in typhoid fever, the bacillus coli invades the tissues very quickly after death, and so rapidly does it multiply that any other organisms present are apt to be crowded out and disappear. The case, however, serves to illustrate a point which I have verified at other *post-mortem* examinations, viz., that this organism is not infrequently the exciting cause of broncho-pneumonia.

Pleural effusions may be divided into three classes: (i.) Mechanical, such as occur in cardiac disease, in some forms of renal disease, and in malignant implication of the pleura. (ii.) Serous effusions of microbic origin. (iii.) Purulent effusions of microbic origin.

The only simple effusion I have examined was taken from a patient suffering from malignant disease of the lung. The fluid was sterile. At the *post-mortem* examination secondary implication of the pleura was discovered. The commonest exciting cause of non-purulent pleural effusion is undoubtedly the tubercle bacillus; fully 75 per cent. of so-called "idiopathic" pleurisies having this origin. Unfortunately it is seldom possible to demonstrate tubercle bacilli by centrifugalisation and film preparations, but if large quantities of the fluid (10 c.c.) be inoculated into guinea pigs positive results will be obtained in a large proportion of cases which would otherwise be styled "rheumatic" or "idiopathic."

Streptococci and pneumococci are also capable of exciting pleurisy, often as a primary disease, and further, if the conditions be such as to permit of the growth of these microorganisms, the effusion will become purulent.

Tubercular effusions seem less liable to become purulent. Of 109 cases of empyema collected by Netter, twenty-nine were associated with pneumococcus, three with pneumococcus and streptococcus, forty-eight with streptococcus, fifteen foetid cases with various saprophytic organisms, and only six with the tubercle bacillus.

I have had the opportunity of making a bacteriological examination in seven cases of empyema. In three the pneumococcus only was found, in one the pneumococcus with staphylococci and streptococci, in two staphylococcus (one aureus, one albus), and in one tubercle bacillus and staphylococcus albus.

The pneumococcal cases all followed attacks of pneumonia.

4

Case 1.—Aged 2 years and 5 months. Had broncho-pneumonia, and subsequent empyema, which was drained. The case terminated fatally, and at the *post-mortem* examination there was found an abscess at the base of the lung on the affected side. The pus from the empyema during life and from the abscess after death showed pneumococci.

Case 2.—Aged 4 years. Said to have had pneumonia one month previously. Pus from empyema showed pure culture of pneumococcus.

Case 3.—Aged 8 years. Lobar pneumonia four weeks previous to operation for empyema. The effusion showed presence of pneumococcus.

Case 4.—Empyema opened six months previously, but still discharging. The pus showed capsulated diplococci, probably pneumococci, also staphylococcus pyogenes aureus.

It is noteworthy that all these pneumococcal cases required operation and drainage. It has been held by some observers that a pneumococcal empyema may frequently be cured by simple aspiration, but this is a point on which there is likely to be much difference of opinion. There can, however, I think, be no doubt that the pneumococcus infection is less dangerous than that due to streptococcus or staphylococcus.

Both the staphylococcus suppurations included in the seven cases were fatal.

Case 1.—Had a history of long-standing pulmonary trouble, dating from an attack of bronchitis thirty years previously. The *post-mortem* examination showed that the left pleura was converted into thick calcified plates, and the contained pus showed staphylococcus pyogenes albus.

Case 2.—Aged 3 months. The empyema was preceded by a broncho-pneumonia. The pus drained off during life showed staphylococcus pyogenes aureus, and the same organism was present in the pus from an abscess cavity in the lung of the affected side, as discovered after death.

It is doubtful whether the following should be classified as a case of empyema :—

Case 5.—Clinically there were signs of fluid at one base, but the exploring needle only brought away thick caseous material, which when examined microscopically was found to contain cocci (which on culture proved to be staphylococcus pyogenes albus) and tubercle bacilli. Such a condition may be regarded as a tubercular pleuritis rather than empyema, but the case serves to raise the question as to whether it is advisable to operate when it is known that the empyema is of tubercular origin.

In conclusion, I may say that the manner in which organisms reach the pleuritic cavity is a matter for conjecture. It would not seem probable that either pleurisy or empyema can be simple primary affections. In health the air in the lungs must be as a rule free from microbic life, or if organisms be present we should not, judging from analogy, expect them to have the power of penetrating a healthy pleura. On the other hand, in diseased conditions of the lungs the neighbouring pleura will certainly suffer, and through a damaged membrane the organisms may pass out just as does the bacillus coli through an injured gut wall. Probably exposure to cold has this injurious effect upon the pleura and thus predisposes to pneumonia and pleurisy.

Our present knowledge of the lesions excited by the pneumococcus and its general infectivity, point to the unsatisfactory nature of our present methods of treatment and to the need for an efficient curative serum.

In the discussion which followed Dr. MICHELL CLARKE said that in cases of empyema information as to the micro-organism concerned might be got from the examination of coverslip preparations. He had not found in four cases of empyema due to the pneumococcus, that simple aspiration cured the patients. They all required incision later. He mentioned a case in which the diphtheria bacillus was abundantly present in the sputum, and in which there were symmetrically seated patches of consolidation in the apex of the lower lobe. There were no throat symptoms. He also alluded to the cases of disseminated broncho-pneumonia which followed influenza.—Dr. CAVE spoke of the value of the bacteriological examination of the blood and of the cerebro-spinal fluid in infection of the system and of the central nervous system in cases of pneumonia; also of the frequent biological association of staphylococci and tubercle bacilli in pleural effusion, so frequent that the demonstration of the former may justifiably excite suspicion of the essentially tubercular origin of the effusion. He also referred to Debove's demonstration of a substance analogous to tuberculin in tubercular effusions, and of his method of demonstrating its presence by injecting tuberculous guinea-pigs and producing a febrile reaction.—Dr. JAMES SWAIN said that suppurative processes produced by the pneumococcus somewhat resembled similar conditions caused by the tubercle bacillus. It was well known that tubercular abscesses rarely needed drainage, and there were also pneumococcal abscesses which had apparently been cured by evacuation without drainage.—Mr. ROGER WILLIAMS thought it remarkable that the pleural fluid was sterile in the only case associated with pulmonary malignant disease, as malignant tumours of any size nearly always teem with bacteria, etc., especially when in direct communication with the external atmosphere. Moreover secondary tumours also nearly always carry microbes with them, and as in this case there was secondary deposit in the pleura, it would seem that the pleural fluid was very likely to have been exposed to infection.

Progress of the Medical Sciences.

MEDICINE.

At the present time the **treatment and prevention of tuberculosis** occupies considerable attention. To pass under notice in this short review the various points bearing upon the subject brought into prominence during the past few months would possibly not be very profitable. It is well, however, sometimes to use our judgment concerning apparently well-established facts, and to consider whether there may not be sources of error causing what appears to be fact to be mixed with fallacy. The members of the medical profession are the leaders of public thought in these matters, and if we lay down the law dogmatically at one time and a few years later formulate rules of different character, we give good reason for those who look to us for guidance to treat our opinions with scant courtesy.

Much blame has been thrown upon **milk,** by laboratory workers and other observers, as a source of infection of tuberculosis in children. Dr. Delépine [1] prefaces his valuable lecture upon tuberculosis and the milk-supply with some rather strong remarks. He says: "The difficulty of dealing with tuberculosis is further increased by the general ignorance of the public. The danger which they incur from a contaminated milk-supply is appalling in its magnitude, yet because this danger is of an insidious nature and its effects are often so gradual that it is difficult to trace their onset they prefer to have their quietude not disturbed. They are also afraid that their purses might have to be opened. Rather than face such possibilities they prefer to believe the few experts who still hold views which numerous most searching investigations have proved to be wrong."

Dr. Delépine's investigations certainly appear to give cause for alarm. He found that of 143 samples of milk 25 gave rise to tuberculosis in guinea pigs. The experiments of Drs. Kanthack and Sladen [2] are perhaps still more striking. Of 90 guinea pigs, inoculated with milk from the dairies in Cambridge, 23, that is 25.55 per cent., died. Dr. Delépine strengthens his attack upon milk by quoting the Registrar's returns of the causes of death at different ages in London, which assign forms of tuberculosis, other than phthisis, to 1,232 cases under the age of one year; whereas later in life, even for so long a period as that between the ages of five and twenty years, there are only 474 in which death is certified as due to these forms of tuberculosis.

Sir R. Thorne Thorne [3] also lays great stress upon the

---

[1] *Lancet*, 1898, ii. 733.   [2] *Ibid.*, 1899, i. 75.   [3] *Ibid.*, 1898, ii. 1289.

Registrar's statistics. He mentions that of recent years the death-rates from most varieties of tuberculosis have greatly diminished, but that "when the death-rates from tabes mesenterica, a form of tuberculosis in which the infection is received into the alimentary canal instead of into the lungs were examined, it was found not only that all the gain attained at other ages had been lost in the case of children and infants, but that in addition to this there had been a very heavy increase in deaths from this cause amongst infants under one year of age." Sir R. Thorne Thorne further states that "this increase had gone hand in hand with a steady increase in the consumption of cow's milk as a food in this country," and that "the danger to man, and especially to the infant population, was one of real gravity, and the loss of child-life due to this disease in milch-cows was appalling."

This is a heavy indictment of milk, and it will be valuable to see what proofs of the truth of the accusation are furnished by the *post-mortem* room. It may be well, however, to pause for a moment to consider peculiarities in the **modes of infection** of children by the tubercle bacillus.

In the adult, as is well known, the apex of the lung is the spot in the body most likely to be first attacked. In the child that is not so. Ordinary phthisical disease of the lung spreading from above downwards is decidedly rare. Infection of the lung is common enough, but the disease enters the lung by a somewhat circuitous course. Tubercle bacilli finding entrance to the lungs are taken up by the lymphatics, and are carried to the bronchial and mediastinal lymph glands. In these glands the disease advances; they enlarge and become caseous, and sooner or later either local invasion of the lung, or general tuberculous infection of the body, usually takes place. Tubercle bacilli finding entrance to the intestines also generally fail to give rise to local lesions. They are first stopped by the mesenteric glands, and finding a suitable soil there may give rise to enlargement and caseation, as in the case of the bronchial glands. Ulcers in the intestines may occur, but when present they are usually of much more recent date than the associated disease of the mesenteric glands.

If the indictment against milk be correct, the *post-mortem* room will furnish us with numerous examples of disease of the mesenteric glands, at the time of life in which children are drinking large quantities of cow's milk. Dr. Sims Woodhead[1] was the first to write upon this subject, and from examination of 127 cases of tuberculosis in children, he found the mesenteric glands caseous in no less than 100 cases. The mediastinal glands were also, however, caseous in 95 cases; but in most of those Dr. Woodhead considered the disease more recent in the thorax than in the abdomen. These statistics taken alone would appear to put the subject beyond the region of dispute.

[1] *Rep. Lab. Roy. Coll. Phys., Edinb.*, 1889, i. 179.

Other observers, however, have not met with the same localisation of tuberculosis of the lymph glands as Dr. Woodhead. Dr. Carr[1] found 79 cases in which tuberculosis in children appeared to start in the thoracic glands, against 20 in the abdominal; and Dr. Colman,[2] after examination of *post-mortem* records at the Children's Hospital, Great Ormond Street, expressed the opinion that, while he did not doubt the possibility of infection of milk in some cases, he was led to attach much more importance to the condition of the thoracic lymphatic glands, as the process was more advanced in them, as a rule, than in the mesenteric glands, and in several they were extensively caseous, when the mesenteric glands showed little or no change.

Dr. Carr and Dr. Colman are not alone in their opinion. Kempner[3] expresses the opinion that tuberculosis, in childhood especially, originates from disease of the bronchial glands. Comby[4] considers that the respiratory tract is always the starting point. In 28 necropsies on children dying of tuberculosis, under the age of two years, the mediastinal glands were affected in every instance. Kossel[5] in 14 necropsies found caseous bronchial glands in 10 cases, and the mesenteric caseous in one; and Weiderhofer[6] found intestinal tuberculosis in only 8 per cent. of cases of tuberculosis in children under the age of two years. But the most striking experience is that of Dr. Emmett Holt.[7] In 119 necropsies upon children dying of tuberculosis, he found caseous bronchial glands in no less than 108, and caseous mesenteric glands in only 38; and in nearly every case of the latter, he considered the abdominal disease had followed the thoracic. He believes that the importance of infection by the intestine has been " greatly exaggerated," and in his opinion does not occur in more than 1 or 2 per cent. of the cases. Dr. Holt quotes Northrup as having had a similar experience to his own. In necropsies on 125 cases of tuberculosis in children, only one case was found in which the disease appeared to have started in the alimentary tract, while in 88 it was clearly through the bronchial lymph glands.

At the Bristol Royal Infirmary the *post-mortem* examinations upon children are not numerous, but those seen during the time I have had charge of the pathological department afford little evidence of primary infection by the alimentary tract. Of ten children of the age of two years and under dying of various forms of tuberculosis, in nine the bronchial and mediastinal glands were caseous. In four of these the mesenteric glands showed a few caseous points, but the disease was much less advanced than in the bronchial glands. In one case, however,

1 *Lancet*, 1894, i. 1177.   2 *Brit. M. J.*, 1893, ii. 740.
3 *Münch. med. Abh., j. Reihe*, Heft 17; abstract in *Brit. M. J.*, 1896, ii. Epitome, p. 52.
4 *Klin. Therap. Woch.*, 1898, v. 604; abstract in *Pediatrics*, 1899, vii. 44.
5 *Kinder-Arzt.*, 1896, vii. 19; abstract in *Pediatrics*, 1896, ii. 356.
6 Quoted in *Med. News*, 1896, lxix. 609.
7 *Med. News*, 1896, lxix. 656.

the mesenteric glands were alone affected; but this was the only case, not only under the age of two years, but at any age, seen in the *post-mortem* room during the past four and a half years, in which infection appeared to have taken place through the alimentary tract.

Another mode of entrance is by the **tonsils**. I have had one well-marked instance of that mode of infection, and some of the statistics quoted above give others; but since the tonsils are open to infection by either the air or milk, examination of such cases has no bearing upon the subject before us.

To return to the question of **infection by the alimentary canal**, the above *post-mortem* statistics must have made it clear that the Registrar's statistics, upon which Dr. Delépine and Sir R. Thorne Thorne laid so much stress, must be, in very great degree, fallacious. The *post-mortem* room shows disease of the mesenteric glands unassociated with tuberculous disease elsewhere to be distinctly rare, consequently tabes mesenterica cannot be of the " appalling " frequency those statistics make it appear to be.

Dr. Carr[1] refers to this point. He says that he has notes of nearly 100 *post-mortem* examinations of cases that clinically might have been called tabes mesenterica, yet in only one of the 100 was any abdominal tuberculosis present. Tuberculosis of the mesenteric glands, however, does exist; but when we find it present, it is not necessary to conclude that the infection was conveyed by milk. In the majority of cases it is secondary to infection of the respiratory tract.

In those cases in which the disease in the mesenteric glands is much less advanced than in the bronchial glands, infection obviously takes place from tubercle bacilli conveyed to the intestines by swallowed infected bronchial secretion. Our experience of early phthisis in adults shows us how the bronchial secretion of bronchitis that precedes local disease may swarm with tubercle bacilli. When tubercle bacilli find their way into the bronchial tubes of children, one can easily understand how, multiplying there and causing increased secretion, the number of bacilli that are absorbed by the lymphatics and enter the bronchial lymph glands must be small, compared with those that, coughed into the mouth in bronchial mucus, are swallowed and finally enter the intestines. There are, however, not only a few cases in which the disease is more advanced in the mesenteric glands than in the bronchial, but occasionally a case occurs in which the mesenteric glands are alone affected. I am not prepared to admit, however, that even these cases are the result of infection derived from cows.

The milk from which babies are fed no doubt frequently stands for the greater part of the day in the dark, ill-ventilated dwellings of the poor, where the dust in many instances contains tubercle bacilli derived from human sufferers from

[1] *Lancet*, 1898, ii. 1662.

tuberculosis. We have seen that it is by air containing such bacilli finding entrance to the lungs that children are generally infected, but we can easily understand how occasionally milk might be so placed as to receive more bacilli than a child's lungs.

There is another way by which children may become infected by the alimentary tract without deriving the disease from cows. The free intercourse of women of the humbler classes, and the attention they pay to one another's babies, introduces an element of risk. The child may be kissed by a phthisical woman, or may have a spoonful of sweetened liquid given to it that has been previously tasted by such a person.

Tuberculous disease in cows may be the same disease as in man, but it does not follow that the tubercle bacilli present in the milk of diseased animals are very virulent towards man. If small-pox in cows assumes a very mild form, in man it might be argued that tuberculosis possibly does also, and that if only a mild attack of tuberculosis protected against the more severe forms of the disease, the best way to protect the younger members of the community would be to feed them on tuberculous cows' milk.

I am not aware, however, that there is yet proof that the tuberculous disease of cows is capable even of communicating a mild form of tuberculosis to man. We cannot, of course, test the power of infected milk on babies, as can be done in guinea-pigs, but Dr. Emmett Holt[1] tells an interesting story that has some bearing upon the point, and may be looked upon as an extensive experiment innocently performed. Near a large American city was a stock farm of Jersey cows, which supplied milk to a large number of the wealthiest families in the city for a period of ten years. At the end of that time, 45 per cent. of the cows were found by the tuberculin test to be tuberculous. They were killed by order of the State Board of Health, and the diagnosis confirmed in every instance by necropsies. Of the many hundreds of children who had taken the milk, in only one could it be found that tuberculosis had developed, and in that case it was not clear that the milk was responsible. The employés about the farm had also been accustomed for several years to drink skimmed milk in large quantities as a beverage in the place of water. Not one, however, developed tuberculosis.

Such a tale does not lend much support to the view of Dr. Delépine, that "the danger from a contaminated milk-supply is appalling in its magnitude." Much as I respect the ability and judgment of the probable author of another statement which appeared recently in one of our local newspapers,[2] I think it rather premature to tell the public that "it is probable the germ of consumption is carried to us most frequently by meat or milk." That milk is a source of danger in many ways none of us doubt.

[1] *Loc. cit.*   [2] *Western Daily Press*, Jan. 30, 1899.

When one learns that as many as 60,000 micro-organisms have been found in a cubic centimetre of milk, one cannot lay too great stress upon the importance of sterilisation. But to arrive at the decision that milk is the most important factor in the spread of tuberculosis appears to me to be an error. If we turn our attention, and that of the public, too strongly in some new direction, we are apt to lose sight of other facts already well established.

There can be no two opinions as to the importance of fresh air and sunlight in destroying the vitality of the tubercle bacillus. Careful regulation of the milk-supply may possibly do a little towards diminishing the death-rate from this disease, but more sunshine and ventilation in the dwellings of the poor will do a great deal more.

(In a recent paper[1] Dr. Leonard Guthrie similarly argues against tuberculous milk being a common cause of tuberculosis in children).

THEODORE FISHER.

SURGERY.

Thrombosis and embolism of the mesenteric vessels, as a cause of acute abdominal affections, has hardly received the amount of general attention it deserves, and it may be worth while, therefore, to draw attention to the signs and symptoms it produces.

The usual result of occlusion of the mesenteric vessels is infarction of the intestine. This infarction may follow occlusion of either the arteries or veins, the effect generally being greater when the latter are obstructed, for in that event there is no hindrance to the supply of blood by the artery but there is hindrance to the escape, and of necessity there is produced intense vascular engorgement and often extravasation of blood in the affected area. When the superior or inferior mesenteric artery is blocked, engorgement also follows, the flow of blood producing it in this case being from the anastomosing arteries and from the veins, the backward pressure of the latter coming into play when the *vis a tergo* is cut off. Litten's experimental ligation of the superior mesenteric artery near its origin, in dogs, always produced this result.

Though infarction of the intestine and mesentery, with gangrene in the severest, and ulceration or simple congestion in the mildest, cases, most frequently follows occlusion of the superior mesenteric artery: yet in 2 cases observed by Virchow, and 1 by Tiedemann, that artery was found obliterated without injury to the intestine.[2] Chiene[3] has also reported a case met with in the dissecting-room, in which there was occlusion of the three anterior branches of the abdominal aorta supplying the viscera.

[1] *Lancet*, 1899, i. 286. [2] Quoted by Elliot, *Ann. Surg.*, 1895, xxi 9.
[3] *J. Anat. & Physiol.*, 1869, iii. 65.

The vitality of the intestine had in no way been impaired, having been maintained by the dilatation of collateral blood-vessels. It appears from these cases that the intestine escapes injury from interference with normal channels of blood-supply if the interference is sufficiently gradually produced to allow of compensatory dilatation of anastomosing arteries.

Councilman[1] remarks upon the probability that small emboli frequently enter the superior mesenteric artery, their entry being favoured by the size of that artery and the angle it forms with the aorta; but that the free anastomosis between its small branches prevents these small emboli impairing intestinal nutrition. He reports 3 cases of embolism of the superior artery which he had met with. One of these is particularly interesting, for clinically the symptoms were those of complete intestinal obstruction, with vomiting finally becoming stercoraceous, great abdominal pain, and tympanites. The patient, who was 85 years of age, died on the twelfth day of illness. The intestine presented a few small ecchymoses, but there was neither intense congestion nor at any place complete infarction. A thrombus attached to an atheromatous patch on the anterior wall of the aorta, just above the origin of the superior mesenteric artery, almost completely occluded the opening of that branch. He thinks it probable that the blood-supply through the obstructed vessel, though sufficient to maintain the vitality of the intestine, interfered with its innervation, leading to paralysis of the bowel and the attendant intestinal obstruction. In a second case, though the entire superior mesenteric artery was obstructed, there was only a beginning of infarction in a small area of the intestine.

Dr. Elliot[2] has analysed the records of 20 carefully reported cases of **occlusion of the superior mesenteric artery,** in which the **abdominal symptoms** were not overshadowed by those of heart disease or by coma. All the cases were rapidly fatal. Pain, often colicky, was the most prominent symptom, and occurred in nearly all. A very notable symptom was the presence of blood in the stools. This was recorded in 13 cases. In 3 the blood was passed without fæces. In 6 the hemorrhage was profuse. In 3 other cases neither fæces nor flatus were passed. Hæmatemesis occurred in 3. Blood is usually found in the intestines at the autopsy, even if not passed during life, and is also frequently found in the peritoneal cavity. In 2 cases there was a palpable swelling, which proved to be infarcted bowel; and in another, a swelling was due to a collection of blood in the mesentery. Subnormal temperature and extreme pallor were noticed in several cases, due no doubt to hemorrhage and peritoneal shock. In nearly half the cases there was diarrhœa. In some there was neither diarrhœa nor other disturbance of the bowels.[3] The source of the embolism is usually

[1] *Boston M. & S. J.*, 1894, cxxx. 410.   [2] *Loc. cit.*
[3] F. S. Watson, *Boston M. & S. J.*, 1894, cxxxi. 555.

vegetations on the cardiac valves, or on atheromatous patches in the aorta. Watson, analysing 8 cases of total occlusion of the main trunk of the superior mesenteric artery, finds that in 1 case there was entire absence of abdominal symptoms, and in 2 others they were very slight, though the infarction affected a large part of the intestines. On the other hand, in a case in which only a small portion of the intestine was in a state of infarct, abdominal pain was sudden and violent, and there was profuse bloody diarrhœa. It is obvious, therefore, that from the clinical signs it is impossible to tell the extent or degree of the intestinal lesion.

It will have been noticed that one of the most characteristic symptoms mentioned above was bloody diarrhœa. If there is evidence of embolism in other parts of the body, producing for example gangrene of the feet, or hemiplegia, hæmoptysis and chest pain, or splenic or renal trouble, the diagnosis of the condition we are discussing will be much facilitated; but this evidence is often wanting. Again, the presence of heart disease and atheromatous arteries will help in the diagnosis. Watson thinks it possible to diagnose about one-fourth of the cases. The affection, perhaps, most closely resembles intussusception, as pointed out by Elliot.[1] In both infarction of the intestine and intussusception there is often diarrhœa and intestinal hemorrhage, and pain and vomiting. The hemorrhage is apt to be more profuse in the embolic affection, but has been recorded as the principal cause of death in both. In intussusception tympanites is rare in the early stages. In that affection too the patients are usually younger. According to Fitz, 56 per cent. of the cases of intussusception are under the age of 10. The characters of a tumour if present would be an important guide to the diagnosis. A few cases are recorded of embolism of the inferior mesenteric artery, but the symptoms do not sufficiently differ from those in which the superior artery is affected to permit of clinical differentiation. It has been said that the presence of fresh blood in the dejections, and the localisation of the pain in the lower part of the abdomen, point to embolism of the inferior vessel.[2]

Elliot[3] has found 14 reported cases of **thrombosis of the superior mesenteric vein.** They were even more rapidly fatal than those of embolism of the artery, nearly all having died on the second or third day with symptoms of intestinal obstruction. The symptoms of this affection are much the same as those of embolism of the corresponding artery, with the exception that diarrhœa has not been recorded as present in any. Blood was vomited or passed in large quantity by the bowel in half the cases. In 5 of the cases there was cirrhosis of the liver, and 2 were syphilitic. In 2 cases a volvulus was considered to be the result of the thrombosis.

It may, therefore, be said that acute abdominal symptoms,

[1] *Loc. cit.*   [2] Elliot, *Loc. cit.*   [3] *Loc. cit.*

associated with the passage of blood and with portal obstruction from cirrhosis of the liver or other cause, would suggest the diagnosis of thrombosis of the mesenteric veins.

The **prognosis** in these affections of the mesenteric vessels is very bad, though, as mentioned above, there are records which show that patients have survived.

Elliot has only found in literature 3 cases which have been operated upon. He reports 2 additional cases of his own. In none was the diagnosis previously made; and 4 out of the 5 died unrelieved.

Laparotomy, and resection of the intestine if it be found to to require it, is the only **treatment** that offers any prospect of success. Watson states that the records of a number of autopsies showed that one-sixth of the cases might have been relieved by such treatment. In the single successful operation for this condition on record, that of Elliot,[1] four feet of intestine, almost gangrenous from infarction, were removed. The open ends of the intestine were sutured to the abdominal wound, and the artificial anus thus produced was subsequently closed by a second operation. The patient was a male, aged 25, and the cause of the infarction was thrombosis of the mesenteric veins. Elliot's second case was one of thrombosis of a branch of the mesenteric artery. An artificial anus was made in the descending colon; but the patient died. At the autopsy four inches of the intestine were found gangrenous and to have been perforated. In most cases the presence of heart disease, atheroma, or cirrhosis of the liver, militates strongly against surgical success.

*　　　*　　　*　　　*

In all cases of **rupture of the kidney**, whether open or subcutaneous, when first seen the question of the advisability of exploring or of performing a primary nephrectomy will arise. Morris[2] and Keen[3] have each written papers, in which this matter is helpfully considered. They are agreed that the symptom of hæmaturia rarely affords help in deciding the question, for it is a very unreliable guide as to the severity of the renal injury. Hæmaturia may be considerable in degree when the renal injury is slight, and slight or absent when the injury is most severe. If, however, hæmaturia is exhausting the patient by its severity, and especially if bloodclots with their attendant septic dangers accumulate in the bladder, then and then only does this symptom afford clear indications that the kidney should be explored. The clots in the bladder must be removed, either by expression (Willard) if laparotomy is performed, otherwise by the aid of a catheter or evacuator, and their further formation must be prevented, either by ligature of the bleeding-points in the kidney or plugging the wound in it, or by nephrectomy. Again, primary anuria does not afford an indication for operation unless it persists for twenty-four or thirty-six hours after shock has passed off, or unless it appears after the lapse of

---

[1] *Loc. cit.*　　[2] *Clin. J.*, 1894, iv. 217.　　[3] *Ann. Surg.*, 1896, xxiv. 138.

some days. In these exceptional circumstances anuria indicates the advisability of exploration, for it may be due to a ureteral clot preventing the escape of the secretion of the only function-ally active kidney present, the other kidney being either absent or diseased. Life in such cases can only be saved by providing an escape for the urine through the loin.

By what **symptoms** or signs then are we to be guided in the majority of cases, in deciding whether to operate or not in these cases of subcutaneous rupture of the kidney? It is "the presence or absence of a distinct and increasing swelling in the loin" which affords the surest guide. As Morris puts it :—"The presence of a distinct and increasing swelling in the renal region makes an early incision through the loin imperative : it is the only way to cut short the progress of the case, to limit the extravasation into the peri-renal tissues, to check or prevent suppuration, to prevent sloughing of the peritoneum, and to save the life of the patient." Having exposed the kidney, it will have to be either removed at once, or dealt with as described above, the degree of injury affording the correct indications.

If in the first instance palliative and non-operative treatment has been adopted, and the case does not progress favourably, and it is obvious that a large hæmatoma has gradually formed, then a secondary exploratory operation, with or without secondary nephrectomy, must be performed. Secondary nephrectomy becomes much more dangerous if postponed until septic com-plications have arisen. The exploratory lumbar incision should be made to anticipate or prevent septic complications if possible. A good instance of a successful secondary nephrec-tomy performed on the above principles is one published by Moynihan,[1] in which the operation was done on the twelfth day after an injury which had torn the kidney from the cortex to the pelvis, almost completely dividing it into two parts. There were no septic complications. Page[2] reports another case of secondary nephrectomy which, though ultimately successful, illustrates the disadvantage of postponing these operations until septic complications have arisen. The patient passed through a long and critical illness, and some months after convalescence there was still slight pyuria, suggesting the possibility of infec-tive processes continuing in the other kidney.

J. LACY FIRTH.

OPHTHALMOLOGY.

The use of a small electro-magnet in extracting **foreign bodies** which have penetrated the eyeball has been resorted to for more than twenty years. In 1892 Haab, acting upon the principle that "He that has the strongest magnet will obtain the best results," invented a larger and immensely more powerful instru-

[1] *Quarterly M. J.*, 1897–98, vi. 246. [2] *Clin. J.*, 1896–97, ix. 65.

ment, which he has since further improved upon. It is now
some twenty-five times as powerful as the ordinary hand electro-
magnet, and weighs considerably over a hundredweight. It is
pivoted on an accurately constructed stand, and is most con-
veniently worked with the street current. Numerous cases of
its success are on record. R. Barkan[1] relates four cases in which
he has used it. In one case the chip of steel had entered the
corneal margin and was lodged in the vitreous, but not visible.
On the eighth day after the injury the patient's eye was
approached to the instrument, and the foreign body gradually
came forward into the lips of the wound, so that it could be
easily extracted with forceps. The lens was not injured, and
in fourteen days the vision was almost perfect. He is so convinced of its utility, that he asserts that no eye clinic should be
without one.

In conjunction with this advance it is important to realise
the progress made in the use of the **X Rays**, more especially
by Mackenzie Davidson. He has devised a very simple and
ingenious apparatus especially for eye work. The Crookes tube
is fixed in a slide, and after the first skiagram is taken, it is
moved a certain distance along the slide before the second plate
is exposed. He draws special attention to the advantage of
having a tube in which the rays emanate from a very small
focus, and he recommends that the terminal should be of
osmium. With such an apparatus two minutes is a sufficient
exposure for each plate, and it should always be possible to
estimate the exact position of any piece of metal not smaller
than a pin's head.

The cost of eye injuries has not been sufficiently recognised.
The nation, to say nothing of clubs and benefit societies, is put
to great unnecessary expense owing to the indifference, we
might almost say the aversion, with which workmen regard
protective glasses. In Cologne the " Quarry-Union " has taken
the matter up. Dr. Hillemanns[2] finds there are defects in all
the protective spectacles in use, whether of glass, quartz, mica,
or gauze. They are either uncomfortable or, owing to obstructing vision, reduce a man's wage-earning power when doing
piecework. He recommends goggles, consisting of a short
truncated cone of open-meshed galvanized-iron gauze, the base
of which fits the face accurately, whilst the summit is closed in
by a disc or lens of glass or, better, rock crystal. Since the
introduction of these protectors at the railway works at Cologne,
five years ago, no eyes have been lost, and the men wear them
willingly. Hillemanns urges the profession to direct the attention of the laity to the advantages of proper protectors.

*   *   *   *

There is not much new to record in the technique of **cataract
extraction**; in fact, some of the later departures are really
reversions to methods abandoned thirty or forty years ago.

[1] *Arch. Ophth.*, 1898, xxvii. 37.   [2] *Ibid.*, 527.

This is mainly due to the introduction of cocaine and antiseptics rendering methods safe and practicable which were formerly often attended with failure. Prof. C. Schweigger[1] advocates extraction of the lens by means of a downward corneal flap— practically the old flap operation of one hundred years ago. This method possesses hardly any advantage, except that the corneal wound is more easily inspected after the operation. But this is rarely necessary after all. Various surgeons have attempted to suture the corneal wound ; but this procedure does not seem to ensure any better results. The most that can be said of it is that it is not so risky as would at first sight appear probable. Secondary operations (needling opaque lens capsule) are not to be lightly undertaken. Schweigger found that in no less than 15 per cent. of his cases, this operation was followed by disagreeable and tedious irritation, lasting weeks or months. This occurred even in cases where there was no traction on the ciliary body during the needling. For the last two years he has used a modification of de Wecker's forceps-scissors, and clipped through the membrane in every case of capsular cataract, and has met with good results.

*　　　*　　　*　　　*

Tho etiology of **pterygium** is still a matter of dispute. Fuchs regards it as intimately connected with pinguecual; others regard them as two entirely distinct conditions. Henry Lopez,[2] of Havana, has had unusual opportunities for studying the two diseases. He estimates that more than half the male population of Cuba suffer from pterygium—we presume he refers only to male adults, because in the next paragraph he says it is very rarely found before the twentieth year. He is convinced that pterygium and pinguecula are but different stages of the same disease. According to him pinguecula grows up to the corneal margin and forms a sharply defined raised lump; foreign bodies lodge in the angle between this lump and the cornea, destroy the corneal epithelium, and render the cornea a prey to the advancing growth. He does not look upon pterygium as being particularly obstinate or necessitating the complicated operations some have devised. Avulsion of the " head " from the cornea, excision of the whole growth, and suture of the gap in the conjunctiva are effective in almost every case.

*　　　*　　　*　　　*

In a very suggestive paper on " **Ophthalmoscopic evidence of general arterial disease,**"[3] Marcus Gunn draws special attention to the "influence of the arterial pressure on the venous blood-stream where the artery and vein cross one another." The appearances that he alludes to are easy to see, now that attention has been drawn to the subject. At first the vein is bent, and consequently loses its central "light-streak" for a short distance on either side of the artery. Later, the venous current

[1] *Arch. Ophth.*, 1898, xxvii. 255.

[2] *Ibid.,* 279.　　[3] *Tr. Ophth. Soc. U. Kingdom*, 1898, xviii. 356.

is markedly impeded and the peripheral portion of the vein is abnormally engorged. His explanation is, that the coats of the artery have undergone a hyaline-fibroid change, the vessel is unduly rigid and tightly distended. He adds: "The result of the increased difficulty in arterial circulation will be to diminish the rapidity of the blood-stream in the capillaries and veins. As a result, there will be a tendency to the escape of *liquor sanguinis* into the surrounding tissues, and this tendency will be much increased where the venous circulation is mechanically impeded, as by an overlying artery." Thus a vicious circle is established, and we get hemorrhages and white patches in the retina. "In the most advanced cases the lines of the folds which radiate from the fovea centralis, due to the œdema, are sometimes eventually marked out by the deposit of white spots of degenerated effusion, so that we get the ophthalmoscopic appearances diagnostic of so-called albuminuric or renal retinitis." Old age does not produce these conditions, and, associated with local disease at any rate, the same appearances may be present in patients of eighteen or twenty.

It would seem that it is not improbable that the formation of this vicious circle may be a factor in some cases of so-called **retinitis proliferans,** but various diseases have been described under this term, and a very different sequence of events is probable in the series of cases mentioned by J. E. Weeks.[1] In twenty-one out of twenty-two cases that he examined after death the retinitis proliferans was due to a fibrinous exudation or hemorrhage into the vitreous, upon which vascular connective tissue creeps up from the retina, thus forming an ophthalmoscopic picture resembling the class of retinitis proliferans first alluded to.

*   *   *   *

In the *Transactions of the Ophthalmological Society* for last year there is a very elaborate report on the question of **excision of the eyeball** and allied operations, from which I extract the following. Removal of a portion of the eye (abscission) is as old as Celsus, but the first recorded case of "extirpation" was performed in 1583 by means of a spoon with cutting edges, and until 1840 a somewhat similar instrument was invariably used. In 1850 the late Augustin Prichard[2] was the first to extirpate an injured blind eye, and he then advocated excision of the exciting eye in all cases of sympathetic ophthalmitis. Evisceration, as practised by von Graefe in 1863 in cases of suppurative panophthalmitis, has not been shown to have any advantages over excision. The relative frequency of sympathetic inflammation, after the introduction of a globe of silver or glass into the emptied sclerotic (Mules's operation) is infinitely greater than after simple excision. It should only be resorted to in such cases as painful blind glaucomatous eyes, or within fourteen days of an injury in a young subject. The only

---

[1] *Tr. Am. Ophth. Soc.*, 1897, viii. 158.   [2] *Prov. M. & S. J.*, 1851, 66.

important objection to the introduction of a similar globe into Tenon's capsule is that it comes out in about a quarter of the cases, and always necessitates for the patient a longer duration in hospital—roughly, twelve days, instead of three days as in excision. Optico-ciliary neurectomy, excision of a portion of the optic and ciliary nerves through an incision over the internal rectus, is only admissible in such cases as painful blind glaucomatous eyes. It has never been known to be followed by sympathetic inflammation except in eyes which had previously been injured in a way likely to cause sympathetic ophthalmitis. It obviates the necessity of an artificial eye; but, unfortunately, the pain for which the operation was undertaken sometimes returns, and in several instances ulceration of the cornea has followed.

* * * *

For **Ophthalmia neonatorum** Prof. Credé, in 1882, advocated as a routine treatment the instillation of a few drops of a 2 per cent. solution of nitrate of silver into the eyes as soon as the child's head was born. Lucien Howe[1] summarises the results of this treatment. The combined experience of a number of obstetricians shows that in a series of more than 40,000 cases ophthalmia neonatorum was fifteen times more prevalent where no treatment was used than when the Credé method was adopted. Solutions of corrosive sublimate, especially the stronger solutions, gave slightly better results; but they cause such excessive inflammation in infants, that the advantage is on the whole in favour of nitrate of silver. He thinks that the Credé method should be made compulsory in all public institutions. Inquiries at 110 of the largest German clinics resulted in the discovery of only four cases in which the method was supposed to have done harm, and in some of these it was doubtful if the nitrate of silver was to blame. Protargol, a protein compound containing 8.3 per cent. of silver, is recommended by Adolf Alt[2] as a substitute for nitrate of silver. It is readily soluble in hot or cold water, and not precipitated by albumin or chloride of sodium. It consequently penetrates much more readily into all the crevices of the conjunctival sac than silver nitrate solution, and its application is much less painful. He uses a 1 per cent. solution, but others have found a 5 per cent. solution more effectual. Largin is another somewhat similar compound which has recently been introduced. Mr. H. G. Parker, the house-surgeon at the Bristol Eye Hospital has obtained good results with a 5 per cent. solution, and judging by the results of a few cases its use can be recommended in all cases of conjunctivitis attended with purulent discharge.

CYRIL H. WALKER.

[1] *Tr. Am. Ophth. Soc.*, 1897, viii. 52; *Am. J. Ophth.*, 1898, xv. 80.
[2] *Am. J. Ophth.*, 1898, xv. 22.

5

An Epitome of the History of Medicine. By ROSWELL PARK, M.D. Pp. xiv., 348. Philadelphia: The F. A. Davis Company. 1897.

It is with very great pleasure that we have read Dr. Roswell Park's praiseworthy book. We congratulate the University of Buffalo on having authorised the delivery of the course of lectures upon which this work was founded, and upon having a Professor who, in addition to the work of his own special department, was capable of undertaking so serious an additional responsibility. A succinct, but fairly complete, history of medicine from the earliest times to the present day has been compiled by the author, special chapters being devoted to the history of the development of antiseptic surgery, American medicine, anæsthesia, and dentistry. The book gives proof of much investigation and study on the author's part, and is written in good nervous English; the author however is obviously more conversant with the history of modern than of ancient medicine, and the hypercritical critic may succeed in discovering an occasional slip; e.g. (p. 34) "Aretæus, who died about 170 B.C., was one of the most brilliant lights of antiquity previous to the Christian era. . . . He came from Cappadocia about the end of the reign of Nero, and lived in Alexandria." It is still a reproach to the Anglo-Saxon nations that so little attention has been paid among them to the history of the medical art, and a really adequate work on the subject does not exist in their language. The author has with much industry done something to remove that reproach, and for his accomplishment we congratulate and thank him.

Inspector-General Sir James Ranald Martin, C.B., F.R.S. By Surgeon-General Sir JOSEPH FAYRER, Bart., M.D., F.R.S. Pp. xvi., 203. London: A. D. Innes & Co. 1897.

This memoir of Sir Ranald Martin, written by a man so well known and appreciated as Sir Joseph Fayrer, is a guarantee for a truthful account of the life of one who was distinguished not only in the position he held in India as a Medical Officer of the Indian Army, but also for his long and honourable career in civil practice both in India and in London, for the admirable work he did as Physician to the Medical Board at the India Office, and also for the excellent literary works on tropical diseases and climates which he has left behind him.

Sir Ranald Martin, like many other distinguished public

servants, hailed from the west coast of Scotland, from the Island of Skye, which is as celebrated for its loyal and patriotic sons as for its gallant and brave though humble breed of wiry terriers.

He came of an ancient and honourable lineage, and, as Sir Joseph Fayrer observes, he not only well maintained the tradition of the stock from which he sprang, but he transmitted his inherited good qualities to a numerous family of sons, some of whom served with distinction in the army and in the Civil Service of India.

Ranald Martin was originally intended for the combative ranks of the army. After he had been educated at the Inverness Royal Academy, a commission was ready for his acceptance in the 42nd Highlanders, the renowned Black Watch. But another career seemed to his father to offer him better prospects. The parental resources were at that time but slender, and the prospect of having to purchase all his steps seemed to his father more than those resources would bear. Young Ranald therefore acquiesced in his father's advice, and although the disappointment was bitter he chose medicine as his future career. He began to study first as an apprentice to a practitioner in Inverness, and in 1813 went to London and entered as a student in St. George's Hospital under Sir Everard Home and Sir Benjamin Brodie; and he also had the great advantage at Windmill Street Medical School of listening to such teachers as Wilson, Charles Bell, and J. Shaw. The period of student life was then very short, for after spending a year at St. George's he passed the College of Surgeons in 1814, which qualified him to practise at the age of 18 years and five months. Guthrie, who became a great surgeon both in military and civil life, passed the College at the age of 16. Truly these men only began to learn their profession *after* they were qualified. They were simply placed on the rails, they did the rest by their own earnest exertions. Two years later, Ranald Martin, having obtained an appointment as Assistant-Surgeon in the East India Company's service, sailed for Calcutta. Immediately on his arrival he was ordered for duty at the Presidency General Hospital for Europeans. The experience he gained in this hospital laid the foundation of his reputation as an earnest worker and close observer of the diseases of tropical climates, a field fresh and unknown to the European physician.

Having been appointed Assistant-Garrison-Surgeon, he was soon after ordered to accompany a force sent to subdue a revolt in Cuttack, in the district of Orissa. Returning to Calcutta, he was ordered to join the Ramghur Battalion for service in the Gondwana campaign. This was at that time a most unhealthy part of India. Here he suffered from a severe attack of malarial fever; but though unable to walk, he had himself carried about in order to make sanitary inspection, and shortly after he forwarded a report to the commanding officer, advising a move of the troops to a higher and healthier situation. This advice was politely declined, as many others of a similar kind were declined in those days, which resulted, as they usually did, in a higher rate of mortality among the troops. Thus, very early in his military career, did Ranald Martin show that he regarded the prevention of disease as one of the greatest, if not the very greatest, of the duties devolving upon a medical officer in charge of troops.

After only ten years' service in India we find this energetic medical officer, although at the time much broken in health, occupying in the great city of Calcutta a position which augured well for his future success.

In 1830 he was made Presidency Surgeon, and soon after was appointed on the staff of the Native Hospital of Calcutta. It was in this institution that he made his great reputation, not only in medical but in surgical cases : here he devised and first performed the operation for the radical cure of hydrocele by injection of tincture of iodine. In short, after his retirement from army service he became a great general practitioner in Calcutta, and attained the largest practice in the city.

But, on looking at his whole career in India and during his residence in London, it is manifest that the two subjects which were nearest to his heart were his devotion to the interests of the service which he had at first entered, and to the great questions of sanitary science which are so important in preserving the health of armies and communities. When we reflect that when Ranald Martin went to India first the death-rate among Europeans in that country was over 60 per 1000 per annum, and that now, chiefly owing to the work of sanitary reformers, of which Martin was one of the pioneers, the mortality has been reduced to about 18 per 1000, blind indeed must be the chronicler of the latter period of the history of India who does not recognise the blessing which has accrued to native and European alike from the improved health of the army and civil population. The change, too, has been brought about in the face of obstinate prejudices as difficult to overcome in the days that are past among educated European officials, as they are at present among the poor and ignorant natives of Bombay and Calcutta, resisting our attempts to remove from their midst a preventible disease which is decimating their families.

As the climate had begun to tell on his constitution, in 1840 Ranald Martin retired from practice in Calcutta and returned to England, after a service of twenty-five years. His reputation followed him to London, where he took a house in Grosvenor Street, with the intention to practise. He met with the greatest encouragement from Sir Benjamin Brodie, from Guthrie, the President of the Royal College of Surgeons, and others. His success was assured from the first, and he soon attained to a large practice, which he carried on until his sudden death in 1874. In 1859 he was appointed Physician to the India Board in succession to Dr. Scott. This brought him into a more prominent official position, and increased his practice.

About this time also the project of establishing an Army Medical School was taken up by Mr. Sydney Herbert, then Secretary of State for War, and Martin was invited by that minister to become a member of the Senate of the School, which was opened at Fort Pitt, Chatham, in the presence of the War Minister, by the late Sir Thomas Longmore, C.B. In recognition of his great services, Martin was made the recipient of several honours. He received the honour of knighthood, and the Companionship of the Order of the Bath.

"As a practitioner," says Sir John Kaye, "he was one of the most popular that ever entered a sick-chamber. His presence was like a gleam of sunshine, and he seldom quitted a patient without leaving him happier than before." He retired from the active work of his profession in November, 1874, and a few days after he was seized with bronchitis, and passed away after a short illness.

Recollections of Thirty-nine Years in the Army. By Sir CHARLES ALEXANDER GORDON, K.C.B. Pp. viii., 320. London: Swan Sonnenschein & Co., Limd. 1898.

This is a record of the services of a distinguished Army Medical Officer, extending uninterruptedly from the year 1841 to 1880. It is a plain statement of facts, without any adornment of style or any attempt at sensational writing. Surgeon-General Gordon has done long and faithful service to his country, and the five medals on his breast shown in his photograph in the frontispiece of his book attest that they were won in many an arduous campaign, and through many dangers from battle besides the risks run in some of the most deadly climates in which British soldiers are called upon to serve.

Sir Charles has purposely avoided all reference to medical or surgical matters in his narrative, although no man is more capable of dealing with them in a masterly manner.

A glance at the page of contents of the book will show the reader what stirring events he has witnessed. Beginning as Assistant-Surgeon of that gallant corps the 3rd Buffs, in 1841, he joined his regiment in India, serving in the Gwalior campaign in 1843. Returning home in 1845, he volunteered for service on the West Coast of Africa, which at that time held out to young medical officers the prospects of early promotion if they survived the risks of the climate. His service there resulted in some damage to his health; but he was back in India in 1852, but only for a short service, as he was compelled to return home again on sick leave. In the bracing air of his native land he soon recovered, and again went to India to find the great Sepoy Mutiny in full force in 1857. Through a great part of the outbreak he served principally with the Jounpore Field Force. He was present at the capture of Lucknow, and returned to England in 1859. While serving at home in 1860 he was suddenly ordered to embark for China, where he served in the stirring events at Tientsin and the Taku Forts, meeting, among others, with General Gordon, of Khartoum celebrity, then a Captain in the Royal Engineers. After a short service at home he returned to India for the fourth time.

In the Franco-German War of 1870 Gordon was appointed Medical Commissioner attached to the French Army, his duties being to report to the War Office on certain specified points relating to military organisation in the field. He remained in Paris during the whole period of the memorable siege, and to the end of the war. His descriptions of the scenes he witnessed are most thrilling.

Subsequently he was again ordered to the East. This time to Burma, and afterwards to the Madras Presidency of India.

It will be seen that in the long service of this most energetic army medical officer he enjoyed very little comparatively of the pleasure of home service, and it is gratifying to know that after so much exposure to the dangers of malaria and to many other risks he returned home in fairly good health. In 1880 his honourable service in the army came to an end, and having received the reward for distinguished military service, he retired as a Surgeon-Major-General; and in the Queen's Jubilee year he received from his sovereign the distinction of K.C.B., which he had so faithfully earned.

We heartily commend this book as very pleasant reading.

Tablets of Anatomy. By Thomas Cooke, M.D., and F. G. Hamilton Cooke. Three parts. [Eleventh Edition.] London: Longmans, Green, and Co. 1898.

These "tablets" are so well known as regards their arrangement and utility that we need not reiterate the many words of praise that have already been bestowed upon them. In Parts I. and II. the newer matter has been interpolated rather than incorporated, and this has led to a somewhat clumsy arrangement of the numbering of the pages and to some unnecessary repetition, which we think might profitably be altered when another edition is provided.

Since the above was written we regret to learn of the death of Mr. Thomas Cooke. While at work in his dissecting room he was seized with an attack of angina pectoris which ended fatally before he could be removed.

The Essentials of Experimental Physiology. By T. G. Brodie, M.D. Pp. xiv., 231. London: Longmans, Green, and Co. 1898.

For some time past we have had most excellent guides for laboratory work in histology and chemical physiology, by Schäfer and Halliburton respectively. Dr. Brodie's is the much wished for companion volume, and will, we think, have the same success. It is written on lines similar to the others—containing a clear account of the main experiments which should be done in such a course, and of the deductions which may be drawn from them. It is admirably done, and will, we hope, be much used.

Hallucinations and Illusions. By EDMUND PARISH. Pp. xiv., 390. London : Walter Scott, Ltd. 1897.

This book, which is one of the "Contemporary Science Series," is an English edition of the German original, which grew out of an examination of the "International Census of Waking Hallu-cinations of the Sane," and forms, in the words of its sub-title, " A Study of the Fallacies of Perception " of great interest.

Psychology is still a very young science, and it is only within the last few years that it has taken its place as an accurate—and to a great extent experimental—study of facts. There is already an extensive literature on the subject, and Mr. Parish is evidently well acquainted with it. In fact, the work is the outcome of a great deal of research and careful reasoning. Dreams, hypnosis, fallacies of memory, association and dis-sociation, after-images, &c., are each dealt with in relation to hallucinations and illusions. From the evidence collected there can be no doubt of the comparative frequency of hallucinations amongst the healthy in a waking condition, and it is stated that it is "impossible in practice as in theory to distinguish between waking hallucinations and those of sleep." Physiology is naturally constantly referred to and modern theories of brain-function are clearly understood; but there are, here and there, allusions to the " subcortical centres " and " basal ganglia," which are perhaps not quite up to date in the *rôle* allotted to these parts.

A powerful case is made out against instances meant to prove telepathy or thought-transference, and this part of the book is of most interest to the general reader, because it is less technical and requires less previous knowledge of the subject.

There is a useful summary in the last chapter, and an appendix with carefully-prepared tables and illustrative cases at the end of the book.

The questions discussed in this "Study" are intricate and abstruse, and great praise must be given to the author for the pains he has taken to sift a large mass of evidence and bring his deductions clearly before the reader.

The Blood : How to Examine and Diagnose its Diseases. By ALFRED C. COLES, M.D. Pp. xii., 260. London : J. & A. Churchill. 1898.

The scope of this book is limited to the examination and staining of the formed elements of the blood. The practical directions for the preparation and staining of blood-films are full and clear enough to enable anyone who carefully follows them to procure good specimens. Dr. Coles advocates the use of hæmatoxylin and eosin as stains, and the plates show that in his hands this method has given good results. We agree that the method of staining with eosin and methylene blue is difficult to carry out, and somewhat uncertain in its results. The author also advises alcohol and ether instead of heat for fixing blood-films. Sections on the pathology of the diseases described are given, but are too short to allow of an adequate treatment of the subject. Generally speaking, the references to the literature are full, and the opinions of other writers given at length. We think that the author might have given his own views more decidedly, and in some cases he has left his statements too vague for a text-book, but this well-printed volume, taken as a whole, gives a satisfactory account of the subject, and will no doubt be found useful for aid in work and for reference. The plates are well executed in colours. An illustration of the Thoma-Zeiss hæmacytometer would render the description more complete.

_____

A System of Medicine. By many Writers. Edited by THOMAS CLIFFORD ALLBUTT, M.D., F.R.S. Vol. V. Pp. xii., 1058. London: Macmillan and Co. Limited. 1898.

An exhaustive account of the diseases of the respiratory organs and of the circulatory system fills up this volume. It is somewhat belated, having waited for Professor Welch's contribution on thrombosis and embolism, which after all did not arrive in time; nevertheless, it well maintains the standard of the four previous volumes.

Dr. William Ewart writes the articles on bronchitis and bronchiectasis, in which many new methods of treatment are described; the most noteworthy of these is the creasote method of Dr. Arnold Chaplin, whose object is to bring about a complete expectoration of the bronchial contents, the vapour inhaled being concentrated to an almost intolerable degree. Whilst the cavities are being cleared and disinfected collateral expansion of the lung is induced by the cough, and the gradual contraction of the sacculations is promoted. This inhalation method has given such brilliant results, that every sufferer should have the benefit of a trial. Treatment by intra-tracheal injection of menthol and guaiacol in olive oil has given good results in inveterate cases of fœtid bronchiectasis, but Dr. Ewart gives a caution as to its use in phthisis. Amongst other methods of treatment are mentioned " (a) The inhalation of an oxygenated and terebinthinated atmosphere; (b) systematic exercise, at first passive only, of the thoracic muscles and of the abdominal muscles, including the use of dumb-bells or clubs, and a variety of postural exercises; (c) systematic respiratory gymnastics, such as deep inspirations followed by deep expirations in various attitudes, reading aloud or singing; (*d*) general massage and passive resistance movements followed by brisk rubbing." It will be seen that Dr. Ewart's article is very complete in its scope, and gives much more encouragement to the chronic bronchial invalid than he commonly receives.

Dr. Pye-Smith's article on pneumonia, and Dr. Percy Kidd's on phthisis pulmonalis, give excellent summaries of what is established with regard to those diseases and their varieties. The former does not lead us to expect a great diminution in the present high mortality of pneumonia, for he remarks that "in the long run the expectant method of treatment, which interferes only as occasion requires, is followed by a far lower mortality than misplaced attempts to 'jugulate' the disease, or than a completely negative treatment." We can scarcely reconcile this statement with the results given by Petresco, whose name, spelt with a final u, does not yet appear to be as well known as his statistics deserve to be, inasmuch as he reports a mortality of 2 per cent. in contrast with the 25.5 per cent. from Guy's Hospital as given by the author in this volume.

A short chapter by Dr. H. D. Rolleston describes a comparatively little known variety of the pneumomycosis of Hughes Bennett, which bears the name "pulmonary aspergillosis," in which the destructive lesions in the lungs are due to their invasion by a fungus, the aspergillus fumigatus. In order to differentiate this malady from other forms of pseudo-tuberculosis it is necessary that cultures should be obtained; without these no opinion as to the identity of the form of aspergillus is valid. The clinical features may resemble either those of chronic pulmonary tuberculosis or those of emphysema, and a secondary infection with tubercle bacilli is not improbable. The prognosis is less grave than that of pulmonary tuberculosis, since the lesion is usually much slower, never sets up a general infection, and tends to undergo a gradual and spontaneous cure.

Dr. Kingston Fowler writes on emphysema and on syphilitic disease of the lungs, and Dr. James F. Goodhart on asthma and hay fever. The account of the diseases of the respiratory organs concludes with articles on intra-pleural tension, on pleurisy and pneumothorax, by Drs. Samuel West, Gee, Herringham, and Finlay.

Amongst the chapters on diseases of the circulatory system, that by the editor on the ubiquitous but little understood chlorosis is one of the most interesting; and other articles by the same author are on functional disorders and mechanical strain of the heart. He makes the remark that "the physician who cannot treat chlorosis successfully with iron should abandon the practice of medicine"; and he has often suspected that incurable chlorosis may mean insoluble pills. He believes that in the sound adult organism the effects of physical stress upon the heart are promptly counteracted by equilibrating machinery, and that the importance of muscular effort as a factor in cardiac disease has been much exaggerated.

A System of Practical Medicine by American Authors. Edited by ALFRED LEE LOOMIS, M.D., and WILLIAM GILMAN THOMPSON, M.D. Vol. III.—*Diseases of the Alimentary Canal —Diseases of the Peritoneum—Diseases of the Liver and Gall Bladder—Diseases of the Spleen—Diseases of the Pancreas— Diseases of the Thyroid Gland—Chronic Metal-Poisoning—Alcoholism; Morphinism, etc.* Pp. 5—9, 19—926. London : Henry Kimpton. 1898.

The list of contributors to this volume comprises nine physicians of New York State, three of Canada, one of Boston, two of Ann Arbor, one of Chicago, one of San Francisco, one of Washington, and one of Philadelphia ; a list which may be looked upon as fairly representative of the North American continent.

Dr. Stockton and Dr. Allen Jones, in their article on diseases of the stomach, give an account of what can be done which is much in advance of the ordinary text-books. Their account of the general examination of the patient and the physical examination of the stomach comprises the use of all modern methods, and their account of the general and chemical analysis of the stomach-contents is especially full and complete. The subjects of hyperchlorhydria, hypochlorhydria, and achylia gastrica are described fully, and the use of the gastric electrode is advocated, both for the correction of defective secretion and in the treatment of the gastric sensory and motor neuroses. In the treatment of gastric ulcer the authors advocate the use of a combination of cerium oxalate, bismuth subcarbonate, and the light magnesium carbonate in large and oft repeated doses, and they do not advise rectal feeding excepting for at least three days after a gastric hemorrhage. It is somewhat of a surprise that they do not peptonise the milk for rectal feeding, and altogether do not give the practice of pre-digestion of milk the attention which its utility appears to demand. In the diagnosis of gastric carcinoma the use of Einhorn's gastrodiaphane is used to "assist in determining the size and location of the neoplasm, as the transillumination shows with less intensity or not at all through the carcinomatous anterior wall of the stomach in contrast to the brighter light transmitted through the rest of the organ." The chapter on gastrectasia and gastroptosis is very complete, and Einhorn's double tube gastric vaporizer has been found to act as an analgesic and slight motor stimulant. The authors emphasise the importance of surgical treatment of pyloric stenosis, especially of the benign kind, in which pylorectomy has been successful in 54 per cent., gastro-enterostomy in 71 per cent., pyloroplasty in 77.4 per cent., and digital divulsion in 59 per cent.

In addition to the topics named at the head of this review, the volume deals with infectious diseases common to man and animals, and with purpura, beri-beri, hæmophilia, diabetes, and insolation.

Lectures on the Malarial Fevers. By WILLIAM SYDNEY THAYER, M.D. Pp. viii., 326. New York: D. Appleton and Company. 1897.

The indiscriminate way in which the term malaria is generally applied to all sorts of febrile and afebrile conditions is an evidence of how backward medical opinion has been in appreciating recent advances in our knowledge of this subject. Professor Thayer's book will be found to contain a full, lucid, and succinct account of Paludism, the various chapters being devoted to history of the discovery of the parasite, methods of examination of the blood, description of the hæmatozoa, clinical description of the malarial fevers, sequelæ and complications, morbid anatomy, general pathology, diagnosis and treatment. A large number of illustrative charts are included, and also plates descriptive of the various phases of the parasites.

Clinically, the author recognises three varieties of malarial fever—tertian (including quotidian), quartan (including double and triple quartan), and æstivo-autumnal, these being respectively the result of infection by hæmamœba vivax, hæmamœba malariæ, and hæmatozoon falciparum. It has been customary to regard æstivo-autumnal fevers as due to a variety of organisms, but these the author is inclined to regard as a single variety of parasite. The crescentic and ovoid bodies, which have given rise to so much discussion, Professor Thayer considers are developed from the smaller forms in the ordinary cycle of development and are incapable of further development in the body. Manson's view, that the flagellated bodies represent the forms in which the malarial parasite exists outside the human body, does not meet with Professor Thayer's support, he himself tending to regard them as degenerate forms. That the mosquito acts an intermediate part he thinks is not proven. "On the whole, it must be said that we are absolutely ignorant of the form in which the malarial parasite exists outside of the human body, and equally ignorant of the manner in which it enters." In the clinical description the fact is emphasised that there may be a special localisation of the parasites in various organs, and thus the attack may take on a special type : thus, with the brain bearing the brunt, there may be coma, or bulbar paralysis, with localisation in the gastro-intestinal mucosa, choleriform symptoms may be the most prominent. The direct exciting cause of the malarial paroxysm Professor Thayer concludes is the liberation of some toxic substance by the specific parasites at the time of their sporulation. The discussion of this point, and indeed the whole chapter devoted to the general pathology, is full of the most interesting and original writing.

Under the head of "Treatment" is discussed the action of quinine on the malarial parasite, and the systematic and scientific administration of this drug is insisted upon, the writer giving it as his opinion that there is scarcely another drug

in the Pharmacopœia, unless it be digitalis, which is more
abused.

Professor Thayer's book promises and deserves to become a
standard work on the subject of malarial fevers.

Diabetes Mellitus and its Treatment. By R. T. WILLIAMSON,
M.D. Pp. xi., 417. London: Young J. Pentland. 1898.

It is rarely that we meet with a work in which an author
not only gives a clear account of valuable observations and
studies of his own, but also a full exposition of the theories
and experiments of other investigators, especially when these
relate to minor branches of the subject where the writer's own
interest is less keen.   Dr. Williamson, however, has carried his
thoroughness not only into his own extensive researches at first
hand, and has not been satisfied with producing a brilliant essay
on the subject from his own point of view, but he has presented
us with probably the best existing abstract of the numerous
papers on every aspect of the subject which have appeared
during the last twelve years.   It was a task much needed, for
the recent literature has been so voluminous and scattered that
reference to it had become practically impossible; and, apart
from the scientific advances which have been made, a large
number of practical improvements have been recorded both in
treatment, diagnosis, and chemical tests.

It is refreshing to read the new light thrown on the usual
tests, and of the errors usually committed.   No precaution
seems too small to notice, but we find that the author relies
chiefly (even in detecting very small amounts of sugar) on
Fehling's solution, phenylhydrazin, and fermentation.   In
difficult cases they are all used successively in the above order,
and Fehling's test again applied to the urine which has gone
through the fermentation process.   The over-sensitiveness of
phenylhydrazin is avoided by boiling for two minutes only, a
valuable improvement which gets rid of the minute crystals
formed from normal urine by the older method.   Dr. Williamson
confesses that the question of traces of sugar in healthy urine
is still unsolved, though he shows reasons for disbelieving
Pavy's estimate of .05 per cent.   In any case, these and other
ordinary tests are unaffected by it.

After discussing some of Pavy's recent controversies, with
a brevity for which the reader will be grateful, he gives us a
summary of the recent work relating to the pancreas, and finds
reason to think that in certain cases diabetes is directly due to
pancreatic disease, though it is not possible to say with certainty
during life whether it is due to this or other causes.

It is important to find that he has rarely failed to find the
tubercle bacillus in the phthisis of diabetes, though he recognises
that rare cases occur where it is absent.

The analysis of the symptoms of coma is especially interesting, and not least the presence of a yellowish deposit in the urine, consisting of enormous numbers of granular casts, which is very often found just before the onset of an attack. Here also the author's test from the blood reaction with methylene blue becomes invaluable for diagnosis if no urine can be obtained.

The chapter on foods and treatment is particularly full and careful. The gain of weight and general condition of the patient is put forward as of more importance than a mere decrease of sugar, desirable as this is. When we come to the question of bread substitutes, the author shows the little value of many of the usual preparations, for which, indeed, a reduced quantity of ordinary bread can be given with more comfort and equally good results. He recommends a cheap and palatable preparation made from aleuronat and cocoanut meal, and having a very low percentage of starch, for use when a rigid diet is indicated. The receipts for the manufacture of this and other articles are clear and practical; and if there is little fresh to be learnt from the chapter on drugs, we feel that the subject is not one on which much can be said at present.

The book is issued in Mr. Pentland's best style, the printing and references are clear and good, and the volume will be of value to every one who is studying the theory of the disease or has to treat it.

Wesen, Ursache und Behandlung der Zuckerkrankheit (Diabetes Mellitus). Von Dr. ALBERT LENNÉ. Pp. iv., 152. Berlin: S. Karger. 1898.

Dr. Lenné has put together a clear and readable account of diabetes for physicians and students. As the outcome of a large practical experience, he finds little success in the use of drugs, though he considers that opium is of some value, and long-continued courses of alkalies when commenced early enough may indirectly produce good results. There does not appear any undue praise of the virtues to be found in the thermal springs of Neuenahr, where the writer practises, though the benefits of a course at a pleasant watering-place are not ignored. Of the value of rest for mind and body and the care of the general health he speaks strongly. As to other treatment, Dr. Lenné seems to rely chiefly on a diet carefully regulated from time to time according to the assimilative powers of his patients, and he prefers whole bread, in quantities such as can be easily dealt with in the body, to any of the artificial substitutes.

A review of modern theories of the pathology of diabetes is given in a succinct form, and extremely full tables of the sugar and starch contents of all possible articles of diet are added.

On the whole it is an interesting and well-written book, and in many points well up to date. Moreover, it possesses the luxury of a capital index, which adds considerably to its value.

A Text-Book of Practical Therapeutics. By HOBART AMORY
HARE, M.D. Sixth Edition. Pp. 758. London: Henry
Kimpton. 1897.

Seated in his editorial chair, Dr. H. A. Hare must see pass
before him in review the vast crowd of therapeutical experiences
and suggestions which is ever being recorded in the medical
journals. That he has long since brought out a successful text-
book of therapeutics is therefore not to be wondered at; this
work in its present edition has been largely re-written, to bring
it up more fully abreast with the present state of the art of
which it treats. The two more important sections of the book
are: (1) A description of the properties and uses of drugs,
arranged in alphabetical order—a plan now adopted in most text-
books of Materia Medica; and (2) A list of the principal recognised diseases, also arranged alphabetically, giving a succinct
yet sometimes fairly full account of the accepted treatment for
each disease. Although Dr. Hare is a Professor of Therapeutics, as well as editor of a journal devoted to the same
subject, he is not unduly carried away by every ephemeral
novelty. In the preface he says: "Only those measures which
have proved useful and reliable in therapeutics are included."
An examination of the text of the book certainly corroborates
this statement, and we should indeed have been not sorry if
some additional suggestions had here and there added to the
well-tried measures enumerated. The article on the treatment
of phthisis is almost depressing in its negations.

The book is excellently printed, wonderfully free from clerical
or typographical errors, and is elaborately indexed. Everything that is affirmed in the book can be accepted as trustworthy, and altogether the work is a bright and worthy
monument of the author's industry and learning.

Outlines of Practical Surgery. By WALTER G. SPENCER, M.B.,
M.S. Pp. x., 694. London: Baillière, Tindall and Cox.
1898.

The practical surgeon of the present day will be much relieved
to find that the author has produced a work of such excellence,
without going too deeply into the details of theoretical pathology
and bacteriology.

The diagrammatic nature of the illustrations with which the
various chapters abound are most clear, and by examining these
"black and white figures" the student of practical surgery can
readily comprehend numerous details in the operative art, which
in some books are not too clearly explained in the text.

We are sorry to see in the pages devoted to bandaging that
no mention is made of the good old method of "reversing" in
spiral bandaging, and we do not quite agree with the text as to

where the spiral bandage may be used. It is certainly doubtful whether (if we except the joints) the commonest method of bandaging is the figure-of-eight. We do not like the description of the suturing of the two ends of the divided intestine round the male and female portions of Murphy's button; the approved method might, in a future edition of the book, be clearly demonstrated by a diagram.

On reading the volume through we find little of importance to detract from its value, and we recommend it as a most useful addition to the library of those wanting a practical book on surgery.

Wounds in War. By Surgeon-Colonel W. F. STEVENSON, M.B. Pp. xv., 419. London: Longmans, Green, and Co. 1897.

It is with great satisfaction and interest that we have read this book of Surgeon-Colonel Stevenson's, and we welcome it cordially, for no one should be more qualified to speak on the subject than the Professor of Military Surgery at Netley. Practically, as Colonel Stevenson points out, the subject is limited to gunshot wounds, those inflicted by sword or bayonet being, at least in warfare between civilised nations, a negligable quantity. Not that our author has by any means omitted to mention other injuries, but he has given them only a small share of his consideration proportionate to their importance. In his clearly printed pages, abundantly illustrated and well furnished with diagrams and tables, he has embodied a vast store of information useful to the military surgeon, and by no means wanting in interest to his civilian *confrère*. Each paragraph is headed with its subject in heavy black type, a plan which increases the value of the book as a work of reference.

The first chapter deals with the mechanism of projectiles, their motion and velocity, and the effects upon them of the resistance of the air and gravitation. It concludes with a description of the Lee-Metford magazine rifle, which has been described as "the best military small arm in existence." We record this fact with some amount of pride, as the part-inventor of this weapon is a Bristol citizen. The second chapter details the characteristics of injuries produced by different projectiles —by the old round bullet, the modern cylindro-conoidal bullet, and by large projectiles and their fragments.

A short chapter is devoted to the primary symptoms of wounds, namely, pain, local shock, anæsthesia, hemorrhage, and the treatment of these conditions, followed by a consideration of the general treatment of wounds in war, with an interesting contrast between the old and new methods, and the bacteriology of wounds. Under the heading "First Field Dressings," great stress is laid upon the importance of the handling of a wound as little as possible, in order to avoid the introduction of septic material.

We are now introduced to the more special subject of the book, namely, gunshot wounds and their treatment. Our author, after again emphasising his remarks on the non-interference with wounds on the field, describes the various means of detecting the extent of injury, and the presence of a bullet or other foreign substance. The finger of the surgeon, Nélaton's probe, or other more clumsy contrivance for diagnosis, will, for the future, be superseded by Röntgen's marvellous discovery, and one incalculable source of danger to the wounded soldier avoided. The risk of secondary hemorrhage, an accident far less common than it used to be, and caused by disintegration of the wall of the vessel by septic arteritis, is minimised by the introduction of the antiseptic treatment of wounds.

From the general consideration we pass to a most interesting and carefully compiled description of the injuries of individual structures of the different joints, the long bones, head, thorax, and abdomen, the indications for conservative treatment, for amputation, and cautions in dealing with penetrating wounds of lung and brain. All these are of great practical value.

The ninth chapter deals with wounds of the abdomen. Penetrating wounds of the abdomen are by far the most fatal of all injuries in war, the mortality running as high as 90 per cent.

It would, we think, be advantageous to found upon the details given in these valuable chapters a small handbook of aphorisms which could be regarded as authoritative, and would, if well put together, be a safe guide and help to the military surgeon in those formidable emergencies with which he may be brought into contact.

The thirteenth chapter is devoted firstly to statistics, and secondly to a description of the duties of bearers in the field, the first dressings, transport of the wounded, and the management of the field hospital, whilst the concluding chapter gives us a *résumé* of the work of the Geneva Convention, and expresses a hope that its suggestions will in time meet with a more general appreciation, and that the Red Cross will be universally recognised as a military badge of neutrality.

An American Text-Book of Genito-Urinary Diseases, Syphilis, and Diseases of the Skin. Edited by L. BOLTON BANGS, M.D., and W. A. HARDAWAY, M.D. Two volumes. Pp. 1—592, 593—1229. London: The Rebman Publishing Co. (Ltd.). Philadelphia: W. B. Saunders. 1898.

The combination of genito-urinary diseases with dermatology, or even with syphilis, is rather astonishing to English readers, but seems to be quite a usual trans-Atlantic practice, as there is an American *Journal of Cutaneous and Genito-Urinary*

Diseases. The articles in this work are by various writers, some of whom are well known for their contributions to the literature of the subject on which they write. Dr. White, of Philadelphia, for instance, writes on diseases of the prostate in conjunction with Dr. Wood, and his recent remarks on the treatment of prostatic hypertrophy by castration and vasectomy are of particular value. It is curious to find "inflammation of the seminal vesicle, the cord, and epididymis, and the testicle proper" as the heading of a section of a chapter, but the author evidently attaches great importance to diseases of the seminal vesicles, and their diagnosis. The subject of diseases and injuries of the ureter is, as might be expected in a modern work, treated in a separate chapter, and by so able a writer as Christian Fenger.

The more recent views about ringworm—including Sabouraud's—are clearly put forth; but ultimately, we feel sure, they will be modified: and the treatment of that comprehensive disease, eczema, is good and rings with common sense. We read: "The successful treatment of eczema is something more than the hasty prescription . . . for internal use and a salve or lotion for external application," and we note with strong approval that all eczemas should be cured. "Internal treatment . . . is not called for in a large proportion of the cases," and "it may be expressed as almost a law that the more circumscribed an eczematous eruption is the less will be needed in the form of general medication ; . . . local eczemas require local applications." We have still the long-standing dispute about lichen ruber acuminatus, lichen ruber, and lichen ruber planus, and it "bids fair to afford abundant material for discussion for some time to come."

The work contains a very thorough and valuable collection of information on the subject of genito-urinary surgery, and the numerous illustrations are good, in this portion particularly those of hypertrophy of the prostate gland, in connection with the article by Drs. White and Wood, while the coloured plates and other illustrations of skin diseases are very faithfully and artistically executed ; some of them are the best we have seen in any similar kind of work. We commend the book very heartily. There are many very useful prescriptions and the classification of skin affections is as good as it can be with the present nomenclature.

Text-Book of Diseases of the Kidneys and Genito-Urinary Organs. By Prof. Dr. PAUL FÜRBRINGER. Translated by W. H. GILBERT, M.D. Vol. II. Pp. vi., 310. London: H. K. Lewis. 1898.

The first volume of this work, which dealt with the medical aspect of the subject, was favourably reviewed by us in March, 1896. Of the second volume, which considers the surgical diseases

6

of the organs in question, it is not possible to speak highly. In fact, the diseases of the genito-urinary organs are now so specialised that it is impossible for one man to deal satisfactorily with the whole of them. It would have been better if the author had confined his information to the diagnosis and medical treatment of those diseases of the urinary organs which fall to the lot of the physician.

The bibliography seems an important feature, but it is arranged alphabetically only according to the authors' names, and not according to subjects. It seems to us that, with Mr. Jacobson's work on diseases of the male genital organs and Mr. Henry Morris's recent book on diseases of the urinary organs, and the very full consideration of the subject in our larger text-books of surgery, there was really no need for the translation of Professor Fürbringer's second volume. To English readers some of the terms used are rather remarkable. For instance, hydrocele in connection with epididymitis, which we should call an acute hydrocele, is spoken of as periorchitis acuta.

The author regrets that pain in the groin is not recognised as common in acute epididymitis. We should certainly have considered that it was known to every observant student. The diagnosis of renal calculus from the other morbid conditions which may readily be mistaken for it receives most inadequate notice, and the reference to the surgical treatment of renal disease is very imperfect and unsatisfactory. Much space is given to an enumeration of the various futile attempts which have been made to discover the condition of the separate kidneys, and yet there is no mention of the work of Howard Kelly in this direction.

We cannot recommend the work either as a concise statement of the leading facts of genito-urinary surgery, or as any approach to an exhaustive treatise on the subject. Some of the information given we even regard as dangerous. For instance, in speaking of the diagnosis of renal cancer, we are told of a case in which aspiration was not only used, but repeated several times for diagnosis, and then after death it was found that the growth was in the "small omentum" and not in the kidney at all! Surely such proceedings are highly dangerous and not to be recommended by illustrative cases. Then again, in speaking of the treatment of stone in the bladder, we are told that the bladder has been opened from the rectum, as if such a proceeding was an approved method of operation.

The Diseases of the Male Urethra. By R. W. STEWART, M.D. Pp. viii., 221. New York: William Wood and Company. 1896.

This is a very useful book, which treats of inflammatory affections of the urethra and their result in the form of stricture. As gonorrhœa is so common it is worth while devoting some considerable time to the study of this disease and its sequelæ. Modern methods of diagnosis, such as the use of the endoscope, are fully described, and the affections of different portions of the urethra considered in separate chapters. The inflammatory diseases of the seminal glands which are connected with the urethra are also considered. We were rather staggered by the word "Cowperitis," which, although not new, is one against which we must enter an etymological protest. There are some good pictures of the anatomy of the urethra and useful representations of instruments employed in urethra diagnosis and treatment, and the book is a decided acquisition to the literature of the subject. The fact that the publishers' work has been done in so excellent a fashion makes it all the more acceptable.

Orthopedic Surgery. By JAMES E. MOORE, M.D. Pp. 354. London: The Rebman Publishing Co. (Ltd.). Philadelphia: W. B. Saunders. 1898.

When another volume upon a small branch of general surgery is added to those which already exist we have a right to claim that it shall be justified by some evidence of originality in the method of treatment, or at least of such care and judgment in examining controversial points, and in fully and accurately setting forth the more recent additions to our knowledge, as shall make it something more than a numerical addition to an overburdened literature. Unfortunately, in both these respects, the work under review, in our opinion, signally fails. For example, in the section on knock-knee nothing is said about the possible *rôle* of the tibia and fibula in the pathology of that affection: pes cavus receives the consideration of only a few lines; while of the important and relatively little-known conditions, termed metatarsalgia and coxa vara the accounts are so meagre and inadequate as to be almost, if not quite, valueless. Nor do we find any compensation in the treatment of the more ordinary portions of the subject, which never rises above mediocrity and is often weak and unsatisfactory.

The publishers' work has been excellently done, and there is no lack of illustrations, well executed, which are liberally scattered through the letterpress.

The Practice of Midwifery. By D. LLOYD ROBERTS, M.D. Fourth Edition. Pp. xv., 585. London: J. & A. Churchill. 1896.

Clear and succinct and quite modern in all its practical part, this book is a very trustworthy manual for students.

The author lays great stress on the proper measures to be used to attain asepsis as far as is possible, and his directions, if followed carefully, will, without being over elaborate, be found amply sufficient.

In describing the mutilating operations for the relief of dystocia he mentions cranioclasm as being the operation of breaking up the base of the skull after craniotomy; we have always been under the impression that this operation was known as basiotripsy while cranioclasm is the operation by which after perforation the vault of the skull is removed piecemeal.

One noteworthy feature is an excellent chapter on symphysiotomy, which gives the completest account of the operation that we have yet met with in any student's manual.

The work, offering a logical and accurate account of the various processes, will form a valuable addition to the student's library. The plates are numerous and well drawn.

Treatise on the Diseases of Women. By ALEXANDER J. C. SKENE, M.D. Third Edition. Pp. xviii., 991. New York: D. Appleton and Company. 1898.

It is six years since the publication of the last edition of this work, and during that period great advances have been made, which have been duly incorporated in the present issue. The treatment of uterine fibroids has been fully brought up to date, but a more clear statement should have been made of the indications for adopting the different methods. The author believes that electrolysis "takes a high rank among the means of treating fibroma of the uterus," but we are not told the class of case in which he considers it desirable to use it. Too much space is given to the "illustrative cases," which, though interesting, occupy a greater part of the book than is warranted by the instruction they afford. The various subjects are handled with such thoroughness and judicious care as the great experience of the author would lead us to expect. A word of praise should also be given to the excellent plates and drawings with which the work is illustrated.

Therapeutics of Infancy and Childhood. By A. JACOBI, M.D. Second Edition. Pp. xvi., 9—629. Philadelphia: J. B. Lippincott Company. 1898.

It is a pleasure to find that some medical man can avoid the stiff and stilted style that is commonly adopted when giving opinions. Dr. Jacobi writes easily—almost conversationally, and frequently forcibly—so that the task of reading a big book like this is comparatively slight. Unless this is a natural faculty an author may, to create a sensation, overstep the bounds of easy writing and become ridiculous and abusive. We regret to say that Dr. Jacobi has sometimes done this; and we think that the author's disapproval of Emil Behring's methods might have been expressed in less severe language with advantage.

Apart from these blemishes, the book is a very useful one, and contains the opinions and experiences of an acute observer, and as such will be of great value to students of children's diseases. There are things which we do not agree with, but that possibly is inevitable. For instance, in this country Rötheln is looked upon as a separate disease, and though acute rheumatism is common among children it is not in our experience frequently seen in infants. Scrofula we generally take to be synonymous with tubercle, but Dr. Jacobi thinks that the bacillus need not be present; and we must express our surprise at ossification of the costal cartilages (and consequent want of expansion of the lung) being a cause of tubercular disease of the lungs.

The Natural and Artificial Methods of Feeding Infants and Young Children. By EDMUND CAUTLEY, M.D. Pp. viii., 376. London: J. & A. Churchill. 1897.

Of the many works that have been produced during the last few years on this subject there is not one that we can recommend more heartily than this. There is little that is new in it, but the author has condensed into a comparatively small space, without undue curtailment, all the recent investigations on the methods of preparing foods for the infant and juvenile stomach. The chapter on proprietary foods is particularly good, and we are in thorough accord with the author in his dictum that in the vast majority of cases in which they are being alone given the child is being deprived of more suitable and appropriate food. We admit with him that several may with advantage be given on occasions: it is the abuse of them that we condemn, and the abuse is more common than the appreciation.

The Study of Children, and their School Training. By FRANCIS WARNER, M.D. Pp. xix., 264. New York: The Macmillan Company. 1898.

The excellence of Dr. Francis Warner's work in connection with the study of childhood is generally recognised; all that is here requisite is, to note the principles and construction of the book under review. Skilful adaptation of the mode of education to the needs of the particular child is the author's contention; and the proposition that all expression of the action of mind is by movement, is adopted as the basis of observation-methods. Thus, says the author, movements, balance, gestures, actions and response indicate the child's brain-state; and it should, therefore, be an object in training children to remove their faulty nerve-signs, or irregular or bad methods in movement, and with them the co-related brain-disorderliness. The earlier chapters deal concisely with the growth and development of the child's body and mind, the points to be considered in seeking indications of normal and abnormal nerve-signs; in later ones are discussed relative mental ability and psychological changes during pubescence. Subsequently comes the practical portion of the book, which deals with the removal of both motorial and mental disorders by physical training and the correction of various unhygienic conditions. Some pithy generalisations are usefully appended in the final chapter. The work should prove of interest and value to all those engaged in the education of children or in the study of them psychologically.

Forensic Medicine and Toxicology. By J. DIXON MANN, M.D. Second Edition. Pp. xiv., 683. London: Charles Griffin and Company, Limited. 1898.

In March, 1894, we noticed the first edition of this work, and considered that it would prove useful for students to peruse before an examination, owing to the condensation of its matter, and help the general practitioner who has no time to refer to the larger manuals. In this second edition improvements have been introduced in many parts. Cases are more frequently given and at more length. Some useful paragraphs have been added in the section dealing with sudden death from natural causes. Under the head of "Life Assurance," something, we think, ought to have been given as the probable duration of life in those suffering from organic diseases: a rather difficult subject, no doubt, but one which is only slightly treated even by the authorities on general disease, to whom we are referred by Dr. Mann. We notice the absence of any account of gunshot wounds caused by modern weapons of precision and the new bullets—for some strange accidents have been caused by them, and suicides effected by their use. Under "Heat-Stroke" there is no mention of how frequently insanity of a dangerous and incurable form follows on an attack. Amongst the poisons, acetylene, now coming so much into use, is noticed, as are also some of the aniline group and poisonous foods.

Epidemic Diphtheria: a Research on the Origin and Spread of the Disease from an International Standpoint. By ARTHUR NEWSHOLME, M.D. Pp. iv., 196. Swan Sonnenschein & Co., Limd. 1898.

This painstaking and valuable contribution to the epidemiology of diphtheria deserves careful study. The first part of the book is taken up with graphic charts showing the behaviour of diphtheria over a long series of years in towns and districts in all parts of the world. The second half of the book contains

Dr. Newsholme's review of the prevalence of diphtheria as shown in these charts, a discussion of the conditions determining pandemics of diphtheria, the relationship of rainfall and of soil to diphtheria, and a review of the position of preventive medicine in relation to the still-increasing prevalence of this . disease. While Dr. Newsholme's conclusions place "waves of diphtheria-prevalence" on a plane above our control, the admission that diphtheria is spread chiefly by personal infection, which is, however, immensely more potent in epidemic than in inter-epidemic years, encourages the hope that present-day methods of control, including bacteriological supervision of throat-cases, should prove effectual in checking its spread.

An Inquiry into the Relative Efficiency of Water Filters in the Prevention of Infective Disease. By G. SIMS WOODHEAD, M.D., and G. E. CARTWRIGHT WOOD, M.D. Pp. viii., 135. London : Printed at the Office of the British Medical Association. 1898.

This is a reprint in book form of a very valuable report upon all classes of domestic filters, with special reference to their power of removing pathogenic organisms from polluted water. A considerable number of filters, representing probably all the numerous types that have been placed upon the market, are examined in detail as regards their permeability both to ordinary water bacteria and to pathogenic forms. The authors arrive at a very important conclusion, already sufficiently recognised by those who have made a special study of the matter, but never perhaps formulated in so complete and authoritative a manner. None of the filters charged with the pulverulent or fibrous media, until lately so universally in use, afford the least protection against the passage of the causative agents of enteric fever or cholera ; but, on the other hand, these filters are likely to prove sources of danger as secondary means of contaminating pure water. Differences in the rapidity of transmission of bacteria were noticed, and were attributed to the varying length of time necessary for washing the organisms through different thicknesses of filtering medium : and it would have added much to the interest of the report if the real efficacy of the sand filter-beds, upon which so much reliance is placed at the present time, had been tested on parallel lines. The only filters that were found to effectually exclude pathogenic bacteria were those in which the media employed were "forms of porcelain, compressed silicious earth and natural stone." In order, however, to bring about a sufficient rapidity of flow through these denser media, it is in general necessary to apply additional pressure, a proceeding which severely tests the mechanical fittings as well as the perfection of structure of the filter itself.

A second deduction from this noteworthy series of experiments is of great scientific interest; namely, that no filter is proof against bacteria capable of growth in the liquid undergoing filtration. No filter, therefore, permanently removes the ordinary water organisms which appear in the filtrate after a lapse of from two to four days, owing to growth along the pores of the filter. A precisely similar result is attained with typhoid and cholera bacilli if as little as one-fiftieth part of ordinary broth is added to the water; no such effect, however, is produced by the addition of sewage, water deposit, or other organic matters likely to occur in natural waters, and it seems improbable, therefore, that risk of this kind would be incurred in actual practice.

The whole report teems with exact and detailed information on many vexed questions; and will well repay perusal by all concerned in the maintenance of the public health.

From Our Dead Selves to Higher Things. By FREDERICK JAMES GANT. Second Edition. Pp. xiv., 185. London: Baillière, Tindall & Cox. 1897.—It is always refreshing to find that a busy surgeon has time to write on matters other than those concerning his profession, and most of us will be the better for reading this expression of the author's inner thoughts. The high-toned morality of the work is unquestionable, but to say with the author that "the veil of 'Agnosticism' is rent in twain from the top to the bottom" depends on the point of view of the reader.

The Determination of Sex. By Dr. LEOPOLD SCHENK. Pp. 173. London: The Werner Company. 1898.—The first half of this book is a discursive account of the various theories which have been held as to the determination of the sex of children. The latter half deals with Dr. Schenk's researches on the subject. They amount to this—that many women, though not considered to be diabetic, pass minute traces of sugar in the urine. Such women generally have female offspring. If these traces of sugar be removed by a diet consisting mainly of proteids and fats, males are produced. The evidence offered in support of this theory is most meagre and unsatisfactory. Some things doubtless are better done in Germany; but it is refreshing, after looking over this volume, to turn to the *Evolution of Sex*, by Geddes and Thomson, who give a lucid account of what is known on the subject.

Rheumatoid Arthritis. By GILBERT A. BANNATYNE, M.D. Second Edition. Pp. xii., 182. Bristol: J. Wright & Co. 1898.—There has been some revision and improvement in this book, which now forms a fairly complete work on the subject. The theory advanced in the first edition as to a microbic origin for the disease is altered in some respects, the author coming to the conclusion that there are at least two forms of rheumatoid arthritis—the one acute and undoubtedly of microbic character, the other chronic and degenerative. No evidence, however, is given as to whether the micro-organisms characteristic of the acute forms are found in the chronic ones, and the relationship of the two is left indefinite. The treatment advocated is much the same as in the former edition. A regrettable point is that the author barely mentions the excellent results which have been obtained by the action of high temperatures, by the hot air or electric radiant baths.

The Extra Pharmacopœia. By WILLIAM MARTINDALE and W. WYNN WESTCOTT, M.B. Ninth Edition. Pp. xxviii., 626. London: H. K. Lewis. 1898.—A work which in a comparatively few years has reached its ninth edition stands in need of no commendatory criticism. The British Pharmacopœia becomes continuously more and more inadequate to fulfil the requirements of practice, and a text-book of information such as this present excellent work is now a necessity. In this last edition have been incorporated all the essential contents of the new B.P., while in addition there is a wondrous store of instruction about the multitude of remedial agents in the use of which the B.P. in its narrow scope does not take notice. A monument of industry, of up-to-date learning, and of usefulness, this book is indispensable to every intelligent practitioner who desires to employ the full therapeutical resources of his art.

Chavasse's Advice to a Wife. Revised by FANCOURT BARNES, M.D. Fourteenth Edition. Pp. 306. London: J. & A. Churchill. [1898.]—We consider that this edition maintains the reputation that previous ones have made for this very useful work. The introductory chapter on the health of the young wife is very good, and can be read with advantage by all women. The portion that follows is more or less pertinent to the subject of pregnancy, and can be recommended as a very good guide.

Chavasse's Advice to a Mother. By GEORGE CARPENTER, M.D. Fifteenth Edition. Pp. x., 430. London: J. & A. Churchill. [1898.]—Few books of this character, we believe, have proved more popular and useful than this, and we are bound to say that it is head and shoulders above the usual manuals intended to instruct mothers on their duties towards their babies. In revising the present edition and relegating the few prescriptions to an appendix, Dr. Carpenter has done well and wisely. About such light and airy conversations as we find here there is a charm which has always attracted us ever since we learnt our first lessons of science from Dr. Brewer's *Guide to Knowledge;* but no book of this kind that we have ever seen has treated us to so many quotations from the poets: Byron, Coleridge, Martin Tupper (1), Shakspere, Barham, Knox, Tennyson, and many others are quoted; while even the author, under the influence of the question of the propriety of sucking one's thumb, breaks out into verse. We commend the advice to the mother on her behaviour to her doctor on pp. 323-5, and only wish we were always treated with so much consideration.

Brief Essays on Orthopædic Surgery. By NEWTON M. SHAFFER, M.D. Pp. v., 81. New York: D. Appleton and Company. 1898.—Those interested in orthopædic surgery as a speciality will do well to read these short essays, which are reprinted from various periodicals. They define the position of the orthopædic surgeon and urge the desirability of conservatism. They deplore the tendency of some specialists—gynæcologists, for example—to commit depredations in the fields of general surgery.

The Diseases of Children's Teeth, their Prevention and Treatment. By R. DENISON PEDLEY. Pp. xi., 268. London: J. P. Segg & Co. [1895.]—Considerable praise is due to the author for his attempt to interest medical students and practitioners in this subject. The book is very readable, not too long, and contains very practical hints. The chapters on oral hygiene and irregularities of position are excellent. It is a pity that the author advocates a proprietary tooth powder. Still, on the whole his book fulfils its aim as well as any work of the kind with which we are acquainted.

Diseases of the Upper Respiratory Tract. By P. WATSON WILLIAMS, M.D. Third Edition. Pp. xvi., 282. Bristol: John Wright & Co. 1898.—This work has evidently met a well-marked requirement. It contains in a small compass much valuable information, and though it is practically a reprint of the previous issue, it is well up to date and forms a handy guide to the subject.

The Johns Hopkins Hospital Reports. Vol. VII. Nos. 1-2 — *Report in Gynecology*. Baltimore: The Johns Hopkins Press. 1898.—The greater part of this report is taken up with a "critical review of seventeen hundred cases of abdominal section from the standpoint of intraperitoneal drainage," wherein the observations of the author, Dr. J. G. Clark, go to show that the drainage-tube is still used too largely in abdominal work. The rest of the book is concerned with "the etiology and structure of true vaginal cysts," written by Dr. J. E. Stokes. Of the merit of these reports we have frequently spoken, and the present work further enhances the solid reputation which they have gained for accurate and painstaking research.

The Middlesex Hospital. Reports of the Medical, Surgical, and Pathological Registrars for the Year 1896. London: H. K. Lewis. 1897.—These reports comprise an elaborate classification of all the cases in the hospital during the year, with abstracts of the more important ones and of *post-mortem* examinations. Attention may be directed to the tables on diphtheria, the classification of cases of hernia, and of over thirty cases of operation on the kidneys. Seven out of sixteen cases of strangulated hernia were fatal, a high mortality now-a-days. Thirty-one cases of appendicitis were admitted to the medical wards, twenty of which recovered, one died, and the rest were transferred to the surgical wards, where twenty-three cases were admitted altogether, five being fatal. In thirty operations on the kidney, two only were followed by death. It is interesting to note that seven of these proved negative explorations, four for nephralgia and three for hæmaturia, *i.e.* nearly 25 per cent.

Clinical Report of the Rotunda Hospitals, 1896-97. Dublin: John Falconer. 1898.—The master and his assistants are highly to be congratulated both on the excellent results obtained, and the manner in which the results are tabulated and presented for perusal. Three thousand four hundred and fifty-five cases were attended, with a total maternal mortality of seven or ·205 per cent. Only two deaths are attributed to sepsis. The number of cases in which the temperature reached 100.8° F. was seventy-eight, but in only fifteen was it considered necessary to wash out the uterus. A review of the work of the gynæcological department contains a very interesting account of the arrangements of the operating theatre, methods of sterilising hands, clothing, instruments, sutures, ligatures, etc. In all plastic operations on the vagina, a preliminary curetting of the uterus is done: this procedure might be more widely adopted with advantage. The lists of operations, the mortality of the same, and the reasons explaining the deaths should all be read in the original paper. The mortality of eleven vaginal cœliotomies, and fifty-five ventral cœliotomies, including nine panhysterectomies, was eight or twelve per cent.

Transactions of the College of Physicians of Philadelphia. Vol. XIX. Philadelphia: Printed for the College. 1897.—The usual obituary notices and presidential address are followed by a selection from the papers read during the year. One of the most noteworthy of these is by Dr. Alfred Stengel on the value of auscultatory percussion in diagnosis. The different methods of stethoscopic percussion are described, and the author gains confidence in the method in accordance with increasing experience: his general conclusions are in accord with other writers, who have learnt the method in one or other of its various forms. A paper by Dr. Charles Winslow Dulles advocates the view " that consumption is not a disease that is now spreading," but that " for many years there has been a comparatively steady decline in the proportion of cases of consumption ": he combats the current views in favour of contagion, and entertains the hope that without spasmodic and violent measures the disease will soon cease to be the scourge and terror that it now is.

Transactions of the American Pediatric Society. Vol. IX. Reprinted from *The Archives of Pediatrics.* 1897.—Several interesting papers will be found in these records; notably a paper by Dr. J. O'Dwyer on retained intubation tubes, based on an experience of over five hundred cases of intubation. Dr. Koplik describes his method of rapid bacteriological diagnosis of diphtheria in two to three hours. There is an interesting paper on several cases of retro-œsophageal (intrathoracic) abscess presenting anomalous symptoms, and on five cases of cerebral abscess in infants. Empyema, pneumonia, and many other interesting subjects are considered.

Transactions of the Dermatological Society of Great Britain and Ireland. Vol. III. London: H. K. Lewis. 1897.—There seems to be life in this Society, for the volume before us contains more than double the matter of the previous one. The address by the President, Dr. J. F. Payne, on "Bacteria in Diseases of the Skin," is well worth perusal; it contains many deep thoughts, and there is no doubt that the "pathology of this organ [skin] is decidedly in advance of that of many other parts in regard to the subject of inflammation." The article on "Yaws in India" by Mr. Arthur Powell is almost exhaustive of the subject; and "The Influence of Light on the Skin," by Dr. R. L. Bowles, shows the competency of the author to discourse on the subject. We should like more pictures of the quality of that which illustrates Dr. Abraham's case of pustular eruption from tar..

The Year-Book of Treatment for 1899. London: Cassell and Company, Limited.—This, the fifteenth annual issue, is excellent in point of merit and general usefulness to the practitioner, and in saying this, we afford it the best recommendation to all those who are not acquainted with this summary of the year's progress. We note one new feature this year in the able article by Dr. Burton-Fanning on "The Open-air Treatment of Phthisis."

Index-Catalogue of the Library of the Surgeon-General's Office, United States Army.—Second Series. Vol. III., C—Czygan. Washington: Government Printing Office. 1898.—The present volume of this monumental work bears the same impress of elaborate care and indefatigable energy which has characterised the previous volumes. It is indispensable to all libraries and writers on medical subjects.

The Journal of Tropical Medicine. London: John Bale, Sons & Danielsson, Ltd.—This is a monthly Journal devoted to medical, surgical, and gynæcological work in the Tropics, and is under the direction of Mr. James Cantlie and Dr. W. J. Simpson, whose long experience of disease in the East entitles them to speak with authority on the subject of tropical medicine. It began life in August, 1898, and has been added to our exchange-list. Amongst noteworthy contributions to the earlier numbers of this periodical are articles—by Sir Joseph Fayrer, "Enteric Fever among British Soldiers in India"; by Haffkine and Bannerman, "The Testing of Haffkine's Plague-Prophylactic in Plague-Stricken Communities in India"; by Rogers on "The

Distribution and Harmfulness of the Anchylostomum"; and by Voorthuis on "Unna's New Method of Treating Leprosy." Space is also devoted to an epitome of recent literature on tropical medicine and to reviews of books bearing upon this subject.

Journal of the Boston Society of Medical Sciences. Boston, U.S.A.—We welcome this Journal as a new exchange. It contains papers of more than local interest, and shows that the Boston Society is doing very good work. With the Medical School of Harvard University and the various other scientific institutions in Massachusetts, its opportunities are great. The opening number of the new volume contains a careful investigation into " The minute Anatomy of the Oblongata and Pons of the Chimpanzee, with special Reference to their Homologies with Man."

Notes on Preparations for the Sick.

Ichthalbin. Ichthyol Capsules. Desichthol. — GUSTAV HERMANNI, Jr., London.—**Ichthalbin** is described as an "insipid powder for internal use, acting as an astringent and disinfectant on the bowels." It is presumably an ichthyol-albumin compound: it is practically tasteless, and should be of service in conditions where intestinal antiseptics are indicated. It does not contain any *soluble* albumin. **Ichthyol Capsules** are described as appetite promoting and nutrition increasing. **Desichthol** is an almost inodorous ichthyol, and is said to be analgesic and antiphlogistic in all forms of painful internal or external inflammation, but we have not been able to verify all these statements.

Granular Effervescent Preparations: Bismuth, Pepsine, and Strychnia; Iron and Arsenic; Salicylate of Lithia. — ALFRED BISHOP & SONS LTD., London.—Bishop's useful preparations are for the most part well known, and have been greatly in use for years. They often do good service in cases of anæmic and other forms of dyspepsia.

Tabloids: Hypophosphites Compound; Zinc Oxide.—BURROUGHS, WELLCOME & Co., London.—These new tabloids should be useful: of the former two strengths are issued, representing respectively half a drachm and one drachm of the compound syrup of hypophosphites. The rapid disintegration of the zinc oxide tabloid when dropped into water ensures its therapeutic activity. The convenience of the tabloid form must increase the utility of an often forgotten but valuable drug in the treatment of summer diarrhœa, gastralgia, epilepsy, chorea, and other results of nerve defects.

Iron Somatose; Milk Somatose. — FRIEDR. BAYER & Co., Elberfeld.—The first of these preparations is a light brown powder, soluble in water, and containing about 2 per cent. of iron. The dose is from 80 to 160 grains three times a day, and as the price is two shillings for one ounce it follows that this must be a very expensive method of giving iron in cases of anæmia. It does not therefore seem to be suitable to the ordinary case, but when other methods do not give satisfactory results this powder may be worthy of trial. The milk preparation contains 5 per cent. of tannic acid; it is therefore somewhat astringent, and more especially applicable to those patients who have a tendency to diarrhœa.

On the Somatose itself we commented in the *Journal* for September, 1895.

Digestive Brown Bread; Diabetic Bread. — J. S. NEWEY, Bristol.—Samples of these breads have been sent to us. They are excellent preparations, likely to be of use both in sickness and in health. The **Digestive Bread** is well named, inasmuch as it is made from malt flour mixed with wheat-meal flour, the malt being stewed for several hours until it attains a heat of 170 degrees. The bread is highly palatable, and it keeps moist and fresh for several days. Being made from whole meal, being well fermented and properly baked, and having the malt digestive intermixed, this bread should be highly nourishing and easily digested.

The **Diabetic Bread** is composed of aleuronat meal and cocoanut flour, mixed with eggs; the meal used in its preparation contains only a small percentage (5 to 7) of starch, and hence the product must be a valuable addition to the dietary of the diabetic patient, who is commonly very intolerant of the various kinds of gluten bread and cannot be induced to persevere with them. If we were diabetic we should feel no hardship in having to take bread like this; we cannot say that we prefer it to other kinds containing starch in quantity, but it is quite agreeable to the palate and retains its moisture well. We congratulate Mr. Newey on having accomplished—what appears to have been a difficulty hitherto—the manufacture in Bristol of an excellent bread for diabetics, which should obtain something more than a mere local reputation.

Harzbach.—BROWN BROTHERS & Co., Glasgow.—This comes to us accompanied with the details of an analysis made by Dr. E. J. Mills, F.R.S. Notwithstanding, or perhaps in consequence of, its manifold composition, it is a very palatable mineral water and it is well aërated. We mixed it with brandy and found in the compound a very pleasant reminder of Apollinaris under similar conditions, and this is giving it high praise.

The "Copeman" Throat and Nasal Spray.—S. MAW, SON, & THOMPSON, London.—This is a simple throat-spray without any indiarubber tubes, specially adapted for use in diphtheria. It is easy to use, and can be kept aseptic. The only objection to it that we can see is that the metal tube would be liable to be acted on by acids, but for many solutions it would be far more simple and cleanly than the ordinary form of throat-spray.

MEETINGS OF SOCIETIES.

Bristol Medico=Chirurgical Society.

December 14th, 1898.

Dr. R. ROXBURGH, President, in the Chair.

Dr. J. MICHELL CLARKE showed a man, aged 60, suffering from acromegaly. The characteristic enlargement of the lower part of the face, hands and feet was well marked. The tongue was very large, and the speech consequently indistinct. The back was bowed, the sternum and chest massive, and the head carried forwards. With the exception of slight deafness, the special senses were normal, and the visual fields were of normal extent. The fundus oculi was normal in each eye. The patient said that neither he nor any of his friends had noticed any change in the appearance of his face or hands, and he thought that his appearance had been as it is now for many years. He had always enjoyed good health, and been able to follow a laborious occupation, and complained only of pains in the loins of two weeks' duration. He had never had syphilis.

Dr. C. ELLIOTT showed a boy, aged 11 years, suffering from a skin eruption which seemed to conform to Hebra's " lichen ruber planus." The disease had existed for over five years, and had begun after an attack of scarlatina for which he had been treated in the Homerton Fever Hospital. The patches, at first the size of millet seeds, have gradually enlarged till now they vary from the size of a threepenny piece to a crown-piece. They are situated on the trunk, both upper and lower extremities, under the chin, on the forehead, and both ears. There is no history of syphilis, but the boy had suffered from hip-disease on the left side about six years. His general health is now good, and he has no trouble with his hip beyond some shortening. Both parents are living and well. Mother has had seven children : four (including the patient) are living; two died of diphtheria, and one was still-born. All treatment had been of little or no benefit. Arsenic, iron, mercury with iodide of potassium, and thyroid extract had been given internally.

Locally, ointments of ichthyol, resorcin, chrysophanic acid and borax, the latter seeming to be the most useful. In the autumn, scarification was tried—"mincemeating" the patches; and although these had not been cured, yet a good effect had been produced, namely, in relieving the constriction felt by the patient and allowing him greater freedom of movement.—Dr. H. WALDO thought it may be a case of what Jonathan Hutchinson calls lichen-psoriasis; but unfortunately he could not discover any papules, the presence of which would make the diagnosis easy. There were only patches accompanied with, perhaps, some pigmentation.—Dr. A. J. HARRISON expressed his doubts about the case being one of lichen ruber planus; but it might be one of the rare forms described by the late Professor Hebra. The papular character is very characteristic in these cases, the angular nature of the papules being well marked. Dr. Harrison showed a photograph of a very remarkable case of the disease.

Dr. E. C. WILLIAMS showed three patients: (1) A case which had been exhibited before the Society[1] thirteen months ago, treated by hot air. After twenty-five baths the boy was able to walk; and now, after the lapse of thirteen months, he is able to walk without difficulty and has no limp. (2) A woman who had rheumatoid arthritis for twenty years. She was unable to dress herself or use her needle. She also had a rash, like psoriasis. She has had forty baths, and the joints are now quite well and the rash has also disappeared. She has had no joint-trouble for the last three months. (3) A child who had had patches of baldness for six months before she came to the Children's Hospital. She was treated with blisters, and also with thyroid extract, without any improvement. For the last five months she has been treated with the oxygen cap, and the hair has grown rapidly. The cure may have been a coincidence.—Dr. B. M. H. ROGERS said that the first case was under his care for some time. The improvement was very considerable —Dr. J. SWAIN did not think that the boy's stiff knee could be called rheumatoid or tubercular. It was most likely traumatic.—Mr. PAUL BUSH was inclined to think that this case might be looked upon as a cure of a stiff knee by movement.— Referring to Dr. Williams's case of alopecia areata, the PRESIDENT advocated the use of pilocarpine internally in this affection, $\frac{1}{16}$th gr. three times a day, together with the local application of the same alkaloid and the weekly shaving of the affected spots. He had seen excellent results from this treatment.—Dr. E. J. CAVE considered it difficult to form an opinion as to the efficacy of treatment in case of alopecia areata, as so many of the cases get quite well under the most various treatment or none at all. He had seen some cases lately which have got well under the local application of formalin.—Dr. C. ELLIOTT could not agree with Dr. Cave that alopecia areata got well without any treatment, although he believed that cases got well under very varied treatment.—Dr. WALDO had found cases of alopecia areata do well with the oxygen cap, but they seem to do equally well with the cap without the oxygen. Saboraud has shown that the disease is caused by a specific bacillus which corresponds to that of the seborrhœa micro-organism.—Dr. E. C. WILLIAMS did not think the knee was tubercular, nor was he prepared to say it was rheumatoid; there was an indefinite history of rheumatism and a history of an injury.

Mr. C. A. MORTON showed a specimen of a large malignant tumour of the kidney, removed by abdominal nephrectomy from a child eighteen months old. It was one of those complex malignant growths

[1] *Bristol M.-Chir. J.*, 1897, xv. 363.

of the kidney which occur in young children—a mixture of sarcoma and new gland-tissue. The upper part of the kidney was not invaded by the growth, but the lower part had been replaced by it. The tumour occupied half the child's abdomen, and projected considerably. In July last, the child was taken to Dr. Cotton for a discharge of blood which was found running down the thighs, but the source of the bleeding was not clear at first. It then became evident that occasional hæmaturia was present, and the abdominal swelling was discovered. Mr. Morton saw the child with Dr. Cotton on August 4th, and operated on the 18th. In the removal of the growth, the posterior layer of the meso-colon was divided, and then the colon drawn forwards. The ureter was divided between double ligatures, but the vessels of the kidney were too much on the stretch to be safely tied, and had to be clamped before division and ligated after. A separate incision was made for drainage in the loin. The amount of shock was moderate, and soon passed off. There were no symptoms after the operation, and primary union took place. At the end of November Dr. Cotton reported that the child's health was not good, but there were no signs of recurrence. Mr. Morton thought that those members of the Society who had perhaps noticed his remarks in the June number of the *Bristol Medico-Chirurgical Journal* might be surprised that he had performed the operation : he had not recommended it, but had placed before the parents the great risk of operation, and the great chance of recurrence ; and they had decided to take the risk for the chance of prolongation of life or the very remote one of cure,—and they had been fortunate in doing so, for at any rate the child's life would be prolonged by several months even if recurrence took place at an early date.—Mr. ROGER WILLIAMS said that hitherto results of such operations had been most unfavourable. Several years ago Newman's statistics [1] showed that three-fourths of those operated on died from the effects of the operation, and of the remaining one-fourth all were dead within a year. A later series showed mortality from the operation of two-thirds, and the after-results were no better than in the foregoing series. Recently, Walker's cases [2] showed mortality from the operation of rather less than one-half, and of the remainder several had survived free from recurrence for upwards of three years. It would require considerable research to unearth, out of the several hundred operated cases on record, a score of " cures " who had survived the operation upwards of three years. This mortality was due to great malignancy of these infantile sarcomata, which exceeded that of corresponding disease in adults ; frequency with which disease is bilateral (50 per cent.), and multiple *ab initio*. Mr. Williams thought that some of these tumours were more malignant than others, the striped-muscle-containing tumours being more malignant than the adeno-sarcomata ; and he remarked on the peculiarity that these two types of sarcoma seldom co-existed, which suggests probable difference of origin. He thought that the best results hitherto attained had been in dealing with the adeno-sarcomata. Renal sarcoma being the commonest form of infantile malignant disease, these cases were of much interest, especially to surgeons.—Mr. T. CARWARDINE suggested the possible origin of the tumour from remains of the Wolffian body, which have been found in the fœtus at the lower and anterior part of the kidney—identical with the situation of this tumour, which appeared rather to invade the kidney secondarily.—In reply to Mr. Roger Williams, Mr. MORTON said the work of Kelynack on *Renal Growths*, and the very important paper by Walker, of the Johns Hopkins

[1] *Diseases of the Kidneys*, 1888.   [2] *Ann. Surg.*, 1897, xxvi. 529.

7

Hospital, of which he had given an abstract in the June number of this *Journal*, gave the most recent information as to the mortality after operation. The one encouraging fact was that it was diminishing. He could not agree with Mr. Williams that there were even a score of cases which had lived for three years after nephrectomy and therefore would be called "cures" according to Volkmann's law. There were two such cases operated on by one surgeon — Abbe, of New York, and two more by German surgeons, and he believed those were all the cases recorded as alive three years after operation. With regard to the bilateral nature of the disease, he called attention to the fact that in the 145 records of cases collected by Walker, the bilateral character of the growth was not marked, though the general view was that it was usually bilateral. Mr. Morton could not agree with Mr. Carwardine that the tumour had arisen outside the kidney. He thought that the fact that the whole organ had not been destroyed by the growth was no reason for rejecting the view that it was essentially a renal growth. A large part of the kidney had been replaced by the tumour. These renal growths of early life had by several pathologists been regarded as arising in remains of the Wolffian body, and the gland tissue when present was thought to resemble more that of the Wolffian body than the kidney.

Dr. JAMES SWAIN showed a specimen of double pyo-salpinx removed from a married but nulliparous woman, who had had severe pelvic pain for two years. The specimen was a good example of large pyo-salpinx, which formed a distinct abdominal tumour—a circumstance which is more infrequent than usual. The operation presented no special difficulty beyond the adhesions which usually exist in these cases, and the patient made an uninterrupted recovery. The pus in such cases is frequently sterile, and that was so in the present case.

Dr. J. O. SYMES showed microscopic specimen and lantern slide of tetanus bacilli in pus. The film was prepared from a suppurating wound of the hand in a patient under the care of Mr. Harsant, at the Bristol Royal Infirmary. Death resulted from tetanus, and cultures of the bacillus were obtained from the wound after death. The number and size of the bacilli were unusually large. Many pyogenic organisms were also present.

Dr. MICHELL CLARKE showed stained blood-films, and lantern slides which showed the various stages of the malaria parasite—tertian variety.

Mr. G. MUNRO SMITH exhibited a series of photo-micrographic lantern slides, prepared by Mr. J. Taylor, illustrating the pathology of rodent ulcer, adenoma of the skin, tubercular ulcer of the tongue, myeloid sarcoma and rickets.—Mr. C. A. MORTON had examined many sections of rodent ulcers, and thoroughly agreed with Mr. Munro Smith that there was not a downgrowth of surface epithelioma, and that they were histologically as well as clinically well differentiated from epithelioma. He objected to the term malignant adenoma which Mr. Smith suggested for rodent ulcer, the type of malignant adenoma of the form of cancer which occurs in the intestine; but here there was a reproduction of gland tissue, whereas in rodent ulcer we found only irregular masses of epithelial cells, and not gland tissue at all. He could not accept Mr. Munro Smith's view that the malignancy of epithelioma consisted in the small round-celled proliferation. He thought the essential condition of malignancy in epithelioma was the invasion of the deeper tissues by the advancing columns of epithelial cells, and he regarded the small round-celled growth as inflammatory, and due to the irritation of the epithelial invasion. He was glad Mr. Smith had shown the slide of tissue removed from the edge of an ulcer of the tongue for purposes of diagnosis, for he had again and again proved the great value of this method in the diagnosis of ulcers on the tongue of doubtful nature. It was much better than taking a mere scraping or than wasting time in giving iodide of potassium. Only cocaine was necessary as an anæsthetic.—Mr. ROGER WILLIAMS thought it could not be maintained that rodent ulcer was exclusively of sebaceous gland origin. It was quite true that hypertrophied sebaceous structures were often concomitant with rodent ulcer; but these were seldom cancerous. The examination of a large number of specimens had convinced him that the disease occasionally arose from the appendicular structures—hair follicles, sweat glands, and sebaceous glands; but he believed that most cases arose from the interpapillary processes of the *rete*, independently of the glands, etc. From the histogenetic standpoint these were different types of rodent ulcer. That the appendicular structures were not essential to the origin of the disease was, he thought, proved by the fact that rodent ulcer sometimes arose from the dermo-papillary membrane lining the *portio vaginalis uteri*, which was skin, without any appendicular structures (sebaceous glands, sweat glands, hair follicles, etc.). He had met with a case of this kind, in which the disease evidently started in the *rete;* and this he believed was its usual origin.—Dr. F. H. EDGEWORTH remarked that the generalisation drawn by Mr. Munro Smith from his section of rickets was probably too wide, as at the last meeting of the Bath and Bristol Branch of the British Medical Association Mr. Flemming had shown sections of rickets in which these appearances were not present.[1]—Dr. MICHELL CLARKE said that he had seen as irregularly-shaped cartilage-cells as those shown on the screen in the specimen of rickets in the normal development of cartilage into bone.

January 11th, 1899.
Dr. R. ROXBURGH, President, in the Chair.

Mr. C. E. S. FLEMMING showed microscopical sections of an angeio-sarcoma from a woman aged 68, who two years before her death fell and hurt her back. A week after the accident she had pain in her sacrum; this continued for nine months before any direct evidence of a growth could be discovered. There was then a pulsating tumour over the right sacro-iliac synchondrosis, with a loud bruit heard down to the femoral artery. The tumour increased steadily in size, latterly causing paralysis of the bladder and pain in the right leg. There was no clinical evidence of any secondary growth. By a partial *post-mortem* examination nearly the whole of the sacrum and a considerable part of the right ilium were found to be destroyed by a large soft mass in appearance like organising bloodclot. Under the microscope this growth was found to consist almost entirely of embryonic blood-vessels, with intervening small collections of nucleated round cells and a few laryngo-myeloid cells. The cells of the blood-vessels were in places markedly columnar, and between the different vessels there could be distinguished in places a fine fibrillar matrix. It appeared probable that the growth might have originated in the cauda equina.—Mr. ROGER WILLIAMS said that though this form of neoplasm was rare, it had now been demonstrated in most parts of the body. If we accept the view that it arose from the peri-epithelium or endothelium of the blood-vessels and lymphatics there was still some difficulty in deciding whether it should be classed with the sarcomata or with carcinomata, because embryologists were at variance as to whether endothelial structures were of archiblastic or of parablastic origin. In their clinical character growths of this kind

[1] *Vide* p. 21 of present number.

generally resembled carcinomata, especially in that they were very prone to disseminate, and he enquired if there were any signs of malignancy in this case. He thought growths of this kind were interesting in connection with Ackermann's hypothesis of sarcomatosis, according to which all sarcomata arose in the immediate vicinity of blood-vessels or lymphatics, every tumour consisting of interwoven neoplastic fasciculi with a central blood-vessel.

Dr. WALDO read a paper on hemorrhoids, which, he said, were always pathological. By far the greater portion of the blood from the plexus of hemorrhoidal veins is carried into the inferior mesenteric vein, and thence into the vena portæ, through the medium of the superior hemorrhoidal vein. The circulation through the portal system is subject to much interference in consequence of hepatic and intestinal obstruction, and in these changes the blood in the hemorrhoidal plexus also participates; and were it not for the provision that exists by which this plexus may free itself to a certain extent from over-distension by its communication with the internal iliac vein, through the medium of the middle hemorrhoidal vein, piles would be much more frequent than they even now are, as a consequence of obstructed portal circulation. All these veins are valveless, and are therefore liable to over-distension whenever the abdominal circulation is sluggish. An invariable accompaniment of internal piles is a greater or less degree of prolapse of the mucous membrane of the rectum, and chiefly on this account the patient should be instructed to have his daily motion at bedtime. The chief reflex phenomena encountered are a dull aching fixed pain at the lower part of the lumbar spine, which may extend down the thighs or round the groins, and irritation in the neighbouring organs. Patients should adopt a rational way of living. The diet should be so regulated as to leave behind the least possible solid residue. Highly seasoned food, or vegetables containing much cellulose and the leguminous vegetables, should be avoided. Meat or fish, rather than much starchy food, is advised. And green vegetables with stewed fruits and preserves, with a fair quantity of diluents, assist the daily action of the bowels. Fat of meat, or cream or butter, may be taken, as oleaginous substances are found to assist the flow of the bile and so indirectly the vascular circulation. Moderate exercise should be taken in various ways. The tendency to bleed after fifty years of age gradually grows less and finally disappears. The tumours may remain, and with them the old tendency to prolapse; but generally they atrophy, leaving little if any future discomfort unless the prolapse is bulky. Treatment by drugs was touched upon, and a mechanical mode of treatment upon physiological principles was explained and advocated. He believed that physicians could assist these patients immensely; but in some cases, whether medical treatment is neglected or not, the only right proceeding is to hand them over to the operating surgeon. A young clergyman from South Africa, who consulted Dr. Waldo a few months ago, told him that two-thirds of the clergy and doctors in that part of the world were operated upon for piles (some of them two or three times), the cause of this being that they averaged fifty miles a day in the saddle.—Mr. MUNRO SMITH suggested that the liver had not so much to do with hemorrhoids as was usually thought. He doubted if obstruction in the portal circulation occurred apart from definite disease of the organ, and if it occurred whether it could be diagnosed.—Dr. AUST LAWRENCE referred to the necessity in all cases of ascertaining by a digital examination that piles really did exist; he mentioned several cases that he had seen treated for piles where the disease was of a malignant character, and often in women all the symptoms were due to uterine displacement.—Mr. C. E. S. FLEMMING objected to the use of glycerine injections, because of their liability to cause painful and troublesome tenesmus and occasionally hemorrhage. He also wished to know in which class of cases anal gymnastics should be adopted, as stretching of the sphincter had been frequently recommended as a method of treatment.—Mr. EWENS had seen many cases of *supposed* piles, which proved to be due either to retroflexed or retroverted uterus, or to an enormous accumulation of fæces in the rectum. Appropriate treatment relieved these cases. He had met with cases of supposed piles which were really malignant disease of the rectum. He had seen much benefit from the administration of hazeline in bleeding piles in connection with mild aperients.—Dr. HARRISON· suggested that hazeline has been long known as efficacious in the treatment of hemorrhoids, invariably as a well-known American popular remedy— Pond's Extract—containing hazeline. Dr. Harrison was surprised to hear that riding on horseback tended to produce piles: of course much exercise would not be advisable where piles were actively asserting themselves, but as a preventative to liver congestion and hemorrhoids the late Lord Palmerston's dictum was a very wise one; viz., " that the outside of a horse was the best thing for the inside of a man." Dr. Harrison also controverted Dr. Waldo's suggestion that pruritus ani was common with piles, Dr. Harrison associating it much more with eczema and fissure of the anus.—Dr. WATSON WILLIAMS considered that while in the less pronounced cases of hemorrhoids medical treatment might be attended with very favourable results, it was well to bear in mind the limitations of medical methods, and in suitable cases to call in the aid of a surgical colleague. He did not think that the advantages of a radical surgical cure were sufficiently often impressed on patients, whose lives were not seldom marred by a condition that could be, and should be, completely removed. —Mr. CARWARDINE pointed out that piles have recently been shown by dissection to be really cavernous angeiomata, fed by the superior hemorrhoidal artery, and consequently not of venous origin,—Dr. ELLIOTT considered heredity an important factor in the causation of piles. He believed bicycling and riding on horseback were of decided benefit to this class of patients. With regard to operation, he begged to remind members that the patient as well as the surgeon had to have a voice in the matter; and when the former heard of death following an operation among his friends, he was not surprised that patients welcomed other modes of treatment. Personally he was acquainted with two fatal cases due to secondary hemorrhage following operation; and knew of a third case, where a fatal result was fortunately prevented by plugging the rectum. Such cases, of course, did not appear in our medical journals.—In reply, Dr. WALDO said, as a large portion of the blood is obliged to return to the heart through the liver, hemorrhoids would certainly be influenced by any obstruction occurring in the latter organ.

Dr. AUST LAWRENCE read a paper in which he urged (1) the necessity of repairing all perineal injuries after labour; (2) the use of catgut with which to repair these injuries, and the non-inclusion of the skin in the operation; (3) the importance of keeping on the forceps until the head is delivered, as this often prevents and ought never to cause rupture of the perineum; (4) the wisdom of telling the husband, etc., that with the use of forceps there may be laceration of the perineum; but it is not caused by the forceps, but by the large size of the child's head and by the small parts of the mother.—Dr. FIRTH mentioned a case in which he had been asked to repair a perineum seven days after confinement.

He had succeeded in persuading the patient to have the operation postponed for at least six weeks.   Dr. Firth asked Dr. Lawrence if he would consent to operate seven days after confinement, and if not, how long he would wait.—Dr. NEWNHAM said that it is perhaps well, in putting sutures into the perineum immediately after the confinement, to be careful not to sew up the rectum entirely.   A case sent to him lately had the perineum and rectum so completely sewn up that ntestinal obstruction was caused ; and, finally, an anus was formed in the posterior wall of the vagina.   It is, therefore, important to see that a direct outlet is left for the fæces after sewing up a bad rupture of the perineum.—Dr. WALTER SWAYNE said that a most important point with regard to the immediate union of lacerations of the genital tract was the prevention of septic poisoning.   In his experience of puerperal septicæmia the most hopeless and intractable cases were those in which lacerations of the vagina and perineum were present.   The raw lacerated surface allows of direct infection of the lymphatic system by septic micro-organisms, and the production of a most acute form of septicæmia.   Then again minor forms of septic infection, in which the general symptoms were more urgent, led to the production of sub-involution of the uterine body and ligaments, and in this way predisposed to displacements such as procidentia.   On these grounds alone the immediate union of all lacerations should be the invariable practice.   He would not criticise Dr. Lawrence's paper, as his remarks should meet with universal acceptance.

Dr. J. LACY FIRTH read a paper on a case of primary sarcoma of the thyroid gland, in which a marked amelioration of symptoms for four months had resulted from partial thyroidectomy, the right lobe having been removed.   The rarity of this form of growth was alluded to, and the almost uniformly rapid fatal result of operations upon them.—Mr. HARSANT referred to a case of primary carcinoma of the thyroid body, upon which he had operated for the relief of dyspnœa; the patient only survived a short period.   He had never met with a case of sarcoma of the thyroid.—Mr. ROGER WILLIAMS said he had made an analysis of all the primary tumours under treatment at four large Metropolitan hospitals during a period of from ten to fifteen years.   Of 7,294 cancers only seven originated in the thyroid, and of 1,266 sarcomas only one started in the thyroid.   He knew of several instances of malignant thyroid neoplasms arising in early life.   Zahn had reported an instance in a fœtus.   In several cases chondromatous, rhabdomyomatous and squamous epithelial structures had been found in these tumours ; and he asked if heterotopic elements of this kind had been noted in Dr. Firth's specimen--Dr. STACK asked whether there was any diminution in the portion of the gland left, as it is said that sometimes malignant disease of the thyroid for a time diminishes after partial operations.—Dr. WALDO asked whether Mr. Firth had administered thyroid extract to patients with non-malignant enlargement of the thyroid gland, considering that the current view was that the system called upon the thyroid body for an increased supply of its excretion, and that the gland responded and as a consequence hypertrophied.   It is said that if the extract is given by the mouth in some of these cases the thyroid body diminishes in size, and the patient recovers.—Mr. MORTON could not quite agree with Mr. Harsant that removal of a portion of the gland was the only method of dealing with urgent dyspnœa in these cases.   He thought an opening into the trachea above the isthmus, and the passage of a large tube such as a wide gum-elastic catheter below the obstruction, might be done in desperate cases.— Mr. PAUL BUSH remarked that in two of his cases of malignant disease of the thyroid gland, in which a partial removal only could be performed, there had been a considerable diminution in the size of the growth following operation, lasting in one case for several months: the growth in this case was undoubtedly a sarcoma; both patients, however, died of the disease eventually.—In reply, Dr. J. LACY FIRTH remarked that microscopical examination showed his case to be one of pure sarcoma of the thyroid. Here and there in the section remains of the thyroid vesicles undergoing destruction were to be seen. In the published drawings of secondary thyroid tumours found in bone and other tissues, there was no appearance of sarcomatous tissue, and they were, therefore, neither sarcomata nor adeno-sarcomata. In his case there had been a very noticeable diminution of the left lobe of the gland for a time after the operation of thyroidectomy on the right side. He had tried the effect of thyroid extract in two cases of enlarged thyroid. The first case was one of sporadic cretinism, and the thyroid gland was the largest he had seen and of the adenomatous type. The extract rapidly produced a marvellous diminution in the size of the gland and amelioration of the symptoms. In the second case, one of ordinary goitre, the effect of the medicine had been favourable, but not to a marked degree.

February 8th, 1899.

Dr. R. ROXBURGH, President, in the chair.

Dr. F. H. EDGEWORTH showed a specimen of abscess of the brain. The patient, a woman aged 43, who had never had any previous illness, was on December 2nd seized with motor aphasia, and paralysis of the right side of the face and tongue and of the right arm, without loss of consciousness. Ten days later the right leg became paralysed and the intelligence blunted, and a week subsequently she died with symptoms of pressure on the left cerebral hemisphere. No lesion or abnormality of the vascular system was detected, and the urine was normal. The *post-mortem* examination showed an old abscess of the left nucleus lenticularis, which had recently invaded the left internal capsule. The rest of the body was intact. The abscess, from its situation, must have been embolic in origin, but no source of septic embolism was discovered. Gross organic lesions of the brain, such as tumour and abscess, may in some instances give rise to suddenly developing symptoms; but there is usually some evidence, such as headache, vomiting, or optic neuritis, which suggests that the lesion is other than a vascular one. Such evidence was wanting in this case.

Dr. SYMES read a paper on "The Bacteriology of some Suppurations complicating Pulmonary Disease." This and the discussion which followed will be found on pp. 30—35.

Dr. MICHELL CLARKE read a paper embodying observations on the temperature in cases of apoplexy, and on the occasional occurrence of painful œdema, and of loss of the knee-jerk in the paralysed limbs in hemiplegia. This will be printed in full in a future number.

Mr. T. CARWARDINE showed microscopic slides illustrating some points in the pathology of Paget's disease of the nipple, from preparations made by Mr. A. L. Flemming. Enlarged axillary glands were present, and they exhibited secondary deposits of epithelium similar to that in the diseased nipple, although there was no tumour in the true breast tissue. Another specimen showed the epithelial change passing down a galactophorous duct (a) as a cellular process passing down the lumen, (b) as a proliferation of and change in the cells of the Malpighian layer around the deep part of the duct.—Mr. ROGER WILLIAMS said the

history of the evolution of our knowledge of Paget's disease showed
at every turn the ill effects entailed by the unscientific use of personal
names for the designation of morbid conditions. The result had been
such mystification and confusion, that it was necessary before discussing
the subject to state precisely what was meant by Paget's disease; for
this term had been applied to so many totally different morbid conditions, that it was now seldom used by two persons in the same sense.
Paget,[1] who first prominently directed attention to the subject, defined
the condition as " disease of the mammary areola preceding cancer of
the mammary gland "—an admirable definition which, had it been
preserved, would have prevented a flood of misunderstanding and
bad practice. It had been repeatedly demonstrated that the areolar
disease referred to was nothing but eczema; and the cancer—which
developed in the substance of the gland, without there being any
obvious connection between the two diseases—was of the acinous
(scirrhus) variety. Paget admitted that the areolar disease might often
be cured, without any ill consequences ensuing; but he thought it
was "very often" followed by the development of cancer in the breast.
In support of this opinion he adduced no statistical data; for none
were then available. Recently the subject had been investigated on
a large scale: and it had been shown that the outbreak of mammary
cancer had been preceded by eczema of the areola, only in about
¼ per cent. of the total cases. We might, therefore, disabuse our
minds of the idea that " Paget's disease " played any important part
in the pathogeny of mammary cancer. Eczematous affections of the
areola were very seldom followed by the development of mammary
cancer: hence the breast should never be extirpated for such conditions, unless there were signs of concomitant malignant disease.
Thin had described as " Paget's disease " cases of cancer of the mammary ducts (tubular cancer) with secondary inflammation of the nipple
and areola by irritant discharges. Another class of cases that had
been described as " Paget's disease " were the so-called " eczema
cancers ": cases in which epithelioma had supervened on eczematous
affections of the nipple and areola. Mr. Williams thought the specimen exhibited this evening was an instance of this kind—squamous
epithelioma, with dissemination in the axillary glands.

Mr. HARSANT read some notes of a case of actinomycosis occurring
in a gentleman living at Taunton, under the care of Dr. Husbands.
Six months ago he had put an ear of barley-straw in his mouth. It
pricked the mucous membrane under the tongue, causing a painful
swelling there which disappeared after a few days. Two or three
weeks afterwards a swelling appeared on the front of the neck, over
the thyro-hyoid membrane; this had gradually increased until it was
as large as a walnut. It presented a semi-fluctuating swelling, the
skin over which was red and œdematous. It was diagnosed as being
probably actinomycosis, and was freely excised. The wound healed
readily and there had been no recurrence. The tumour contained
numerous yellow granules, which under the microscope showed the
characteristic ray-fungus. Microscopical specimens were shown by
Dr. Symes; and a photo-micrograph, prepared by Mr. James Taylor,
was thrown on the screen.—Dr. WALDO asked Mr. Harsant if the glands
in the neighbourhood of the growth were affected in his case. He
considered this a very important point, as the fungus was too large
to pass along the lymphatics, and unless pyogenic microbes gained an
entrance and set up suppuration the glands remained healthy. The
disease spread through the blood-vessels. He remarked that it was

[1] St. Barth. Hosp. Rep., 1874, x. 87.

singular that the bone was nearly always affected when actinomycosis attacked the lower animals, whereas in man it was quite the exception. On the other hand, suppuration was the rule in man and never occurred in animals. He said there were some well authenticated cases in which the internal administration of iodides seemed to cure the patient, and also when an iodide solution was injected into the tissues. Electro-chemical treatment was also well spoken of, the solution being injected and then a current passed through to decompose the substance, and so utilise the antiseptic power of iodine in its nascent state.

Prof. FAWCETT showed through the lantern some sections of the cord, medulla, and midbrain, stained by a modification of the Weigert-Pal method.

J. PAUL BUSH, Hon. Sec.

The Library of the Bristol Medico-Chirurgical Society.

The following donations have been received since the publication of the list in December:

February 28th, 1899.

Clinical Society of London (1) ... ... 1 volume.
Laryngological Society of London (2) ... ... 1 ,,
B. M. H. Rogers, M.D. ... ... 3 volumes.
Royal Academy of Medicine in Ireland ... ... 1 volume.
Surgeon-General, United States Army (3) ... ... 14 volumes.
James Swain, M.D. ... ... 1 volume.
Caleb Trapnell (4) ... ... 1 ,,

Unbound periodicals have been received from Dr. B. M. H. Rogers, Dr. R. Shingleton Smith, the Surgeon-General, United States Army, and Dr. B. W. Walker. Dr. Shaw has presented a framed picture; and unframed pictures have been received from the Surgeon-General, United States Army, and Dr. De Forest Willard.

THIRTY-FIRST LIST OF BOOKS.

The titles of books mentioned in previous lists are not repeated.

The figures in brackets refer to the figures after the names of the donors, and show by whom the volumes were presented. The books to which no such figures are attached have either been bought from the Library Fund or received through the *Journal.*

Aarons, S. J. ... ... *Golden Rules of Gynæcology* ... ...[1898]
Bannatyne, G. A. *The Thermal Waters of Bath* 1899
Beasley, H. ... ... *The Pharmaceutical Formulary.* 12th Ed. (Ed. by
J. O. Braithwaite) 1899

Bell, J. ... ...   *Notes on Surgery for Nurses.* ... ... 5th Ed.   1899

Burdon-Sanderson, J.   *Ludwig and Modern Physiology*   1898

Catalogue (Index) of the Library of the Surgeon-General's Office, United States Army. 2nd Ser., Vol. III. ... ...   (3)   1898

Children, An American Text-Book of the Diseases of. (Ed. by L. Starr and T. S. Westcott.) 2nd Ed. 2 parts   1898

Copeman, S. M. ...   *Vaccination : its Natural History and Pathology...* ...   1899

Dowse, T. S. ...   *The Treatment of Disease by Physical Methods*   1898

Engelmann, G. J.   *Accouchements chez les Peuples primitifs.* (Étude français par P. Rodet) ... ... (4)   1886

Fenwick, E. H. ...   *Golden Rules of Surgical Practice.* ... ... 5th Ed. [1898]

Foster, M. ... ...   *Recent Advances in Science*   1898

Fothergill, W. E.   *Golden Rules of Obstetric Practice* ... ... [1898]

Gage, S. H. ... ...   *The Processes of Life revealed by the Microscope*   1898

Glycerine, The Properties and Uses of Pure ... ... [1898]

Gowers, Sir W. R.   *Diseases of the Nervous System.* 3rd Ed. (Ed. by Sir W. R. Gowers and J. Taylor.) Vol. I. ...   1899

Grünwald, L. ...   *Atlas and Abstract of the Diseases of the Larynx.* (Translated. Ed. by C. P. Grayson)   1898

Guy de Chauliac...   *La Grande Chirurgie, 1363.* (Revue par E. Nicaise)   1890

Gynecology, An American Text-Book of. (Ed. by J. M. Baldy.) 2nd Ed.   1898

Haviland, A. ...   *The Geographical Distribution of Disease in Great Britain.* ... ... 2nd Ed.   1892

Haydn, J. ... ...   *The Book of Dignities.* 3rd Ed. (Ed. by H. Ockerby.)   1894

Hewlett, R. T. ...   *A Manual of Bacteriology*   1898

Hillemand, C. ...   *Organothérapie ou Opothérapie*   1899

Hofmann, E. von   *Atlas of Legal Medicine.* (Translated. Ed. by F. Peterson and A. O. J. Kelly)   1898

Keen, W. W. ...   *The Surgical Complications and Sequels of Typhoid Fever*   1898

Kingscote, E. ...   *On So-called Spasmodic Asthma*   1899

Lexicon of Medicine and the Allied Sciences. (New Syd. Soc.) Part XXIV.   1898

Liaras, E. J. Moure et G.   *Traitement chirurgical de quelques Paralysies faciales d'Origine otique*   1899

Longmore, Sir T.   *Richard Wiseman*   1891

Macilwain, G. ...   *Memoirs of John Abernethy.* 2 vols.   1853

M'Keown, W. A....   *" Unripe " Cataract*   1898

Méric, H. de ...   *Dictionary of Medical Terms—English-French*   1899

Mondeville, H. de   *Chirurgie, 1306 à 1320.* (Traduction française, avec des notes, par E. Nicaise)   1893

Moure et G. Liaras, E. J.   *Traitement chirurgical de quelques Paralysies faciales d'Origine otique*   1899

Mracek, F. ... ...   *Atlas of Syphilis and the Venereal Diseases.* (Translated. Ed. by L. B. Bangs)   1898

Myxœdema, Report of a Committee of the Clinical Society of London on... (1)   1888

Nahm, [—] ... ...   *The Erection of a Consumptive Sanatorium for the People.* (Tr. by W. Calwell)   1898

Nisbet, W. W. Van Valzah and J. D. [Eds.] *The Diseases of the Stomach*   1899

Pathology, An Atlas of Illustrations of. (New. Syd. Soc.) Fasc. XII. ...   1898

Powell, Sir R. D....   *Treatment in Diseases and Disorders of the Heart* ...   1899

Prichard, J. C. ...   *Physical History of Mankind.* Vols. I., 4th Ed., 1841; II.–IV., 3rd Ed., 1837-44; V.   1847

Robinson, H. B. ...   *Traumatic Birth Paralyses of the Upper Extremity* ...   1899

Roth, B. ... ... *Lateral Curvature of the Spine.* ... ... 2nd Ed. 1899
Schweinitz, E. A. de *The War with the Microbes* 1898
Thorne, W. B. ... *Observations on Cardio-Vascular Repair* 1898
Thurston, R. H. ... *The Animal as a Prime Mover* 1898
Tirard, N. ... ... *Albuminuria and Bright's Disease* 1899
Tweedie, Mrs. A. [Ed.] *George Harley*... 1899
Van Dieren, E. ... *Beri-Beri en Voeding* 1898
Van Valzah and J. D. Nisbet, W. W. [Eds.] *The Diseases of the Stomach* 1899
Vierordt, O. ... ... *Medical Diagnosis.* (Tr. by F. H. Stuart.) 4th Ed. 1898
Walters, F. R. ... *Sanatoria for Consumptives* 1899
Williams, W. R. ... *Cancer* 1898
    ,, ... *Sarcoma* 1898
Zuckerkandl, O. ... *Atlas and Epitome of Operative Surgery.* (Translated. Ed. by J. C. DaCosta) 1898

TRANSACTIONS, REPORTS, JOURNALS, &c.

American Journal of the Medical Sciences, The... ... ... Vol. CXVI. 1898
Annual and Analytical Cyclopædia of Practical Medicine ... Vol. II. 1899
Archives de Neurologie ... ... 2e Sér., Tomes V., VI. 1898
Birmingham Medical Review, The ... ... Vols. XLIII., XLIV. 1898
Brain ... ... Vol. X. 1888
British Almanac, The 1899
British Journal of Dental Science, The... ... (3) Vols. XVII.—XIX. 1874–76
British Journal of Dermatology, The ... ... Vol. X. 1898
British Medical Journal, The ... ... Vol II. for 1898
Brooklyn Medical Journal, The ... ... Vol. XII. 1898
Cincinnati Lancet and Observer, The (3) Vols. IX.—XIII., 1866–70, XV. 1872
Directory of Booksellers, The International 1899
Dublin Journal of Medical Science, The ... ... Vol. CVI. 1898
Edinburgh Medical Journal, The ... ... N.S., Vol. IV. 1898
Edinburgh Obstetrical Society, The Transactions of the... Vol. XXII. 1897
Epidemiological Society of London, Transactions of the N.S., Vol. XVII. 1898
Glasgow Medical Journal, The ... . Vol. L. 1898
Hazell's Annual 1886–91, 1893, 1899
Hospitals—
    Guy's Hospital Reports ... ... Vol. LIII. 1898
    Johns Hopkins Hospital Reports, The ... ... Vol. VII., No. 4. 1898
    Saint Bartholomew's Hospital Reports ... ...Vol. XXXIV. 1899
    Saint Thomas's Hospital Reports ... ...N.S., Vol. XXVI. 1898
Journal of Cutaneous and Genito-Urinary Diseases ... ... Vol. XVI. [1898]
Journal of the Sanitary Institute ... ... Vols. XV.—XVIII. 1894–97
Lancet, The... ... ... Vol. II. for 1898
Laryngological Society of London, Proceedings of the ... (2) Vol. V. 1898
Medical Directory, The 1899
Medical Press and Circular, The ... ... [Vol. CXVII.] 1898
Medical Record ... ... Vol. LIV. 1898
Medical Repository, The (New York) ... ... (3) Vols. III.—VI. 1800–1803
Medical Society of London, Transactions of the ... ... Vol. XXI. 1898
Medico-Chirurgical Transactions ... ...Vol. LXXXI. 1898

Mercy and Truth ... ... Vol. II.   1898.

Mexico.   Informes Rendidos por los Inspectores Sanitarios de Cuartel y por los de los distritos al consejo Superior de Salubridad, [1896], 1897, 2 vols. ... ...   1898.

Michigan State Medical Society, Transactions of the ... Vol. XXII.   1898.

Odontological Society of Great Britain, Transactions of the N.S., Vol. XXX.   1898.

Philadelphia Medical Journal ... ... Vol. II.   1898.

Practitioner, The ... ... Vol. LXI.   1898.

Retrospect of Medicine, Braithwaite's ... ... Vol. CXVIII.   1899.

St. Louis Medical and Surgical Journal, The   Vols. LXXIV., LXXV.   1898

Scottish Medical and Surgical Journal, The ... ...Vol. III.   1898

West London Medical Journal ... ...Vol. III.   1898

Whitaker's Almanack ... ...1876–82, 1884–92,   1899.

Who's Who ... ...   1899.

Year-Book of Treatment, The... ... ...   1899.

Local Medical Notes.

BRISTOL.

HOSPITAL SUNDAY.—The second annual collection in places of worship on behalf of the Medical Charities of this City has been more productive than the first. This is partly due to better organisation, and partly to the fact that the recipients of the notes given for the collections found that they got more for their money by contributing through this Fund. The principle on which the distribution of notes was made was so arranged that the donors of small amounts received more in proportion than those who sent large ones, on the theory that the smaller subscriptions came from the poorer congregations. With very few exceptions the plan seems to have given satisfaction. It is hoped that next year, by arrangement with the Institutions, more notes will be at the disposal of the Committee. We cannot help expressing the great loss the Committee has experienced by the appointment of the Rev. Canon Cornish to the see of Grahamstown. It was largely due to his indefatigable exertions that the Hospital Sunday Fund was put upon its present sound basis, and the Committee will find it difficult to fill his place with a man of equal calibre, organising power, or enthusiasm.

THE CONVALESCENT HOME.—This will soon, we hope, be opened for the reception of inmates. All the legal formalities have been concluded, and the necessary alterations are being pushed forward. No date has as yet been mentioned for the opening, but we believe that when the doors are opened the building will be found to be replete with every convenience.

THE PREVENTION OF CONSUMPTION.—A movement has been started to form a local committee or branch of the National Association for the Prevention of Consumption and other forms of Tuberculosis. Several meetings have been held to discuss the matter, and a provisional committee of medical men has been formed, of which Dr. E. L. Fox is the chairman; Dr. D. S. Davies, vice-chairman; Dr. Michell Clarke, honorary secretary; and Dr. P. Watson Williams, honorary treasurer. It is to be hoped that the citizens of Bristol will give their cordial assistance in this important matter, and that some practical results will follow.

UNIVERSITY COLLEGE.—Dr. G. Parker has been appointed Joint Lecturer on Medical Jurisprudence in place of Dr. A. J. Harrison, resigned.

EYE DISPENSARY.—Dr. Alex. Ogilvy has been appointed Surgeon to the Eye Dispensary in the place of Mr. Cyril H. Walker, resigned.

FEVER HOSPITALS.—Dr. D. S. Davies has been appointed Medical Superintendent of the City of Bristol Fever Hospitals at Ham Green and Novers Hill.

Congress of Gynæcology and Obstetrics.

The Third Session of the International Congress of Gynæcology and Obstetrics will be held at Amsterdam, from the 8th to the 12th of August, 1899. The questions arranged for discussion are as follows:—1. The surgical treatment of fibro-myoma. 2. The relative value of antisepsis and improved technic for the actual results in Gynæcological Surgery. 3. The influence of posture on the form and dimensions of the pelvis. 4. The indication for Cæsarean section compared to that for symphysiotomy, craniotomy, and premature induction of labour.

SCRAPS

PICKED UP BY THE ASSISTANT-EDITOR.

The **Misericordia.**—The Roman correspondent of the *Lancet*, writing in the issue of February 25th, says:—"When the 'Romance of Outdoor Relief' comes to be written it will owe some of its most touching, most picturesque, chapters to the Misericordia—a brotherhood peculiar to Tuscany, seen at its best in Florence, though also admirably *en évidence* at Siena, Pisa, Leghorn, and Lucca, and not unworthily represented in the minor provincial towns, inland or maritime. Ecclesiastical in origin, it was founded in 1244 by Pietro di Luca Borsi and its *personnel* is drawn from every social rank, all and individually bound to serve whenever summoned, without fee or reward. The Grand Duke himself, when presiding at a State banquet in the Pitti Palace, has had to rise and leave his guests when his turn came and to bear a hand with tradesmen, nobles, mechanics, professional men—with the company, in fact, promiscuously improvised to transport some victim of an accident or to carry a patient from the sick bed to the suburban lodging indicated by the physician. The service is not one of 'unskilled labour.' The members of the brotherhood have all been previously trained to lift the sufferer from the street, to turn the patient in bed, and put him on the 'bara' or stretcher with the minimum of pain or of risk to compromised limbs or organs, and thereafter to bear him through the thoroughfares to his destination with the least possible vibration, friction, or disturbance. As often happens, the particular company told off on sudden duty is composed of men as various in altitude as they are in social position, so that in carrying the 'bara' shoulder high they employ for the first part of the journey those of them who are as nearly as possible of the same height, and when these are tired they lower their burden to the less tall without interruption of movement or alteration of pace and so continue the shifting process till the sufferer is at his journey's end and laid down in bed with scarcely the consciousness of having been transported at all. Few sights or sounds are more impressive in the Florence of to-day than the 'measured march' of the Misericordia through its crowded streets, as robed in black gowns and hooded in black cowls with

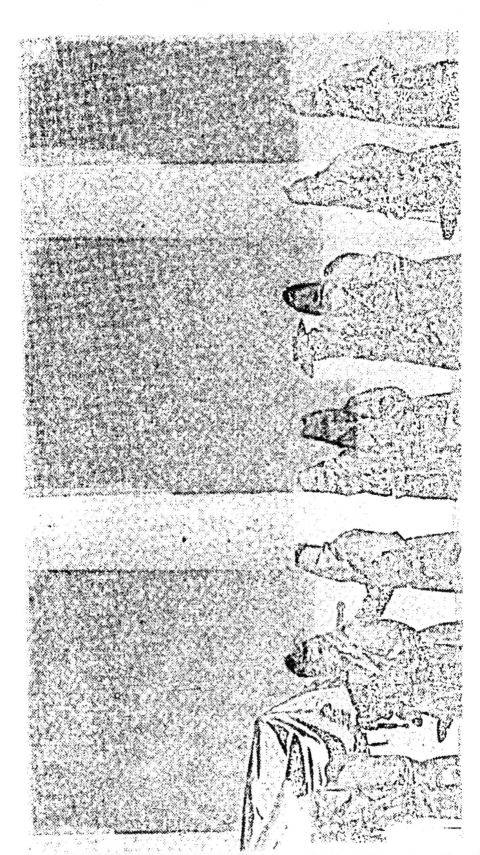

openings for the eyes the brotherhood wends its way with its burden, the bystander lifting his hat sympathetically, the traffic reverently falling aside, and the street noises subdued to a momentary hush in presence of

' The still, sad music of humanity.'

Queen Victoria, it is well known, took profound interest in the Misericordia during her successive sojourns in Florence, and one of its highest office-bearers, the late Cavaliere Cesare Barsi, was deputed by the Arci-Confraternità to visit the Villa Palmieri, there to set forth to Her Majesty its origin and constitution, the nature of its service, the resources at its command, and the more striking incidents in its experience. As I have said, the brotherhood is peculiar to Tuscany, though other cities have their equivalents, each in its own way rendering similar service; few if any of them, however, being able to point to the same antiquity of origin, to the same large resources, or to the same admirable discipline and organisation. I have been led to give this brief notice of the Misericordia from the funeral obsequies just celebrated in Florence of the Provveditore (or general provider and administrator) of the Brotherhood, Signor Giuseppe Bronzuoli—a singularly imposing and pictur-esque pageant composed of 300 members of the Arci-Confraternità, 50 'capi di guardia' (chiefs of the guard) and 35 priests. The procession included many citizens among whom were not a few surgeons and physicians, those of them who immediately followed the hearse bearing lighted torches."

Canon Wallace, who kindly lent me the photograph from which the picture on the opposite page has been reproduced, sends me the following information, for the authenticity of which he does not vouch, but which he got from apparently good sources :—

In the 13th century, the porters in the piazza of the Duomo, Florence, were a gambling, swearing set. In 1240, Pietro Borsi, one of their number, set on foot a system of fines for bad language, and suggested that the accumulated money should be used for litters and bearers for the sick.

Under the present system, which has been developed out of Borsi's idea, at the sound of the campanile bell, day or night, the members on the roster for that day repair at once to the hall of meeting. The summoning official turns an hour-glass to mark the interval between their summons and arrival. In assigning their task the Captain says: "Brethren, prepare for a work of mercy," then kneeling prays: "Mitte, Domine, nobis caritatem, humilitatem et fortitudinem." They reply: "Ut in hoc opere Te sequamur." He then bids them say a Paternoster for the sufferer. Four take up the litter. The captain leads and four follow. They relieve each other. As they change one set says, "God reward you ;" the other replies, "Go ye in peace." Some of the sick nurses are trained specially to move sufferers and patients in accident cases, and are called "Mutanti." They receive no pay, and are allowed to accept only cold water. In sickness a physician is provided for them. They are of "all sorts and conditions of men," and when the official dress is slipped on over their ordinary clothes the rank or occupation of the brother can only be guessed from his boots.

Clinical Records (26).—The house-surgeon of a London hospital was attending to the injuries of a woman whose arm had been severely bitten. As he was examining the wound, he said: "What sort of animal bit you ? This is too small for a horse's bite, and too large for a dog." "Oh, sir," replied the patient, "it wasn't an animal. It was another lydy."

Medical Philology (XXIX.)—The following is to be found in the *Promptorium* : "Deffe, or dulle. *Obtusus, agrestis.*" Mr. Way's note says: "Jamieson observes that deaf signifies properly stupid, and the term is transferred in a more limited sense to the ear It is also applied to that which has lost its germinating power ; thus in the North, as in Devonshire, a rotten nut is called deaf, and barren corn is called deaf corn, an expression literally Ang.-Saxon. An unproductive soil is likewise termed deaf. The plant lamium, or archangel, known by the common name, dead or blind nettle, in the *Promptorium*, has the epithet DEFFE, evidently because it does not possess the stinging property of the true nettle. "

Jamieson's statement is not quite accurate. Although the word was used with the general meaning to which he refers, it was also employed in its ordinary restricted sense from very early times. The *New English Dictionary* gives 9th and 13th century instances; and it will be remembered that the Wife of Bath, described by Chaucer, long before the compilation of the *Promptorium*, was "som-del deef, and that was scathe."

The *Promptorium* in another place gives *surdus* as an equivalent of "deffe."

Readers who may be interested in the forms which are figurative or now dialectal will find several quotations in the *New English Dictionary*.

La Médecine en quatrains.—Quelqu'un pensa, dit-on, à mettre l'histoire de France en madrigaux. Ce n'était pas une tâche plus extraordinaire que de découper la médecine en quatrains, et plus d'un s'y est essayé.

Il y a les *Aphorismes d'Hippocrate*, mis en vers françois, par le sieur de Launay, chirurgien; Paris, 1642. Il y a les *Quatrains anatomiques des os et des muscles du corps humain*, par le sieur Claude Binet; Lyon, 1664.

La chimie elle-même s'est, parfois, ingénieusement et agréablement alliée à la poésie. En doutez-vous? Lisez ceci:

> Voulez-vous fair' de l'hydrogène?
> Prenez un tub' de porcelaine;
> Mettez-y du fer et de l'eau:
> Placez le tout sur un fourneau,
> En vapeur l'eau décomposée
> Est promptement analysée:
> L'oxygène s'unit au fer,
> Et l'hydrogèn' s'en va dans l'air.

De la musique d'Hervé là-dessus et ce serait charmant !—*La Revue médicale.*

Hebrew Therapeutics.—From a periodical called *The Old Paths*, in which the Rev. Alexander McCaul, D.D., compared "the Principles and Doctrines of Modern Judaism with the Religion of Moses and the Prophets," I extract from the number for July 1st, 1836, the following:—

"Wisdom is a test of true religion, and folly of a false one. Let us then apply this test to the religion of the oral law. Does it commend itself to the understanding by its wisdom, and the wisdom of its teachers? It is true, that it speaks well of itself, and calls all its doctors 'wise men'; but the histories which the Talmud gives of the Rabbinical practice with regard to charms lead to the inevitable conclusion that wisdom is not one of the characteristics of the oral law. Take for example the following: 'For a bleeding at the nose, let a man be brought who is a priest, and whose name is Levi, and let him write the word Levi backwards. If this cannot be done, get a layman, and let him write the following words backwards—"Ana pipi Shila bar sumki," or let him write these words—"Taam dli bemi keseph, taam li bemi paggan." Or let him take a root of grass, and the cord of an old bed, and paper and saffron, and the red part of the inside of a palm-tree, and let him burn them together, and let him take some wool, and twist two threads, and let him dip them in vinegar, and then roll them in the ashes, and put them into his nose. Or let him look out for a small stream of water that flows from east to west, and let him go and stand with one leg on each side of it, and let him take with his right hand some mud from under his left foot, and with his left hand from under his right foot, and let him twist two threads of wool, and dip them in the mud, and put them into his nostrils. Or let him be placed under a spout, and let water be brought and poured upon him, and let them say, 'As this water ceases to flow, so let the blood of M., the son of the woman N., also cease."' (Gittin, fol. 69, col. 1.) Now we ask any Jew of common sense, whether this passage savours most of wisdom or folly? Vinegar and water may be very useful in such a case, or even mud, if used in sufficient quantity, might stop up the nose, and therefore stop the bleeding too, but what manner of benefit can proceed from the word Levi written backwards, or from the words which Rashi pronounced to be magical? Why is the mud of water flowing from east to west more efficacious, and why is it to be taken with the right hand from under the left foot, and with the left hand from under the right foot? Plainly because the authors of this passage thought there was some charm or magic power, and their minds were so overpowered by superstition as to lead them to disregard the plain words of Moses forbidding all magic. It cannot be pretended that this is a rare case, the Talmud abounds in such remedies, all equally wise."

The Bristol
Medico=Chirurgical Journal.

JUNE, 1899.

ON THE TEMPERATURE IN CÀSES OF APOPLEXY,

AND ON THE

OCCURRENCE (1) OF ŒDEMA AND (2) OF LOSS OF THE KNEE-JERK IN THE PARALYSED LIMBS IN HEMIPLEGIA.

BY

J. MICHELL CLARKE, M.A., M.D. Cantab., F.R.C.P.,

Professor of Pathology, University College, Bristol, and Physician to the Bristol General Hospital.

THE following cases illustrate some of the more interesting points with regard to the temperature of the body in vascular lesions of the cerebral hemispheres. Briefly stated, the chief facts known are—that in cases of cerebral hemorrhage there is an initial fall of the body-temperature; that in rapidly fatal cases this subnormal temperature is maintained, but in others which live for some hours it may be succeeded by a rise to a high level; that in cases which prove fatal after a few days the initial fall is followed by a stationary period of return to the normal or near it, ending in a rise of the temperature before death; and in cases which recover, the temperature after an initial fall and rise returns to normal, or, rather, remains somewhat subnormal for some time. In softening due to thrombosis,

8

there is no initial fall, or it is very slight; the temperature rises, and this is followed by secondary oscillations of considerable amplitude.

Dr. Dana called attention to the fact that in cases of cerebral hemorrhage, accompanied with hemiplegia, the temperature upon the paralysed is higher than that upon the sound side, and that in acute cerebral softening from thrombosis or embolism this difference in temperature is not present.   He says: "There are exceptions to this rule which I have laid down, but these exceptions are rare, and are to be explained either on the ground that the hæmorrhage is very small or the acute softening is very extensive." [1]

This difference of temperature on the two sides in hemorrhage may be of practical use in the diagnosis from softening due to thrombosis or embolism.   Dr. Dana further says that he has never found any perceptible temperature-disturbance in hemiplegia due to embolism, no matter how severe and pronounced the central disturbance was.

CASE 1.—The first case that I wish to report in illustration of the temperature changes in cerebral hemorrhage is that of a man, aged 48, who had had two attacks of rheumatic fever.   There was a history of loss of power in the left side and muffled speech on December 9th, 1898, since which day patient had been confined to bed.   On admission, December 17th, patient had left hemiplegia, and was in a dazed, heavy mental state.   Early on December 19th he passed into a condition of profound coma, in which he died.   The urine contained a considerable quantity of albumin.

The necropsy showed that there was subacute interstitial nephritis, the heart was much dilated, and both ventricular walls were hypertrophied and showed patches of fibroid degeneration.   The right cerebral hemisphere was enlarged—the convolutions flattened—and so soft that it was removed with difficulty.   The white and grey matter of all the parts of the hemisphere corresponding to the distribution of the middle cerebral artery, with the exception of a narrow zone on the ventral aspects of the optic thalamus and nucleus lenticularis, were yellow, softened, and broken down.   A clot was found obstructing this artery, and its branches were thrombosed.   A large recent hemorrhage had ploughed up the white substance of the frontal lobe and extended to the surface, about the middle part of the second frontal convolution.   The other parts of the brain were normal.

The chart indicates the very high rise of temperature which accompanies the fatal termination in a large cerebral hemorrhage, the temperature on the paralysed side being regularly

[1] *Post-Graduate*, 1896, xi. 316.

a degree higher than that on the sound side, and the interesting fact that thirty minutes after death the temperature on both sides was 106°—that is to say, the temperature on the paralysed side ceased to rise after death, whilst that on the sound side rose one degree. Does this indicate that the healthy side of the brain exerts to some extent an inhibiting influence on the rise of temperature on the opposite side of the body, this inhibition ceasing, of course, with death?

Case 2 was that of a woman, aged 44, a heavy drinker, who was admitted with right hemiplegia and partial right hemianæsthesia. She was in a very dull, stuporous mental condition. She had had an apoplectic seizure five days before admission.

At the necropsy a large hemorrhage was found to have taken place into the left optic thalamus, and this had later ruptured into the left lateral ventricle, which was filled with bloodclot.

The chart shows the temperature disturbances due to the initial hemorrhage into the thalamus, the temperature on the paralysed varying from half to two degrees higher than that on the sound side; and this difference between the two sides was maintained in the rise of temperature which immediately preceded death, which was due to the effused blood bursting into the lateral ventricle.

Case 3.—A patient admitted (aged 57) with left hemiplegia and hemianæsthesia, which had come on during the night seven days before admission. He was sensible on admission, but gradually became more dull, and could give no account of himself. After a short period of quiet delirium he gradually became deeply comatose, and so died. Pupils small and contracted. A marked feature in the case was the paralysis of the muscles of the left side of the abdomen, which caused the abdominal wall to be flaccid and bulged out.

P.M.E.—The white matter of the right hemisphere was extensively softened and diffluent (white softening). This was most marked in and around the internal capsule, lenticular nucleus, and optic thalamus, extending a little way into the posterior part of the hemisphere and for a considerable distance into the frontal lobe.

The chart shows a rise of temperature before death, with a fall at death; the temperature of the paralysed side was two degrees above that of the sound side on admission, and for the most part slightly above the latter until just before death, when the temperature on each side fell together to the same level. In this extensive softening the temperature difference between the two sides rather resembled that of hemorrhage, but was more irregular.

CASE 4.—A man, aged 46. The symptoms of his illness began with tingling in the left hand and arm, and twitchings of the muscles of this arm and the left leg for a few days. Six days before admission he had a fit, in which he became unconscious, and in which there were twitchings of the muscles of the whole of the left side of the body. This fit was followed by left hemiplegia. After admission he had two or three fits of the same kind, and twitchings of the left arm and calf-muscles were frequently observed. He was dull and drowsy on admission, but subsequently slightly improved; he had very little power of movement of either left arm or leg. Drowsiness was markedly increased on the twelfth day of the illness, and on the fourteenth day deepened into coma, in which he died on the eighteenth day.

A large area of softening was found in the region of the right lenticular nucleus and optic thalamus.

The chart shows that the temperature is irregular, and that on the paralysed and sound side fairly correspond with each other.

CASE 10.—Hemorrhage into the pons Varolii. The chief symptoms were fits, consisting of twitching of the muscles on both sides of the body, with stertor, frothing at the mouth, and cyanosis. Apart from the fits, in the intervals between them convulsive twitchings of the muscles occurred. All four limbs were paralysed, and the motions and urine passed unconsciously. There was drowsiness at first, which passed into coma. There was no oculo-motor paralysis, and the pupils on admission were equal and not contracted. On the last day of life there were irregular, horizontal, oscillating movements of the eyeballs, and alternating contraction and dilatation of the pupils, which were, however, never strongly contracted. The face was slightly drawn to the right; the abdomen was retracted. The superficial reflexes were normal on admission, and there was double ankle-clonus.

Post mortem the kidneys were contracted and granular. Two hemorrhages were found in the pons—one on the left side, about ½ inch in long (transverse) diameter, just above upper end of fourth ventricle, in the tegmental region, dorsal to the fillet; the other, about ⅛ inch in diameter, a little lower down, close to the raphe, at the same level in the pons as the first hemorrhage and on the right side.

The temperature was persistently subnormal and identical on both sides of the body. It is interesting to note the subnormal temperature in the presence of frequent convulsions.

As to the mode of production of a high temperature under such conditions, one must premise that it is not due to muscular convulsions, for these are often absent. Although the subject is an obscure and difficult one, it is hardly to be doubted that the thermo-taxic mechanism is the one at fault. The arguments for the location of the thermo-taxic mechanism in the central nervous system need not be recapitulated; they are well known. This localisation has been further established by numerous experiments to be probably in or near the corpus striatum. Thus Hale White,[1] experimenting on rabbits, found that "lesions of the corpus striatum, if not large enough to cause shock and hemorrhage, lead to a considerable rise of temperature, on the average equal on the two sides of the body, even if only one corpus striatum is damaged." Although lesions of the septum lucidum and posterior part of the upper surface of the cortex in rabbits also caused a rise of temperature, his experiments showed that injuries to the corpus striatum were by far the most important.

The normal regulation of heat is effected by variations in the loss of heat—for a greater amount of heat is produced than is actually necessary—" the heat-producing activities of the organism tend to exceed . . . . its requirements."[2] The heat - regulating mechanism being disordered in cerebral lesions, the temperature tends to rise. The observation that although the temperature rises on both sides of the body, it remains lower on the side of the lesion, is difficult to explain; possibly the sound hemisphere, although much disordered, may still exert some controlling influence on the temperature of the opposite side of the body. In this connection the fact that in the first case the temperature on the sound side rose one degree—to the level of that on the paralysed side—after death is interesting.

In the remaining cases recovery took place, and therefore the diagnosis was not confirmed by *post-mortem* examination; but the cases were selected as being ones in which the diagnosis from clinical symptoms appeared reasonably certain. The first, No. 5, illustrates again the difference between the temperature on the two sides in hemorrhage; No. 7, a similar, but slighter, difference in a case of cerebral syphilis, probably from occlusion of a vessel; No. 8, the subnormal temperature which may persist some weeks in hemiplegia; and No. 9, a want of correspondence between the temperature in the axilla and the surface temperature.

[1] *Brit. M. J.*, 1891, i. 150.

[2] Burdon-Sanderson, "The Doctrine of Fever"; Clifford Allbutt's *System of Medicine*, 1896, vol. i., p. 150.

CASE 5.—In this case, although there was no autopsy, the lesion was almost certainly a hemorrhage into the right cerebral hemisphere. The chart shows the difference of temperature on the two sides (paralysed highest) seven days after the apoplectic stroke; after another week the temperature became normal on both sides. Another point of interest was the marked diminution of the knee-jerk in the paralysed leg; it could only be obtained with great difficulty. At the same time rigidity came on in the usual way, and was quite marked one month after the fit. The leg became very tender on movement, and the left knee-joint was swollen and tender.

CASE 7.—From a case of hemiplegia due to syphilitic occlusion of a branch of the right middle cerebral artery. The chart shows a difference between the two sides of at first one to two degrees, the temperature on the sound side being markedly subnormal; then follow, as recovery proceeds, a number of rather wide oscillations lasting for about a week, subsequently the temperature on both sides returned to normal.

CASE 8.—This chart is taken from a case of hemiplegia seven weeks after the onset. The subnormal temperature on both sides of the body is noticeable at so long a period after the initial lesion; as the patient only came under observation some time after the seizure and recovered, the exact nature of it could not be ascertained. It was probably a hemorrhage. There was no albuminuria.

In some cases of hemiplegia which are associated with disease of the kidneys, a persistent low temperature may be noted, but there was no such reason for it in this case.

CASE 9 was one of hemiplegia probably due to softening from thrombosis in the course of chronic Bright's disease. The chart shows that the difference in temperature between the two sides is slight and inconstant. On the 5th August, when the temperature in the axilla was half a degree higher on the paralysed than on the sound side, the surface-temperature was nearly 1½ degrees lower on the former than on the latter. This case presented another symptom sometimes met with in hemiplegia— excessive tenderness to touch or movement of the paralysed limbs. The patient screamed loudly if they were moved or touched. This was not attributable to rigidity of the limbs, as the rigidity was only slight. Another symptom she suffered from was well-marked œdema of the paralysed side of the body only, especially of the arm and leg. Associated with this appeared trophic disturbances in the shape of a sore on the heel and a blister if the skin was thrown into a crease or fold anywhere by her position in bed.

The presence of this unilateral œdema is, I think, to be attributed to a change in the innervation or nutrition of the vessel-walls, and may be compared to the experimental œdema in the leg produced after division of one sciatic nerve in the leg after the production of artificial hydræmia.

When albuminuria is present the above seems to be the most reasonable explanation of œdema of the paralysed side, and is in accordance with known factors in the production of œdema. But in other cases the etiology is not to be thus

explained, for a similar œdema may occur in hemiplegia in cases in which albuminuria is absent, and there is no reason to suspect disease of the kidneys. Thus in a woman who suffered from mitral disease, and in whom left hemiplegia was presumably due to thrombosis followed by softening, but who had no albuminuria nor other evidence of kidney-disease, five weeks after the attack œdema of the paralysed arm and hand came on, and the limb became painful to the touch, and there was at the same time marked rigidity. Indications of vaso-motor disturbance were found in cold sweats and lividity confined to the hand and forearm, and this limb was always colder than the right. The leg was less affected, and began to recover power early. There was, of course, no evidence of local pressure upon or of disease of the vessels of the left arm.

In both these cases the appearance of œdema was accompanied by pain, which was more or less constant, but much increased by movement. This pain was not the same as that which is aroused by forcibly moving the parts of a rigidly-contracted limb, and was apparently not connected with the rigidity present. The appearance of this painful œdema is an unfavourable sign in the prognosis as to recovery of power in the limbs, and is difficult to relieve by treatment. The first of the above two cases (case No. 9) exhibited also another phenomenon which I have observed in three cases of hemiplegia—a marked diminution or sometimes loss of the knee-jerk in the paralysed leg, the exact contrary of what usually obtains. I append brief notices of the two other cases.

A man, aged 71, was admitted three days after onset of a seizure, probably due to thrombosis, which occurred in the night, and was accompanied by twitchings of the right side of the face, right arm and leg, but not by complete loss of consciousness. Right hemiplegia resulted, and was at first accompanied by anæsthesia of the whole of the right lower extremity, which was soon reduced to a patch of anæsthesia in the area of distribution of the N. cutaneus femoris. There was slight concentric contraction of the right visual field and a moderate amount of albumin in the urine. He recovered power gradually, and was able to walk out of the Hospital four weeks later. The right knee-jerk was completely absent, and could never be obtained by any method or by reinforcement, whilst the left knee-jerk was active and the superficial reflexes normal. The leg became moderately stiff, but was never very rigid; it was not, however, flaccid. Subsequent examinations showed the right knee-jerk to be always absent.

In the case of a man, aged 65, with left hemiplegia, partial, not complete, hemianæsthesia, left hemianopsia, and with slight movements of athetosis in the left hand, the left knee-jerk was also absent. On the right side it was normal. The other reflexes were normal, and the amount of rigidity present in the paralysed limbs was only moderate.

I cannot give any explanation of the loss of the knee-jerk on the side of the hemiplegia; especial care was taken to ascertain that it was really absent. In two of the cases there was also some anæsthesia on the affected side; but in the other the sensory disturbance was in the opposite direction, consisting of increased pain and tenderness.

FRACTURE OF THE PATELLA.

BY

A. W. PRICHARD, M.R.C.S.,
Surgeon to the Bristol Royal Infirmary.

IN a case of fractured patella there is often some difficulty in knowing what treatment it is best to recommend to the patient and his friends, and there are many points to be considered. I do not mean to go into all details; these are best left to the judgment of the surgeon in charge of the case. I will briefly mention the five methods of treatment that are now in fashion, and offer some remarks on each.

Firstly, the plan without operation. This, the old one, consists of rest with the application of splint and bandages. There are various excellent ways of drawing the fragments together, and perhaps in almost the majority of cases this method is the one to be recommended, and it often gives fair results; but the best result that can be hoped for is a ligamentous union with more or less impairment of extension, and the probability is that the individual will never be able to run or climb a ladder.

Secondly, subcutaneous silk ligature, by surrounding the knee-cap either laterally or vertically by a stout silk cord. In the latter case the ligature is passed by means of a strong needle right into the joint, and is left in, resting on the condyles. I have had no personal experience of this plan, but I cannot imagine that it would be successful in many cases when the tilting of the fragments and the indipping of the fibrous covering are considered. The tilting is present in most cases, as seen in Fig. 1, and is sometimes remarkable, as in one case which I wired, where the fractured surface of the upper fragment was directly forwards. The dipping in of the fibrous covering has been present and has given some trouble in all cases that I have seen operated on.

Thirdly, the recently recommended method of massage of the thigh muscles, and passive movement of the knee from the commencement of the case. This is advocated by those who think that the cause of bad results in cases that have not been operated on is to some extent atrophy of the quadriceps, and contraction of the fasciæ from want of use. I cannot say anything about this treatment from my own experience—I want to see it tried—but it can never result in bony union if the fragments have been separated, and a ligamentous union can never give the support that a bony one gives.

Fourthly, the method of an open operation and sewing up the fibrous covering and split lateral expansion of the quadriceps by buried sutures. This has, to my mind, little to recommend it in comparison with wiring, as the operation would be as severe, and the result not so secure.

Fifthly, wiring. It is usual to make a longitudinal incision and then carefully to scrape away all material between the fragments, to bore and pass the wire, then to irrigate the joint, washing out all clot, then tighten the wire. I always put a drainage tube into the joint on the outer side, and remove it in twenty-four hours. One can generally rely upon a single stout silver wire. A good plan, when the lower fragment is small, is to pass two wires through one hole in the lower, and separate them to pass through two holes in the upper. This gives a very firm hold. The method was suggested by my colleague, Mr. Paul Bush.

Wiring the patella should not be done too soon after the

accident, the joint should be allowed at least forty-eight hours to begin to recover from the immediate effect of the injury. I have seen a disastrous result from the operation being done on the same day as the fracture. Certainly the operation should not be undertaken by any one who has not complete confidence in his antiseptics and in his carpentering skill, nor in cases where the general health is not good; but as far as my experience and my ideas go, it is the right thing to recommend in young adults who have to use their legs in earning their living, or who wish to be able to indulge in a fair amount of active exercise.

I briefly mention two special cases :—

CASE 1.—F. A., aged 40. When playing hockey on November 27th, 1897, slipped and sustained a transverse fracture of the left patella.

November 30th. Patella wired with a single silver wire, joint washed out with boracic lotion and drained. Wound healed well.

Sixteen days later passive movements were begun. Patient went home January 7th, six weeks after the operation.

He played cricket all the following summer, and on September 10th, 1898, whilst bowling in a match the right knee-cap gave way. He was found to have a transverse fracture just below the middle.

September 19th. Right patella wired—one silver wire   (*Vide* skiagram, Fig. 2.)

October 11th. Twenty-two days after operation passive movement was commenced—about fifteen degrees from horizontal.

Patient went out well six weeks from the operation, well able to bend both knees.

He is playing cricket this season.

CASE 2.—C. W. In December, 1892, fractured left patella. This was treated at the Bristol Royal Infirmary with back splints and cross-bars, the fragments being pulled together by strapping. He wore a leather splint for some months. Six months later he was readmitted for stretching of the union, and was treated as on the previous occasion.

March 2nd, 1899, was admitted for a similar accident to the same patella—the interval between the fragments was fully one inch. (*Vide* skiagram, Fig. 3.)

March 14th. I cut away the dense fibrous tissue between the fragments, and freshened the ends of the bones and brought them together with two wire sutures passed through one hole in the lower and two holes in the upper fragment. (*Vide* skiagram, Fig. 4.)

March 29th. Wounds were quite healed—passive movements were begun sixteen days after operation.

April 24th. Patient went out, able to walk easily without a splint, bending his knee fairly well with no separation of fragments.

Fig. 1.

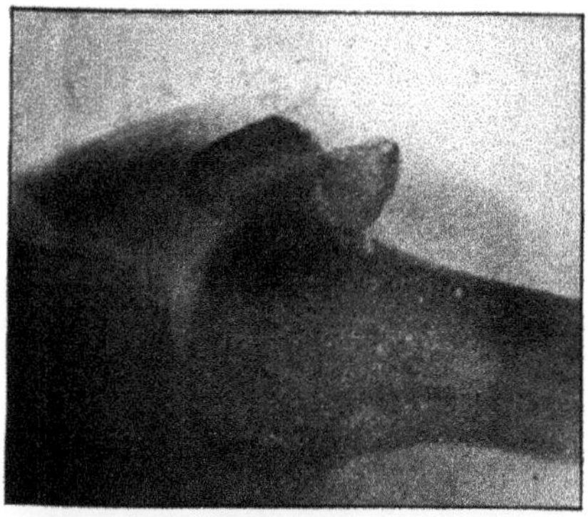

Fig. 2.

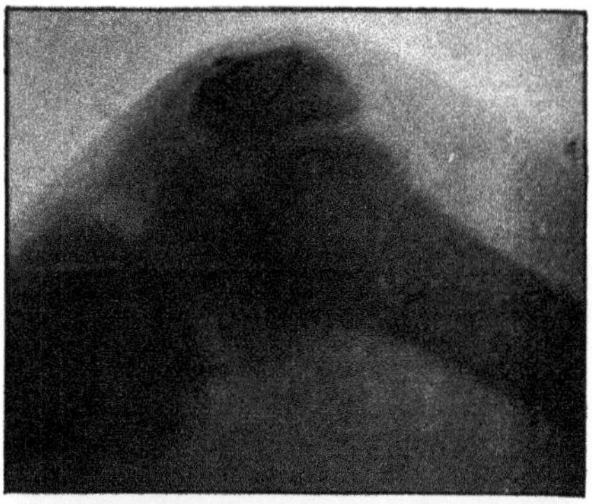

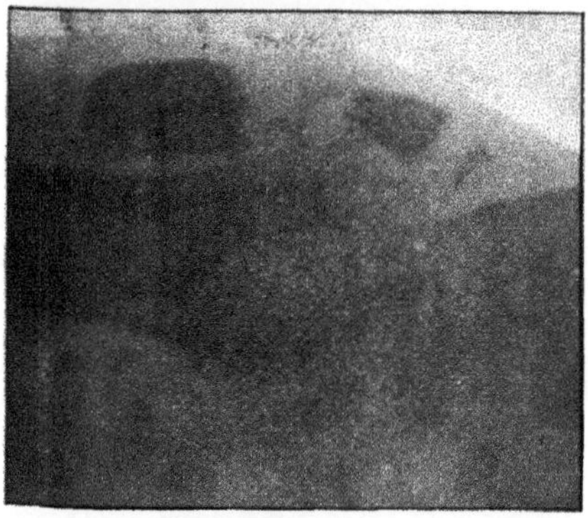

Fig. 3.

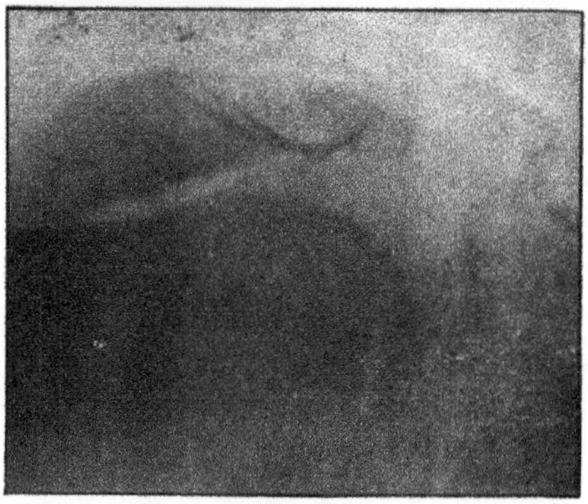

Fig. 4.

IDIOPATHIC THROMBOSIS OF THE PORTAL AND CONTRIBUTORY VEINS.

BY

BERTRAM M. H. ROGERS, B.A., M.D., B.Ch. Oxon.,

Physician and Pathologist to the Royal Hospital for Sick Children and Women, Bristol.

CASES of thrombosis of the portal vein, other than those caused by some septic influence, are of such rare occurrence that the subject is hardly to be found in text-books on medicine, and in the enormous mass of medical literature that now exists only some dozen cases comparable to the one to be related are to be found.

The history and course of the case which was recently under my care at the Children's Hospital is singularly complete, and consequently interesting, for the boy was under the observation either of my colleagues or myself for eight years. It is as well, perhaps, to admit at the beginning of this paper that the condition which was found *post mortem* was not diagnosed during life, but in this I do not find myself without good companions; for not only did my colleagues not recognise the true nature of the case, but in all those that I have collected from various medical publications the state of affairs was recognised but once, and that by Sir William Jenner. Whether the line of treatment adopted would have been modified had a correct diagnosis been made is another matter. This I shall refer to later.

Herbert R. was first admitted to the Hospital in October, 1891, at that time being under the care of Dr. Edgeworth, who has kindly supplied me with the notes he made at the time. The child was then 4 years and 9 months old, and had been ill for three months with increasing size of the abdomen. He was the fourth child of eight, three of whom were dead; and he is stated to have wasted from birth (a statement one often hears, but which is difficult of belief). There was no history of paternal syphilis. Examination revealed a small quantity of free fluid in the peritoneal cavity and an enlarged

[1] Read at the April Meeting of the Bristol Medico-Chirurgical Society.

spleen, whose lower edge was three inches below the costal margin.
There appeared to be no disease in any other organ. There were no
enlarged lymphatic glands, and no albumin in the urine. The bowels
were open rather freely, the motions being a dirty yellow colour
and acid in reaction. The red corpuscles were 70 per cent., the
proportion of red to white 200 to 1, and the hæmoglobin 75 per cent.,
though a few days after the percentage was less. In December he was
discharged; but in February, 1892, was re-admitted, with a history of
having vomited up some blood. Examination showed that the spleen
had not altered in size, but the liver was two inches below the costal
margin. There was no ascites. As no hemorrhage occurred, he was
sent home again in March.

In October, 1895, he was again admitted, his parents stating that he
had passed some blood by the bowel. He was sick several times soon
after admission, but it was not till November 9th that he brought up
five ounces of pure, bright, alkaline blood, and a few hours later six
more. This reduced the hæmoglobin to 20 per cent. On the 17th he
brought up twenty-four ounces of blood and passed a black motion,
and on the 18th, in another attack of hæmatemesis, he vomited eight
ounces. This reduced him to an extreme state of anæmia, but he
recovered so far that the hæmoglobin rose as high as 60 per cent., and
the red corpuscles from 1,080,000 to 5,250,000, and he went on till
January 13th, 1894, when he vomited twenty ounces of mixed blood and
food. This was the last attack during this stay in the Hospital, and
he improved so much that he went home in May. On leaving, his
spleen was observed to have reached to within half an inch of the
umbilicus.

In June, 1898, he came in again for a month; but keeping quite well
all the time, though rather anæmic, he went home again. In November
he again was admitted, after having, it was said, vomited "two
quarts of blood." Whatever amount this really represents cannot be
certain; but on the following day, the 9th, he brought up altogether
thirty-three ounces, reducing him to such a collapsed condition that he
was only brought back to life by transfusion with saline solution and
inhalations of oxygen. (I may parenthetically remark that of the
number of times I have employed oxygen, I believe this is the only
case in which it did good, and here it was probably assisted greatly by
the transfusion.) After this attack he slowly but gradually improved,
and there was no evidence of hemorrhage till December 5th, when he
passed black motions for two days. This hemorrhage, whenever it took
place, did not seem to affect him, as his improvement continued till the
19th, when, after a very restless night, he vomited four pints and seven
ounces of blood-stained fluid in the twenty-four hours. How much of this
was blood cannot be said; but after the first symptom of hæmatemesis
no fluid, except ice, was allowed, so that the actual quantity of blood
must have been large. The next day, the 20th, he passed some bright
blood—five ounces—by the bowel, and vomited thirteen ounces of pure
blood. Till January 16th he was free, but on that day he began to
bring up small quantities of blood, amounting in all to ten ounces.
This was almost entirely clotted. He also brought up eight ounces of
clear fluid, alkaline in reaction and containing a trace of albumin, the
source of which I cannot explain. The following day, for the first
time, his temperature rose, reaching 101°, and he passed some black
fæcal matter. On the 22nd he again vomited, this time twelve ounces
of bright red clotted blood. These repeated attacks of hæmatemesis
reduced him to an extreme state of collapse, and, with repeated small
vomits and passing of small black motions, he died on February 4th.

During all this time the physical conditions did not vary. A small amount of fluid was always present in the abdomen, which appeared to increase just before an attack of hæmatemesis came on. The spleen reached to within half an inch of the umbilicus, but the liver apparently recovered its normal size. A trace of albumin was observed at times in his urine, and his anæmic condition gave rise to hæmic murmurs.

One peculiar fact I noticed about the boy, and that was a curious earthy smell. I do not remember ever to have noticed this in any other patient, and on my calling attention to it others who happened to be with me also observed it.

The necropsy was made by me the following day. The body was very pale, and there was only slight rigor mortis. On opening the thorax a small quantity of fluid was found in each pleural cavity. The lungs were healthy; the heart was small, the right side flaccid and empty, the left full of clot; there was no pericardial fluid. No disease of the valves was present. The abdominal cavity contained several pints of clear fluid; the intestines were in a natural position, and there were no adhesions except those to be mentioned later round the spleen. The only abnormality noticed was the greatly enlarged spleen. The upper surface of this organ was firmly adherent to the diaphragm in one place, and the rest had a dull grey colour, and looked as if its surface was covered with lymph, in reality being due to the thickening of the capsule. On moving it, it was found to be also firmly adherent to the stomach, so that the two organs were removed together. Unfortunately, I did not then recognise the condition, and cut through the veins, which were thrombosed, and only removed a short portion of the duodenum. The liver, which was slightly smaller than one would have expected for a boy of this age, was pale, but otherwise normal; the gall-bladder was very large, and full of bile. The pancreas and mesentery were found to be much overgrown with fibrous tissue, and about two feet down the small intestine a deeply-congested patch, with hard knotted veins leading to it, was found and removed. The only other pathological matter of interest found was a horseshoe kidney, the second I have found while acting as pathologist to the Children's Hospital. On examining the spleen and stomach more closely, it was found that the splenic vein was full of hard discoloured clot, and that a new set of vessels had developed, which led into the spleen at various points. Tracing the vein forwards, the clot was found to extend to the vein in the small curvature of the stomach, the coronary, while, to compensate for this obstruction to the flow of blood, large veins, which were easily seen in the recent state, coursed across the stomach from the right gastro-epiploic vein. The coronary vein was blocked as far as the duodenum, but the venous communications there seem to have been sufficiently good to have prevented any engorgement. In the small intestine this did not hold good, and a branch of the superior mesenteric, which had become involved in the clot, produced a deeply-congested patch about four inches long. Here the walls of the intestine were much thickened, and the mucous membrane of a deep chocolate colour. Round the pancreas there was a considerable overgrowth of connective tissue, and the plexus of veins known as the pancreatico-duodenal and its branches were all filled with firm discoloured clot. The portal itself, as it entered the liver, was hard and cord-like, but on cutting into the liver substance it did not appear that the clot extended to any depth, nor did I find any compensatory branches. The inferior mesenteric vein was not affected.

From the cases I have found reported elsewhere, I conclude that the symptoms in this case were not unusual, but were, in fact, those seen in this condition. Hæmatemesis of more or less severe type—melæna, enlargement of the spleen, and ascites were present in every case. Osler[1] records a case in which there were hemorrhoids and no ascites, the spleen was much enlarged and adherent to the stomach and diaphragm; the liver small, and the veins of the spleen and the rectum were thrombosed. The portal vein was represented by a fibrous cord; there was no calcification of the walls, but some at the junction of the splenic and superior mesenteric. His opinion was that the primary thrombosis was portal and not splenic. In his *Principles and Practice of Medicine*, in 1892, p. 429, he says it is rarely seen except in cases of cirrhosis. These cases are rare no doubt, but from the cases I have found I should say cirrhosis was a rare cause of thrombosis, as its absence is remarked in every case except one. In Sir William Jenner's case,[2] though the patient was admittedly a heavy drinker, no cirrhosis was found. This case is a peculiar one, from the fact that the abdomen burst. This came about in the following manner: The patient was tapped for ascites, and the puncture ulcerated, and an ulcer in the intestine, caused by thrombosis of the mesenteric vein, perforated, allowing gas to escape into the peritoneal cavity, and so causing the explosion. In this case the spleen was large. Dr. Lyons[3] mentions the case of a woman aged 45, who was tapped to the extent of 500 quarts in eight months for ascites, in whom at the necropsy a clot was found in the portal vein. He particularly remarks on the absence of cirrhosis, and mentions that the liver was small. Another one is reported by Dr. Goodhart[4] as a case of cirrhosis of the liver, probably originating in phlebitis of the portal vein. Microscopical sections of the liver were shown from a woman aged 21, who in May, 1883, vomited a large quantity of blood. Diminution of the size of the liver, with splenic enlargement, came on; but on death following, only a partial examination of

[1] *J. Anat. & Physiol.*, 1882, xvi. 208.
[2] *Lancet*, 1874, i. 1.   [3] *Dublin J. M. Sc.*, 1877, lxiv. 457.
[4] *Tr. Path. Soc. Lond.*, 1889, xl. 134.

the body appears to have been made, for "the portal vein trunk was not examined." It certainly seems strange to ascribe the cirrhosis to a thrombosis which possibly was never present, and certainly was never looked for.

Dr. Moorhead [1] records the case of a man aged 57, who died of hæmatemesis, and at the *post-mortem* examination the liver was normal in size and appearance—the spleen enlarged to three times its natural size. T. B. Peacock [2] remarks on the atrophy of the liver in a case of his—a man aged 52, who died of ascites, diarrhœa, and vomiting,—and believes that the condition was due to the thrombosis. S. West [3] makes much the same remarks on a case of his—a young woman with much the same symptoms as the other cases mentioned.

I think it is evident from these facts that cirrhosis from thrombosis of the portal vein is rare. That to a large amount the liver depends on the blood of the portal vein for nutrition is, I believe, a well-known fact, and should this supply be withdrawn a shrinking of the organ takes place, with impairment of function; the liver is, in fact, starved. The causes which lead to thrombosis are very obscure. In all of the cases except one I have found no reason for the condition is given, possibly because none existed. The only one solitary cause, given in one case, is indulgence in alcohol. The disease comes on apparently from no assignable cause, and usually attacks adults. My case is the youngest patient recorded; most of the others are between thirty and fifty. The course of the disease is towards a fatal issue—no case, so far as I can discover, has been recorded of a recovery. The length of the illness varies, too, considerably. Mine again holds the record for nearly eight years, most of the others are of only a month's duration or only five weeks. The longest after mine is a case recorded by G. Balfour and Grainger Stewart [4] of a young woman who, after a history of ascites for five years, died seven weeks after coming under observation. She probably, from the state of the organs found *post mortem*, had suffered from the disease all that

[1] *Tr. Path. Soc. Lond.*, 1867, xviii. 61.
[2] *Ibid.*, 1873, xxiv. 122.   [3] *Ibid.*, 1878, xxix. 107.
[4] *Edinb. M. J.*, 1869, xiv. 589.

time.   I see a difficulty in my case, and that is, that the periods of illness were interrupted by months of improving health. What was the condition of the boy's veins during that time cannot be said with certainty; but it is highly probable that the thrombosis existed all that time, and that from some unexplained cause, possibly some extension of the thrombosis, certain symptoms appeared at intervals.   It is a point worth noting that no fever existed in any of the cases.

The question of treatment must now be considered, for it is evident that most who saw a case such as this—one with blood being vomited by the pint — would give hæmostatic drugs. As the patient is suffering from rather too much hæmostasis, that hardly appears to be right, yet I believe most would give them.   I think we might say this, that drugs which are believed to cause hæmostasis by clogging the blood at the orifice of the vessel might be given with advantage; but those that are intended to act on the vessels, such as ergotine, or on the blood itself, increasing its coagulability, such as chloride of calcium, are counter-indicated.

The blood that was passed by the bowel no doubt came from the congested patch in the intestine, as well as from the stomach.   It would be rather a matter of surprise if the veins of the mesentery were not thrombosed when the splenic, into which the superior generally empties its contents, was affected. In my case the inferior was not affected, but in one recorded by Barclay and Holl [1] from the duodenum downwards there was much extravasation of blood, and part of the superior and inferior mesenteric vessels were thrombosed.   In Osler's case mentioned before the hemorrhoidal veins were blocked with clot, and in Payne's [2] case the superior mesenteric, and this, according to him, was the oldest part of the clot.   The diagnosis, as Osler says, is rarely made, and must always be obscure.   I thought in my case that the hemorrhage probably came from an ulcer in the stomach, but I could not account for the ascites or enlargement of the spleen.

[1] *Med. Times*, 1851, n. s., ii. 36.
[2] *Tr. Path. Soc. Lond.*, 1870, xxi. 228.

In the discussion which followed the reading of Dr. Rogers's paper, Dr. F. H. EDGEWORTH said that the chief difficulties of the case lie in the causation of the first thrombosis, which cannot have been due simply to the chlorotic condition of the blood or to the excess of the white corpuscles, but rather to some cause which produced both this and the thrombosis. It is a little remarkable that the thrombosis began in the splenic veins, for the spleen is probably an organ where a certain amount of disintegration of blood-cells goes on, and it was shown that tissue-fibrinogens will, if injected into the blood, cause an intra-vascular coagulation limited to the portal area. It is possible then that the thrombosis in the splenic veins was due to substances produced in the spleen by excessive or abnormal disintegration of blood-cells, brought about by the same cause which produced the alteration in the constitution of the blood. The changes in the blood and lymph-glands which have been observed as a result of excision of the spleen were not present in this case, unless the excess of leucocytes can be so regarded. This is probably due to the fact that the spleen was only slowly and incompletely put out of circulation owing to the opening out of new channels.—Dr. T. FISHER stated that he had seen a case diagnosed during life by Dr. Goodhart. In that case, in addition to hæmatemesis and ascites, there was a venous hum over the spleen. Dr. Fisher asked Dr. Rogers if there was any sign of re-establishment of the circulation through the thrombosed vessels to account for the temporary improvement.—Dr. ROGERS, in reply, stated he had not come across the report of Dr. Goodhart's case. There did not appear to be any attempt to compensate for the thrombosis except in the spleen, to which he had called attention.

A CASE OF EXTREME BRADYCARDIA.

BY

R. GEORGE FENDICK, M.R.C.S., and GEORGE PARKER, M.D. Cantab.

WITH NOTES ON THE EYE-SYMPTOMS
BY F. RICHARDSON CROSS, M.B. Lond., F.R.C.S.

ALTHOUGH instances of abnormally slow pulse are by no means rare, we think that the following case has some special features of interest which justify our recording it; especially as so little is known of the pathology of this phenomenon, that it is desirable to collect as fully as possible the actual facts observed in well-marked cases.

It is generally granted that bradycardia is a symptom of

9

various affections, and not one peculiar to a single disease.
These affections may be either extra-cardiac, or those of the
heart itself, or there may be a combined lesion such as the
arterio-sclerosis of the heart and medulla oblongata postulated
by M. Huchard[1]; and there is often extreme difficulty in
deciding where the cause of the condition really is, a difficulty
which was felt by us in the present case. Most remarkable,
too, is the slowness of reaction to cardiac stimulants.
Alexander Morison mentions that no effect was noticed for
some hours after he injected about twenty minims each of
liq. strychninæ and of the tinctures of digitalis and stro-
phanthus, besides nine minims of tincture of belladonna.[2]
We noticed a similar lack of response to doses or injections of
ether and strychnia, though we could find nothing in the
cardiac sounds or the area of dulness to indicate a degenerate
muscle, and the rate would rise to the normal of itself after a
varying period. Yet in such instances no one can lightly
regard the serious alternatives of letting a patient die at once
from cerebral asphyxia, or of administering almost fatally
strong stimulants. When the heart-beats sink, as in our patient,
to 11 or 12 in the minute, it is clear that little is needed
to put an end to them altogether. An extremely slow pulse,
however, is not always incompatible with prolonged life if
due care be taken. Occasionally it seems to be the normal
condition in persons who otherwise enjoy good health, and,
putting aside the perhaps doubtful cases of Napoleon and
Colonel Townshend, instances may be found of individuals
who have lived for a long period with pulses of 30 or 40.
We know one man now living whose pulse for some time
remained about 28.

It is curious how little effect on the general health may be
caused by the bradycardia. In the present case there was
for a long period neither œdema nor dyspnœa; the colour of
the face, the general nutrition, and the mental faculties
remained unaltered. He was seen at various times by different
consultants, none of whom observed any certain signs of

[1] *Maladies du Cœur*, p 324; quoted by Morison, *Treatment*, 1899, ii. 97.
[2] *Loc. cit.*

cerebral tumour or detected any valvular disease. The notes of the remarkable eye changes, including altitudinal hemianopsia, have been kindly given by Mr. Richardson Cross, whose diagnosis of the brain condition was verified *post mortem.*

The following is a brief history of the case :

A. G., 58, a civil engineer, a man of stout build, looking older than his years, but of temperate habits, had served in the North-Western Provinces of India in early life, and was still engaged in business at home. He was of fairly active habits, and usually enjoyed good health, though we noticed afterwards a gummatous cicatrix in the liver. For ten or twelve years he had complained of failing vision and attacks of giddiness, and showed a marked arcus senilis. In April, 1894, he suffered from sudden vertigo with severe syncopal symptoms, from which he did not recover sufficiently to return to business for some weeks. After this his health was never quite as good as before. Any prolonged strain on the eyes brought on minor attacks of vertigo, but careful and repeated auscultation about this time revealed no valvular lesion or change in the pulse. There was never any trace of albumin in the urine, the lungs were normal, and the liver seemed a little enlarged. In February, 1897, he sent for Mr. Fendick, his usual attendant, early one morning complaining of faintness. His pulse was found to be only 40 beats to the minute; but within two hours it rose to 80, and fluctuated for the rest of the day between 35 and 88. He was kept in bed for some days, and gradually recovered so far as to be able to get out of doors.

On April 19th his pulse was found to be as low as 30 at 8 a.m., and about this time a very slight transient epileptiform convulsion was noticed after each slowing of the pulse. This was at first limited to the muscles of the throat; but later on it spread to the face and upper part of the body, and was accompanied with momentary unconsciousness. Later in the day of the 19th of April the pulse sank to 24, and remained at an average of 30 till 5.30 p.m. on the 20th. It was intermittent, and this increased whenever he attempted to sleep. For some days he remained restless, breathing heavily, with an average pulse of 68. Throughout the illness no difference was observed by either of us between the rate noted at the wrist and over the cardiac region. Scarcely a day passed at this period without epileptiform convulsions more or less severe, sometimes during sleep, and accompanied by a marked slowing of the pulse and intermittency.

On May 13th, at 1.30 p.m., the pulse fell to 24, and by three o'clock rose to 94. During the night there were frequent convulsions, and the pulse fell to 20 for some hours, becoming markedly irregular. The next day the rate fell to 16, and again showed intermittency, rising to the normal on the 15th, but it fell again to 20 the day after. He remained in bed, but fairly well, till the 27th May, when other attacks followed with a rate of 24.

During June he was practically free from trouble; but a fresh series of attacks commenced on the 10th of July, and lasted for some days, with a pulse varying from 20 to 72. The patient then gradually improved, and went to the seaside for some months, returning sufficiently well to resume the management of his business. He persevered with this for the first six months of 1898.

In July the old condition returned; the pulse varied during the latter half of the month from 16 to 80, with a large number of epileptiform attacks of greater or less severity. Many of these occurred immediately upon waking, before he rose in any way from the recumbent posture, and for some days the seizures came on hourly. The mental faculties were perfectly clear, but he was very anxious and apprehensive of approaching death. He took food fairly well, and the body appeared well nourished. The bowels were regular, but he was troubled with considerable flatulency and distension. Occasionally laboured respiration was noticed during sleep. Numerous drugs were tried with little or no success, including various cardiac stimulants, as well as bromides and iodides in large doses, which he had also taken in former years.

He improved for the first ten days of August, the pulse remaining at 70; but he continued weak and very fearful of moving lest another attack should come on. Afterwards mental confusion and wandering began to appear. The pulse fell to an average of 22 on August 11th, and on the 13th it sank to 16. Some difficulty in swallowing was experienced, and definite Cheyne-Stokes respiration followed. After a pause of fifteen seconds, five deep inspirations would be succeeded by twice the number of shallow ones.

On the 15th, after a period of normal pulse-rate, fresh attacks came on, while the heart varied from 15 to 30 for twenty-four hours. Some twitching now occurred in the left hand; the patient began to refuse food, and became excited and slightly delirious. On the 18th the pulse again fell to 22, then to 14, and finally reached 11 beats per minute before midnight. It remained at nearly the same rate for four hours. Respiration was laboured, cold sweats appeared on the face, and neither injections of ether or other measures had any effect. Rectal feeding had to be resorted to, and the urine was drawn off by a catheter on the 19th for the first time. The pulse ranged from 14 to 30. On the 20th several seizures took place; but the pulse improved slightly, and even reached 70 at one time. The patient was evidently sinking; breathing became rapid and the temperature febrile. This was as high as 101.6° on August 21st, when the respiration rose to 60 and the pulse ranged from 25 to 60. He became gradually comatose, and died the same evening.

A necropsy was kindly permitted, and carried out under some difficulties. The body was well nourished; the digestive organs, the kidneys, and the lungs presented nothing of interest except the cicatrix on the liver and some degree of emphysema in the lungs. In the brain there were marked patches of atheroma in the vessels of the base, but otherwise the conditions were normal. No tumour, softening, or trace of hemorrhage could be found. A portion of the medulla was hardened, and examined microscopically. The walls of the vessels were considerably thickened, but no definite changes were observed in the other tissues. The heart was of normal size, and the valves perfect; but the walls showed two or three areas where fibroid degeneration was present. One of these in the ventricular septum near the base formed a nodule readily perceptible to the finger. The aorta was healthy; the coronary arteries were affected by atheromatous degeneration to a slight degree, but there was no thrombus or obliteration of their channels. Microscopically the muscle varied, being quite normal in one place, while in another advanced fibroid changes were present. Thus in part of the septum healthy muscle fibres had almost disappeared.

NOTES BY MR. F. RICHARDSON CROSS.

I saw Mr. A. G. with Mr. Fendick on April 1st, 1886. His right eye was sound and the vision good. In the left there was well-marked optic neuritis, and the very unusual phenomenon of altitudinal hemianopsia. The lower half of the field of vision was lost, central vision was useless. He could see no objects with this eye except by lowering his head and getting them in the upper part of the field, where he could still see them. This was due to a lesion in the upper part of the optic nerve, not to a cerebral condition. Large doses of iodide of potassium somewhat improved the vision. On July 23rd I found the left nerve atrophied. There was loss of the lower half of the field of vision now in both eyes, and the patient saw very badly indeed. The right eye had well-marked optic neuritis.

October 20th.—Both optic nerves showed post-neuritic atrophy; vision—R $\frac{6}{24}$, L $\frac{6}{24}$.

April 19th, 1894. I saw the patient at his house. He had been very ill for a fortnight, with difficulty in walking, giddiness, and nausea. The hemianopsia had scarcely altered. The function of the macula lutea of the right eye was active, that of the left impaired. Each eye saw $\frac{6}{15}$. Double optic atrophy, no neuritis; patient walked with difficulty, the knee-jerks were exaggerated, otherwise all objective symptoms except vision were normal.

April 13th, 1897.—The patient felt very ill. Pupil movements were normal. Vision—R $\frac{6}{24}$, L $\frac{6}{36}$. Hemianopsia as before, optic atrophy, but no fresh neuritis. There was no special sense trouble except the eyesight. The knee-jerks were exaggerated, cardiac weakness with flushing of the face and faintness. I considered that there was no gross cerebral lesion, but defective cerebral circulation and probably degenerate vessels.

REMARKS BY DR. G. PARKER.

I first saw the patient in consultation with Mr. Fendick in July, 1898, and afterwards at his request took charge of the case during his absence. It might be said that in the absence

of more definite pathological changes we are left in the dark
as to the exact production of the symptoms.   The case,
however, is clearly one of paroxysmal bradycardia occurring
in a patient who had fibroid changes in the ventricles and
diseased coronary arteries, while the exciting causes of the
attacks were probably changes in the cerebral circulation,
eye-strain, and digestive disturbances.   Thus, in 1897, I find
on three occasions attacks were noted as coming on after
reading or using the eyes at his office.   In the later stages
indeed the tendency to seizure was so strong that it is difficult
to discover the exciting causes, but the patient dreaded the
slightest noise or excitement for fear of a recurrence.   In the
classical instance related by Holberton,[1] the heart-rate sank
to an average of 33 for some years after an injury of the cord
and medulla ; but upon an attack of dyspepsia or mental excitement this would fall till it reached even 7½ to the minute, and
violent convulsions followed.   It was in one of these after-
dinner attacks that the patient finally died.   Sansom,[2] indeed,
seems to think that the influence is often in the other direction,
and that the dyspeptic cases seen in paroxysmal and sometimes
in persistent bradycardia may be caused by extension to other
vagus branches of the disturbance existing in the cardiac area.

Now, bradycardia may be temporary or it may be
permanent, or it may be paroxysmal, and the question arises
whether any one of these is part of a definite group of symptoms,
and always dependent on one and the same cause.

It is clear that permanent bradycardia may be found in
perfect health, perhaps more often in very tall men, as Seymour
Taylor[3] notices, and again in diseases, such as uræmia and
chlorosis, where a high-tension pulse exists.   It used to be the
fashion to ascribe it to fatty degeneration of the heart, and
again to fibroid changes, disease of the coronary arteries, or
dilated heart, but all of these may be absent in a well-marked
case.   Austin Flint regards it as due to a brain lesion, others
hold that it is often caused by atheroma of the cerebral vessels.
Certainly disease of some part of the nervous system, such as

---

[1] *Med.-Chir. Tr.*, 1841, xxiv. 76.
[2] *Lancet*, 1897, ii. 523.   [3] *Ibid.*, 1891, i. 1247.

an injury to the medulla or cord, is often the only lesion we can discover, and it has been said with some probability that the effect is produced by "an accentuation of inhibitory action coming to the vagus by spinal accessory fibres from the medullary centre" (S. Taylor, *loc. cit.*), since it has been shown that permanent slowing is never caused by the vagus alone.

Temporary bradycardia may also be physiological as in parturition, or it may follow after fevers, in various blood states, or from poisoning. Thus Lewin records a rate of 12 in plumbism. In shock or great pain, and in the last stage of organic heart disease, it is also seen, though how caused is doubtful.

Finally, we may have a paroxysmal form as in this case, with some analogies to paroxysmal tachycardia. Generally, however, there is a permanently infrequent pulse, becoming at times extremely slow, as in Holberton's case. It is very rare to find, as in our patient, a rate of 60, 70, or 80, falling in a short time to 20 or 12, and rising as suddenly. Hodgson's[1] showed an average rate of 29, falling at times to 6, with an occasional gap of thirty seconds, ending in convulsions. This appears to have gone on for six months, after which he recovered and remained fairly well for years. Kinnicutt[2] mentions another with a rate of 30 or 40, falling to 13 and 7; Jacobi one of 12, dropping to 7. R. T. Bruce[3] reported one recently where the pulse was about 20, but for two days before death attacks came on with an interval of forty seconds between the heart-beats followed by convulsions. The breathing showed similar intervals, which curiously resembles Col. Townshend's condition. Adams's celebrated case must be included here.[4] For seven years the rate was usually 30, but a further fall would occur, followed by convulsive seizures, from time to time. There were atheromatous and fatty changes present, but their importance is uncertain.

It is possible that all cases of the Stokes-Adams pheno-

[1] *Brit. M. J.*, 1891, i. 760.
[2] *Tr. Ass. Am. Physicians*, 1889, iv.   [3] *Scottish M. & S. J.*, 1898, ii. 330.
[4] *Dublin Hosp. Rep.*, 1827, iv. 353.

menon have this temporary fall of rate, but many reports omit the pulse - rate before and after the seizures. I find only the permanent rate given by Stokes himself,[1] so that it is impossible to say whether his instances were paroxysmal or not.

The phenomena in question may vary from simple vertigo or syncope to strong convulsions and prolonged unconscious-ness. True epilepsy is occasionally followed by a very slow pulse; but these convulsions are caused by the slowing through the cerebral anæmia induced by it. One of Stokes's patients could stop them by going on his hands and knees and hanging down his head — the Indian fashion of stopping a fainting attack.

Another point is the long duration of these cases. Mr. Fendick noted pulse-changes for two years and vertigo for ten, and I have given other instances of even longer periods above. Hodgson's patient was alive four years after the attacks, and seems to have recovered from them entirely, though the pulse remained at about 32. The combination of Cheyne-Stokes breathing with paroxysmal bradycardia has been referred to both in our own history and in Bruce's, while Seymour Taylor mentions an instance where the same rhythm was seen in the pulse as in the breathing, and passed away when that improved. Stokes supplies no data as to the pulse in the case which has given the name to the affection, though it appears in his paper on slow pulses. As the com-bination is so rare, I cannot think that any strong argument can be based on it in favour of the cause of paroxysmal brady-cardia lying in the central nervous system, though on the whole the evidence seems to point in that direction. Grasset and others [2] assert that the Stokes-Adams phenomenon may be due to changes in the cerebral vessels alone. Cardiac disease probably plays a part in some cases. Thus the fibroid infiltrations in our case are curiously like those detailed by Ogle [3] in four instances of bradycardia, one of which

---

[1] *Dublin Q. J. M. Sc.*, 1846, ii. 73.

[2] Clifford Allbutt's *System of Medicine*, 1899, vol. vi., p. 341.

[3] *Lancet*, 1897, i. 296.

suffered from convulsions.   Masses of fibroid infiltration were found in the septum and bases of the ventricles; but there is, after all, no proof that the intra-cardiac ganglia were weakened by them, and that unusual effect was thus given to the inhibitory impulses of the vagus.   Such changes are, I think, found in many cases where the pulse is unaltered.

A CASE OF DISLOCATION OF THE HAND AND CARPUS BACKWARDS.

BY

Trafford Mitchell, M.D. Glasg.

On 23rd August I was called to see M. J., a boy aged 13 years. Whilst crossing an earthen embankment five feet high on his way to fetch water, his foot had caught in a wire on the top of the embankment, and he had fallen to the ground with his right hand under him, the back of the hand being downwards. When he got up again he found himself unable to catch hold of the tin vessel he had been carrying. He then returned home, and fainted on account of the pain. I found both bones of the right forearm perfectly sound, of normal shape, and free from crepitus; but on the dorsal aspect I found an abrupt projection, which, I soon discovered, was due to the carpus overlapping the lower end of the radius, whilst the lower part of the latter bone projected on the palmar aspect. There was shortening of the limb below the elbow. By traction on the hand and gentle pressure on the carpus, all deformity disappeared, and the pain immediately ceased. There were a few abrasions on the back of the hand, and a little discolouration was subsequently visible in the neighbourhood of the wrist. The treatment employed consisted only of the application of a little liniment and a narrow flannel bandage, splints being found unnecessary. The wrist is now as strong as ever, and free from deformity.

Progress of the Medical Sciences.

MEDICINE.

In continuation of our former report (pp. 36-41) on the *rôle* of milk in the production of tuberculosis, a paper by Dr. Leonard G. Guthrie[1] is of interest.   The following is a synopsis of his

[1] *Lancet*, 1899, i. 286.

conclusions :—1. Thoracic tuberculosis in children is more common than abdominal in the proportion of three to two. 2. Tabes mesenterica, as a cause of death in young children, is practically unknown. 3. The preponderance of thoracic over abdominal tuberculosis is not necessarily and solely due to the direct entry of bacilli into the air passages. In addition to this mode of infection, the lungs may be affected—(a) by bacilli entering the thoracic glands through the lymphatics of the pharynx, tonsils, and œsophagus above, and through the lymphatics of the intestines and the abdominal glands below ; and (b) by the entry of bacilli through the thoracic ducts into the pulmonary circulation viâ the right heart. 4. Primary infection through the alimentary tract does not prove that food has been the sole source of evil ; therefore tuberculosis in children is not likely to be materially checked by purification of the milk-supply alone. 5. The alleged increase of tuberculous meningitis of late years is probably due to pulmonary tuberculosis set up by severe epidemics of measles. Sims Woodhead [1] reports a large number of experiments in which it had been shown that milk had set up tuberculosis of the tonsils. It had been known for a very long time that pigs fed on tuberculous milk invariably developed a swelling under the jaw, but it was some time before attention had been drawn to the fact that apparently the invasion of the tubercle bacillus was through the tonsils. This mode of invasion had, perhaps, more to do with pulmonary tuberculosis than was sometimes imagined.

A year ago we directed attention to Gardiner's researches [2] on the **immunity from phthisis at high altitudes**, and from a perusal of such books as that of Solly [3] and of Weber, [4] we were almost led to the belief that high altitude is the one thing needful for the cure of tubercular diseases of the lungs ; but now all this is changed. *The Practitioner's* new crusade (June, 1898) has been taken up so vigorously that now **sanatorium treatment** is everything, and altitude is nothing. Allusion was made to this matter recently, [5] but I make no excuse for again recurring to the topic, in which at present the whole world is keenly interested.

A publication of the views of a non-medical Nordrach patient, in the *Nineteenth Century*, [6] has been followed by a reply from Dr. Sinclair Coghill, [7] and again by a rejoinder from Mr. James Arthur Gibson. [8] These have been widely read, and all the world now inclines to the belief that medicinal treatment and climatic treatment are nothing in comparison with the methods associated with what is known as sanatorium treatment. These have been summarised in an excellent monograph, [9] and

[1] *Brit. M. J.*, 1899, i. 1038. [2] *Bristol M.-Chir. J.*, 1898, xvi. 127.
[3] *Medical Climatology*, 1897. (See p. 145 of this number.)
[4] *The Mineral Waters and Health Resorts of Europe*, 1898. (See p. 146 of this number.) [5] *Bristol M.-Chir. J.*, 1898, xvi. 235.
[6] 1899, xlv. 92. [7] *Ibid.*, 304. [8] *Ibid.*, 389.
[9] *Sanatoria for Consumptives*. By F. R. Walters. 1899.

here we find an account of some forty or more sanatoria, in various parts of the world, in which more or less successful results have been obtained at various altitudes, and some of them at comparatively low levels.

The essential and one common factor of treatment in all these results is the **open-air treatment,** and this has been well described by Dr. Burton-Fanning.[1] He admits that there is nothing new in the idea that a large percentage of phthisis cases should be curable, nor is there anything new in the vaunting of an open-air life for consumptives; but he adds, "We have failed in our management of phthisical cases through lack of insistance and perseverance." It is claimed that the elevation of the method into a complete system has become needful, and that the essential feature of the "cure" is the perpetual existence of the patient in the open air. "The whole *raison d'être* of these establishments is the practice of this particular cure, and not only do patients go prepared to submit themselves to it, but the whole spirit of the place and its equipment make the adoption of the routine an easy matter. The same broad principles govern the treatment at all these Continental sanatoria for consumption. . . . The *rationale* of this treatment lies in the removal of the patient from those conditions which favour the activity of the tubercle bacillus, while at the same time his constitutional resisting powers are sought to be increased in every conceivable way, to the end that he may successfully repel the attacks of his destroyer. . . . Seeing that the greater number of sufferers from consumption cannot avail themselves of the treatment which is offered abroad, and that in the case of those more fortunately situated banishment to a foreign land often involves many unnecessary hardships, the necessity for establishing sanatoria at home is manifest."

A writer in the *Medical Magazine* (April, 1899), on the *régime* of the Victoria Hospital for Consumption, Edinburgh, remarks: "The usual type of a tuberculous case is quite modified by open-air treatment. In an uncomplicated case the temperature remains subnormal. Night sweating is absent, cough is absent, dyspepsia is absent. Dr. Philip explains the usual cause of cough to be **irritation from vitiated air.** The same cause is to be assigned to the night sweating, CO_2 stimulating the sweating centre. It seems a very rational treatment to avoid the presence of the CO_2 in the air by plenty of fresh air in the room, rather than to be obliged to give a respiratory stimulant such as the usual picrotoxine, to get rid of the CO_2 in the body. Instead of having *dyspepsia*, patients begin to lay on weight rapidly. One patient had been in but three days who had already gained $1\frac{1}{2}$ lb. In connection with weight, two types of patient were shown—the thin patient who put on flesh rapidly, and the fat, flabby patient who did not gain weight, but whose muscles

[1] *The Year-Book of Treatment,* 1899, p. 55.

began to feel firmer to the touch.   The gaining weight was
the good symptom in the former, the firming up the good
symptom in the latter."

Dr. Pott describes the usual routine as follows[1] :—A
patient comes for treatment. He has come shivering from
his fireside, where he has been treated like an exotic, subject
to chills and draughts, and breathing bad air. The first thing
to do is to acclimatise him to live in a room in which there is a
brisk fire, but in which the windows are gradually opened wider
and wider, until at length he is accustomed to them being wide
open all day. Having arrived at this stage, a fine day is
chosen, and the patient, warmly wrapped up, is taken out into
the balcony, and lies on a couch in a horizontal position,
sheltered from the wind and rain, and basking in the sunshine.
He is kept warm, plentifully fed with stimulating food, and
provided with light occupation and congenial society. At first
the period in the open-air is short, but it is lengthened until the
patient is quite accustomed to spending the whole day in that
way. The bedrooms are light, roomy, and well ventilated, and
numerous well-thought-of ideas for the thorough continuance
of the treatment and care of the patient are carried out under
constant supervision. Breakfast is taken with open windows,
and there are no special restraints or fussy rules to vex the
residents. Caps and overcoats are worn indoors if required,
and in fact, to use Dr. Pott's own words, "The regulated daily
life of each patient is ordered with a view to getting well and
learning to keep well." "The objects of the treatment are to
combat the wasting and fever of the malady by the use of an
excess of pure air, hygiene, a suitable and very full diet,
regulated exercise, and rest."

It is admitted by Dr. Walters that "those who try to live
in the open air in a climate like our own will meet with many
difficulties, owing to the absence of special shelters and contrivances for warding off rain and wind while admitting fresh
air." The credit of showing how this may be accomplished
belongs mainly to Brehmer, Dettweiler, and their followers, and
the essence of their methods is the elimination of haphazard
treatment and the prescription of absolute repose or of various
degrees of exercise, according to definite medical indications.
" Patients who are febrile muts be kept at rest ; if persistently
febrile or with high temperatures at night, absolute rest in
bed is needed, windows being kept open, or the bed wheeled
on to the balcony according to weather and season and other
indications." [2]

In spite of all the difficulties in carrying out open-air
treatment in this country, Gibson says,[3] "As to a site for
the sanatorium. Go to the highlands of Scotland, the low-
lands of England, or to the bogs of Ireland, and plant your

---

[1] *Guardian*, January 21, 1899.
[2] Walters, *op. cit.*, p. 38.   [3] *Loc. cit.*, p. 400.

sanatoria there—it is of little consequence where. I see many doctors, leaders of public thought on matters of health, still coquetting with climate.' *Climate has nothing to do with the matter.* All that is *absolutely* necessary is (1) a spot in the country where *pure* air is to be had, (2) well away from smoke, dust, traffic, and excitement, where the patients may lead the quiet unconventional lives so necessary to their well-being; (3) the proper treatment, and (4) (but most important) the man to honestly carry it out. *These four things are indispensable,* nothing else is. . . . When it has been proved beyond doubt that consumption is quite as curable at home, on these lines, as it is abroad, it will be the duty of the State to undertake such measures as may be necessary for the cure, prevention, and final eradication of this disease." We fear that this time is yet far distant, and that the views of the enthusiast must as yet be accepted with some reservation. The diet in the sanatorium is one of the most essential elements of what Walther speaks of as the **proper treatment.** " *The movement in this country will succeed only in so far as it follows Nordrach lines,*" says Gibson. All writers are agreed as to the necessity of good food, and a special kind of feeding is adopted at the different sanatoria on the Continent. The weight is usually taken every week regularly, and " if the patient does his duty, gains of from one to four pounds should be made weekly."

The method of forced feeding—the Debove method—was in frequent use some fifteen years ago, but now we hear little of it. This method is advised by Wilcox,[1] more especially for cases of tuberculous laryngitis. Wilcox recommends the separation of the meals into those containing the bulk of the starchy food and meals containing the bulk of the proteids. As a rule, the object at the various sanatoria is to get the consumptive to eat the maximum amount of nutritious and fattening food that can be tolerated, but the end is gained in slightly different ways at different places. The ingestion of this large quantity of food is helped by force of precept and influence, but the great promoter of appetite is fresh air.[2]

The results of sanatorium treatment appear from the published statements to be eminently satisfactory. They have been summarised by Walters,[3] but it is very difficult to make any comparison between institutions so variously situated. "Generally speaking, one may say that from one-fourth to one-third of the patients treated in sanatoria are practically cured, or a still greater proportion if they are treated in an early stage. Probably systematic and prolonged treatment from an early stage would restore to health from one-half to two-thirds of our consumptive patients, even without the advantage of an Alpine or other high altitude station. Unfortunately, it is quite out of the question to expect patients to submit to more

[1] *Med. News,* 1898, lxxii.' 586.
[2] *Year-Book of Treatment,* 1899, p. 58.   [3] *Op. cit.,* p. 49.

than a few months' treatment in a sanatorium, so that we must trust to the educational influence of the sanatorium to complete the recovery of those treated in it. . . . The good results of treatment are permanent in a large proportion of cases."

Gibson claims for Nordrach that the type of cases taken comprising all stages and including many failures from other sanatoria, the percentage of cures amounts to 30, that of nearly cured 65, leaving a balance of only 5 per cent. not improved. . . . "Of the twenty-two cases that I have known who went out to Nordrach from this country within the last four years, twenty were cured of consumption, one died from another cause, and the remaining one might have been cured if an operation on the lungs had been consented to by the patient's friends. . . . I have erred, I think, on the safe side in saying that Walther cures 90 per cent. of his cases." [1] These are the words of a grateful enthusiast who has been cured of his disease, but it yet remains to be demonstrated whether results like this can be achieved under any conditions. in the climate of the British Islands.

In spite of the generally accepted view that the notification of phthisis is impracticable, a paper by Dr. Newsholme [2] points out that, so far as the patient is concerned, notification need imply, and ought to imply, nothing beyond sending him a precautionary circular, and that small difficulties of detail need not embarrass us. "If notification is desirable in the interests of the public health it should be adopted and a desirable principle is never impracticable." Hitherto the Local Government Board has not been convinced, and hence there is no need as yet to determine what limits to official action after notification are desirable.

R. SHINGLETON SMITH.

SURGERY.

The best method of dealing with the **pedicle** after the **removal of uterine fibroids** by cœliotomy is still undecided.

Mr. Bland Sutton, in a paper read before the Obstetrical Society of London,[3] on 28 cases of hysterectomy with intra-peritoneal treatment of the pedicle, strongly advocates that method. His results—only 2 deaths in 28 cases—are very good; but we must remember that he lays it down most distinctly that all fibroids should be removed just as all ovarian cysts ought to be, and therefore he is likely to have a series of less formidable tumours than those who only operate when the tumour is growing very large, or causes considerable distress or serious hemorrhage. His contention that his mortality in these cases is as low as after ovariotomy is hardly correct, for—as pointed out by one of the speakers in the debate on

[1] Loc. cit., p. 396.   [2] Lancet, 1899, i. 279.
[3] Tr. Obst. Soc. Lond., 1898, xxxix. 292.

his paper—7 per cent. for ovariotomy is rather high at the present time, and if operating in all cases gives a mortality of 7 per cent. it would probably be considerably higher with surgeons who only operate on very large tumours, or those causing pressure symptoms and hemorrhage, and it is only on such tumours that the majority of surgeons and gynæcologists operate.

Moreover, Mr. Meredith (one of the surgeons to the Samaritan Hospital), at the same meeting of the society, referred to [1] his own results with the extra-peritoneal method, and they give a lower mortality than Mr. Bland Sutton's. Mr. Meredith had a run of 30 cases treated by the extra-peritoneal method without a death, and two series of 40 and 47 cases respectively with but two deaths in each, and 83 recoveries out of a total of 90 cases—results which, he says, " have not as yet, so far as I know, been equalled by advocates of the intra-peritoneal method ; " and Mr. Meredith is not a surgeon who operates on uterine fibroids without special reason, and therefore would not have such simple cases to deal with as Mr. Bland Sutton. Mr. Knowsley Thornton (also surgeon to the Samaritan Hospital), in an article on hysterectomy,[2] says that, putting on one side cases in which large fibroid tumours burrow in the broad ligament or under the parietal peritoneum as a specially difficult and dangerous class of cases, in his practice cases treated by the serre-nœud had a mortality of only 8 per cent., as against 50 per cent. in cases treated by the intra-peritoneal method.

There is always a risk of injury to the ureter in the intra-peritoneal method ; and, if the uterine arteries are not efficiently secured, of hemorrhage also, and the ligation of the uterine arteries may not be an easy matter in cases in which the tumour burrows in the broad ligament, and in such cases the ureters would be in special danger. Although in the extra-peritoneal method a slough is produced by the wire of the serre-nœud, yet this slough is not offensive, but tends to dry up if properly treated, nor is there any risk of peritonitis from it, for if it is rightly placed with regard to the peritoneum the peritoneal cavity is safely shut off before suppuration begins around the constricted portion of the pedicle. There certainly is no evidence that peritonitis has ever been produced by dragging on the pedicle. Hemorrhage after the operation, from slipping of the wire, would be an accident due to its improper application. In the intra-peritoneal method there is always a possibility of infection of the peritoneum from the opened uterine cavity, and some surgeons have applied the cautery or strong antiseptic to the cervical canal to prevent this. For in writing of the intra-peritoneal method, I refer to that originally practised by Baer,[3] and now employed by Bland Sutton, in which

[1] *Tr. Obst. Soc. Lond.*, 1898, xxxix. 306.
[2] Clifford Allbutt and Playfair's *System of Gynæcology*, 1896.
[3] *N. York J. Gynæc. & Obst*, 1892, ii. 986.

the cervix is left without ligation, and the bleeding from its surface controlled by previous ligation of the uterine arteries. Complete removal of the uterus, with its greater risk of injury to the ureters, seems unnecessary. But the extra-peritoneal method necessitates a more tedious recovery than the intra-peritoneal method, and this is really the chief objection to it. On the other hand, to rapidly complete an operation for the removal of a very large tumour, or to avoid the risk of injury to the ureters in cases in which the tumour has opened up the broad ligaments near the cervix and thus left little room for ligation of the uterine arteries, the extra-peritoneal method has distinct advantages.

The publication of one case treated by either method is, of course, of little value as an argument for its general adoption; but to show that the results of the extra-peritoneal method are not so dreadful as some writers have represented, I will briefly refer to some details of one of my own cases.

The tumour reached across the abdomen from one anterior spine to the other, and extended two inches above the umbilicus. After removal it weighed five pounds. It was complicated with a small ovarian cyst. The body of the uterus was buried in the tumour, and I applied the serre-nœud two inches above the vaginal attachment. The operation was performed on July 18th, in the Hospital for Children and Women. She never had a bad symptom. By the 21st the constricted portion of the pedicle was getting quite hard and dry, not "hanging out from the abdominal wall with foul pus discharging from the stump," as the usual condition of the pedicle has been recently described.[1] The serre-nœud handle was removed on the 21st, and the wire and pins later. On September 4th she was discharged; the sinus had not healed, but it closed some time after.[2]

The more recently published results of **operations for the removal of malignant tumour** are of much value, especially with regard to the breast and the tongue, and they may be said to be distinctly encouraging; indeed we are now able to speak of long periods of non-recurrence after the removal of malignant tumour in certain parts, in a way never thought of some years ago. This is due to early and free removal.

The average duration of life in **cancer of the breast** not operated on is 2½ years from the time when it is first noticed. The risk of operation is very small. Watson Cheyne[3] has operated on 61 cases with a mortality of only 1.6 per cent., and Halsted on 50 with no death. All these operations were

[1] *Bristol M.-Chir. J.*, 1899, xvii. 9.

[2] Another case, also treated by the serre-nœud, is referred to in my remarks at the May meeting of the Bristol Medico-Chirurgical Society.

[3] *Brit. M. J.*, 1896, i. 390.

extensive ones, including removal of glands. They were, of course, all aseptic. With a very thorough removal of the disease together with the glands, whether palpable before operation or not, out of the 61 cases operated on by Watson Cheyne up to three years ago no less than half are cured.[1] Although the term "cure" as applied to these cases only means absence of recurrence for three years or longer, the further history of the eleven "cured" cases which Watson Cheyne reported in 1896 shows that in only one has there so far been any recurrence of the disease, and in that case it was probably a fresh development, as the patient is reported to have died of cancer of the intestine six years after the breast operation. Halsted (who is Professor of Surgery in the Johns Hopkins Hospital, Baltimore) has recently given us [2] the results of his operations for cancer of the breast up to April, 1898. He says that "of the 76 cases operated upon three or more years ago, 31 (41 per cent.) are living without local recurrence or signs of metastases." His method of operating is even more extensive than Watson Cheyne's, for he removes the greater part of the pectoralis major muscle in every case. Mr. Butlin has practised the method for the last few years, and has had a remarkably successful series of cases, for he had eight cures out of thirteen cases operated on.[3] He regards this as a very fortunate series, and says that he does not expect "that the next or many future series of thirteen cases will yield nearly such good results"; but it shows what operation can do for cancer of the breast, especially when we note that Butlin says that the cases were not obtained early for operation; "there is scarcely one in which the disease was not known to have existed several months, and there are many in which it had existed for one, two, three, or more years. There were many in which the axilla was full of cancerous glands, and several in which the primary tumour was ulcerated." Warren [4] has also had 17 cures in 72 operations, or about 25 per cent. I have not yet followed up the histories of all the patients I have operated on for cancer of the breast—and I have always operated in the thorough way that Watson Cheyne does,—but I know of a few cases free from disease more than three years from the operation. In one case, after three years from the operation, there has twice been very slight local recurrence in the neighbourhood of the scar. These recurrent growths have been removed.

The chance, then, of prolongation of life, and even cure of the disease, is so good, that we can unhesitatingly advise operation, which must be of the thorough or so-called "complete" kind which Watson Cheyne practises, and which he has described in his Lettsomian Lectures,[5] and has more recently referred to his paper in the *Lancet*.[6]

[1] *Lancet*, 1899, i. 756.   [2] *Tr. Am. Surg. Ass.*, 1898, xvi. 162.
[3] *St. Barth. Hosp. Rep.*, 1899, xxxiv. 49.
[4] *Boston M. & S. J.*, 1898, cxxxix. 186.   [5] *Loc. cit.*   [6] *Loc. cit.*

10

The only question which remains to be considered is, What are the **contra-indications to operation**? Watson Cheyne gives them as follows:[1] 1. Cases of cancer *en cuirasse*. 2. Cases where there is a large mass in the axilla involving the nerves. 3. Cases where large glands can be felt above the clavicle. 4. All cases where secondary cancers already exist elsewhere. He has removed a portion of the axillary vein several times when involved in gland growth, and once a portion of the artery and vein, without any harm resulting. I have myself also more than once removed portions of the axillary vein with the gland-growth without any harm resulting. Halsted[2] does not now consider enlargement of the supra-clavicular glands a contra-indication to operation, and he clears out the supra-clavicular region thoroughly in every case. He has records of two cases on which he operated for removal of supra-clavicular glands which appeared after the breast and axillary contents had been removed, in which there was no recurrence three and a half years after the supra-clavicular glands were excised. Halsted says: "In one of these latter cases I considered the prognosis desperately bad, at both the infra- and supra-clavicular operations. At the first operation the cancer had infiltrated the axillary fat diffusely, and could with difficulty be separated from the subclavian vein; at the second operation the same desperate state of affairs was encountered in the neck."

The results of operations for **cancer of the tongue** have been considered in recent papers by Watson Cheyne[3] and Butlin.[4] Watson Cheyne, from a study of the statistics of some Continental surgeons, comes to the conclusion that the mortality of excision of cancer of the tongue may be estimated at 15 to 20 per cent., but some surgeons have had a much lower death-rate in a certain series of cases. Thus Kocher had only one death in his last series of 28 cases, and Volkmann only two deaths in 91 cases. Kocher's cures amounted to 18 per cent., Koenig's to 12 per cent. Mr. Butlin's results are particularly encouraging. He has operated on 102 cases, with a mortality of 10 per cent., and 20 per cent. of cures. His private operations—or in other words his operations on cases at an earlier stage than the hospital ones—give the splendid result of only one death in 49 cases, and 13 cures. These operations are included in the 102 already given, and this result is an illustration of the desirability of operating for cancer at the earliest possible moment.

In cancer of the tongue we have a disease which proves fatal without operation in a year to eighteen months, and towards the end is a terribly painful and distressing disease. At a moderate risk—5 per cent. mortality in early cases limited to

[1] *Brit. M. J.*, 1896, i. 387.　　[2] *Loc. cit.*
[3] *Brit. M. J.*, 1896, i. 449.　　[4] *Ibid.*, 1898, i. 541.

the tongue, but with 15 to 20 per cent. mortality in extensive cases, in which the disease has extended to the floor of the mouth, palate and tonsils—the disease can be removed with a chance of cure in 20 per cent. of cases (and even more in earlier cases), a chance of prolongation of life by many months in almost 95 per cent. of early and 80 to 85 per cent. of extensive cases.

If recurrence takes place after operation, in many cases it is not in the mouth, where the disease is so distressing, but in the glands of the neck, and such recurrence in most cases admits of removal.

The lesson which a study of recent literature on the treatment of cancer of the tongue teaches most emphatically is, that at the very earliest moment the growth should be removed, and that weeks must not be lost in treating an ulcer of doubtful nature by iodide, when the diagnosis can be established in a few days by the microscopic examination of a portion of tissue snipped off the edge of the ulcer under cocaine.

C. A. MORTON.

OBSTETRICS AND GYNÆCOLOGY.

Post-partum hemorrhage is truly described as *the* obstetric emergency in which prompt and proper action on the part of the attendant is of vital importance to the patient, as the issue will be determined before assistance can be obtained or complicated measures carried out. The rules for treatment therefore should be as simple and widely understood as possible. Too much stress cannot be laid on prophylactic measures. The third stage of labour should be left to nature, but not to nature unwatched and unassisted, the fundus being carefully controlled by light manual pressure until and for some time after the third stage is completed. Unnecessary hurry in this stage is to be deprecated ; half an hour is quite an average time. Secondary uterine inertia from exhaustion by prolongation of the second stage and the withholding of nourishment should not be allowed to occur. If extractive manipulations are necessary, they should be conducted in a manner as much like the natural process as possible. In no case should the uterus be emptied between the pains, and the fundus should be followed down by the hand as the contents are expelled. Should inertia be dreaded, strychnia and ergotin, the latter in ½-grain doses thrice daily, should be administered during the last month.

Delee[1] gives some novel methods of treatment in cases where *post-partum* hemorrhage occurs in spite of all precautions : in the first place, if the third stage has not been completed, and this will usually be the case when the hemorrhage is partly or entirely caused by laceration, the placenta must be at once

[1] *J. Am. M. Ass.*, 1899, xxxii. 802.

expressed or removed by the hand; the uterus being empty, firm bimanual compression is employed, doubling the uterus on itself and closing the cervix. He also recommends compression of the aorta. He then suggests, supposing that by compression the uterus is under control, that it should be plugged with iodoform, sterilised, or borated gauze; in order to do this the anterior and posterior lips are seized with vulsella and the uterus drawn down to the outlet: this proceeding itself is a valuable remedial agent, since traction on the cervix straightens out the vessels in the broad ligament and by putting the tissues on the stretch compresses them: three to four yards of the packing, which should be a yard wide, are then introduced into the uterine cavity until it is filled tightly; if after this proceeding any oozing takes place, he stitches the lips of the cervix together so that the uterine cavity is completely closed. He states that he has found this proceeding of great value.

He mentions the use of the hot douche at 120°F. after it has been ascertained whether the hemorrhage is due to atony or to laceration. We would prefer to reverse the order: the hot douche will almost invariably either stop or cause a great diminution of hemorrhage from either or both of these causes, especially that due to atony; the action of the douche is much increased by the use of half an ounce of ordinary vinegar to the pint; should this not cause cessation, lacerations are probably present, and the uterus should be packed while the lacerations are sewn up. The packing may be left in for twenty-four or forty-eight hours; but if iodoform gauze is used, watch must be kept for the symptoms of iodoform poisoning—namely, headache and rise of temperature, which, if present, will disappear at once on removing the packing.

The suture of the lesion seems rather a refinement: the slight oozing which occurs after packing is often due to uterine contractions squeezing out serum and blood that has been already absorbed by the packing, and if the latter is done sufficiently tightly the hemorrhage will infallibly cease. This method is undoubtedly of the greatest value, and should be employed more frequently as an emergency measure: the hot douche is preferable, as it can be used without removing the supporting and compressing bands for more than a moment, and does not require assistants in addition to the nurse usually present; in any case manual compression and the hot douche will give time for further skilled assistance to be obtained, when the packing can be done.

The sense of security in the mind of the attendant when he has packed the uterus tightly is most gratifying; there need then be no anxiety about recurrence of the bleeding, a state of things which under other circumstances will keep him in a state of anxiety for several hours. In the obstetric department of the Bristol Royal Infirmary this method is looked upon as a routine measure to be adopted in all cases where artificial emptying of the uterus is resorted to if hemorrhage occurs after it, especially in cases of abortion and miscarriage after the use of the curette. Not only is hemorrhage prevented, but involution is more rapid owing to the securing of the complete evacuation which occurs when the gauze is removed.

The **uterus** is one of the commonest organs to be attacked by **malignant disease**; in fact, one-third of the total cases of cancer occurring in the female consist of those in which this organ is attacked.

The nature of the treatment to be adopted depends on several factors in each case, the most important of which is the stage at which the disease has arrived when the question of the treatment to be adopted first arises, since on this depends very largely its success or failure. As regards treatment, we may at once exclude all other than radical operative measures except in those cases in which the disease is so far advanced that obviously no radical measures will give more than temporary relief, owing to the impossibility of removing the whole of the affected tissue. As regards operative measures, the broad lines of procedure may be briefly laid down as follows: Radical operation should not be undertaken unless there is a reasonable hope that all affected tissue can be removed without causing damage to vitally important organs, or without subjecting the patient to an operation of such severity as to render her immediate recovery unlikely.

Another most important point for consideration is the **prospect of cure**, or the length of time which will elapse after recovery from the operation before recurrence takes place. This practically depends on several conditions: firstly, the possibility of complete operative removal; secondly, the method of performance of the operation; and thirdly, the nature and situation of the growth. As regards operative treatment of these cases considered generally, the prospect here is apparently quite as good if not better than that in cases where other organs are affected which can be subjected to radical treatment, *e.g.*, the breast, tongue, lip, penis, or rectum. Recurrence, after operations on the uterus, does not take place any sooner than, if as soon as, after operations on the above, which are considered the most favourable situations for operative treatment; the immediate mortality is if anything lower than after operations on the above - named other organs; therefore operation may be undertaken under favourable conditions quite as readily.

Even in those cases where after radical operation undertaken for uterine cancer early recurrence takes place, unless this occurs in the peritoneum, the fatal termination is attended with less suffering, while in the interval the patient may be restored to comparative health by the removal of the sloughing mass, which causes a severe form of septic absorption, with its attendant wasting anæmia and pains.

Halliday Croom,[1] in a paper on **vaginal hysterectomy**, gives a very unfavourable account of his own results from this operation. He is so impressed with the rapidity of recurrence and the great pain suffered by those who die after this operation with secondary peritoneal infection, that he goes so far as to state that although in certain favourable cases recurrence may not occur, or only occur after some years, yet as a general rule recurrence occurs early, and if in the peritoneum the patient's exitus is much more painful than if the growth had not been attacked. It appears to me, however, that it is impossible to say how any given case will terminate; and while it is quite true that in certain cases the rate of progress of the growth is slow, and that the patient may live many months in a greater or less degree of discomfort, at the same time we cannot prophecy as to whether secondary infection of the peritoneum will not take place even if the growth is left alone, and while the fatal result is ultimately certain if the latter plan is adopted, it is equally certain that in cases subjected to radical treatment a certain number will live perhaps for several years in comparative health and comfort. Croom states that of the cases operated on by him, fourteen in number, all were dead within the year—a truly sombre picture, and gives a most gloomy view of the results of surgical intervention in these cases; he quotes the following results from the practice of others, thus: from the statistics of the Dresden Klinik forty-five cases out of eighty were free from recurrence two years after operation; thirty-four out of fifty-eight were without recurrence three years after; twenty-five out of forty-two, four years after; eighteen out of thirty, five years after; six out of nine, six years after; two cases who had survived seven years were quite well; while in Leopold's practice we are informed that seventy-two out of seventy-six of his cases were well and without recurrence from one to five years after operation.

It would appear that Croom takes too gloomy a view of the case, and that it is not justifiable to augur, as he does, that the operative treatment of cancer of the uterus is to be condemned because in a limited number of cases such as his the result as regards recurrence has not been good.

At the eleventh annual meeting of the Southern Surgical and Gynecological Association, held at Memphis, U.S.A., McMurtry[2] read a paper on the same subject, which has a striking similarity to that of Halliday Croom, and described five cases on which he had operated by vaginal hysterectomy during the past year, two of which had recurrence within five months, one in the bladder and one in the vagina; all five appeared to be typically suitable cases for the operation. He

[1] *Edinb. M. J.*, 1898, N.S. iv. 489.   [2] *Am. J. Obst.*, 1899, xxxix. 217.

considered it doubtful whether one of the three remaining would be alive three years after operation. He advocated as a preferable measure the removal of the uterus by abdominal section, with a liberal removal of adjacent structures, especially the vaginal wall; he did not, however, advocate removal of the sub-peritoneal glands, as their enlargement was often due to inflammation.

In the subsequent discussion, which brought out strongly the opinion that the negro race is not so little susceptible to cancer as is generally supposed, Howard Kelly expressed surprise at the author's conclusions, and stated that his experience —a by no means small one—led him to quite an opposite opinion, many of his cases of vaginal hysterectomy for cancer having completely recovered and remained well for several years.

Against the gloomy views taken by McMurtry and Croom we may place the opinions and records of F. B. Jessett,[1] who publishes one hundred and seven cases distributed over seven years. We gather from his statements that nine died as the immediate result of operation. He prefaces a very interesting table with some instructive remarks on diagnosis and pathology; he lays great stress on the necessity for the vaginal examination of women who suffer from irregular hemorrhages apart from parturition and pregnancy, and especially of those who so suffer when past the climacteric, or who have any watery or fœtid discharge in addition to the hemorrhage: while this necessity is not recognised, a very large number of cases must go untreated until surgical intervention is useless except as a palliative. He regards malignant disease in its inception as being purely local, and considers that until cellular tissue is invaded the lymphatics are unaffected. As previously stated, nine operations had a fatal termination, not a large number considering the gravity of the operation, and this includes complicated cases. He considers that operation should be limited to those cases in which the mobility of the uterus is not impaired and the broad ligaments not invaded. He does not consider that invasion of the vaginal wall is an absolute contra-indication, nor that it is necessary that the cervix should be able to be drawn down to the outlet, a condition considered essential by some operators. He considers that affection of the iliac glands occurs late in the disease. As regards technique, he is of opinion that the union of the vesical and rectal peritoneal edges by suture is very important, and prefers to use the ligature for securing the uterine and ovarian vessels. He gives the following as the **indications for advising operation**: coloured and offensive discharge occurring in a patient at or past the menopause, and the passing of the sound causing bleeding; if after vaginal examination no growth is felt, dilatation of the cervix, exploration of the uterine cavity, curetting and careful microscopical examination of removed structures; if malignant growth is felt on

[1] *Brit. Gynæc. J.*, 1899, xiv. 541.

vaginal examination, or if the portions removed show malignant tissue under the microscope, he advises hysterectomy.

Of his 107 cases, nine died and recurrence took place in fifty-one, which number includes those lost sight of; forty-seven remained free from recurrence for periods varying from two years in the case of the last series to seven years in the case of the first; his figures as regards recurrence show a striking similarity to those of the Dresden Klinik mentioned above, the percentages being nearly the same. This seems to be, to a certain extent, an answer to Croom's statement, that cancer of the uterus in England and Germany must be two different things.

In the same way that the operation for removal of cancer of the breast has been extended so as to include the clearing of the axilla and removal of the subclavicular glands and tissue, with a marked improvement as regards delaying recurrence, operators are now seeking to apply the same principles to the uterus. To this end Freund's operation is being increasingly performed, with the additional procedure of removing a large part of the pelvic peritoneum together with the glands in the pelvis and the whole of the broad ligaments.

Ries [1] reports fifteen cases treated by the Ries-Clark operation, with three deaths. The technique of the operation, which is essentially a panhysterectomy by the combined method, is as follows:—The patient is prepared by a preliminary curetting and cauterisation under anæsthesia, while at the same time the whole pelvis is carefully explored for infected glands. If the growth is within the cervix, the cervical lips are sewn together to prevent contamination; if without, a vaginal cuff is raised and sewn over the cervix. Fresh assistants, instruments, sponges, etc., are provided for the next steps. The patient is placed in steep Trendelenburg position, incision from pubes to umbilicus, and the pelvis palpated carefully to exclude enlarged and immovable glands; these being found absent, the infundibulo-pelvic ligament is ligatured and cut close to the pelvic wall. The peritoneum is then incised along the common iliac artery, and the vessels exposed by dissection until the ureter is reached; the ureter is then exposed in the whole of its length in the pelvis —i.e. from the brim to the base of the bladder. Bleeding points are clamped as cut, or ligatured. When the uterine artery comes into view it is ligatured close to its origin, but outside the ureter and by sight; then the whole of the cellular tissue and glands lying between the external iliac artery superiorly, the pelvic wall laterally, the base of the bladder anteriorly, the pelvic floor inferiorly, and the meso-rectum posteriorly, is removed; the last lifted up and freed from all accessible glands. This procedure, begun on the left side, is repeated on the right. Adhesions between uterus and rectum are now divided if present. The round ligaments are secured, and the peritoneum of

[1] *Am. Gynæc. & Obst. J.*, 1898, xiii. 570.

Douglas's pouch incised close to rectum, and the vagina opened; the anterior space being already accessible as far as the peritoneum, the uterus is now free all around and is removed. The pelvis is now closed in by suturing the anterior edge of the peritoneum, which extends from the lateral wall across the vesico-uterine pouch, to the posterior which extends from the lateral wall across the pouch of Douglas; the abdomen is then closed in the ordinary way.

Werder[1] has devised a somewhat similar procedure, with this difference, that instead of by a prolonged dissection removing cellular tissue and glands, although he mentions this as an advantageous procedure, he removes the whole of the upper part of the vagina. He commences in the same way as Ries, but without freeing the peritoneum from the lateral walls of the pelvis, the anterior and posterior cul-de-sacs being opened and the lateral fornices separated from them. Recurrence is known to have taken place in forty-six cases; in twenty-four cases the average time before recurrence was nine months, and the average time before death sixteen months.

The result of an examination of the foregoing appears to be—(1) That the immediate mortality of all cases from the operation may be taken roughly as less than 10 per cent. if vaginal hysterectomy is chosen, but may be expected to be more if the more extensive operations of Ries, Clark, and Werder be undertaken; but if only the most favourable cases be selected, the mortality will not be higher than 7 to 8 per cent. (2) That a restoration to health of a certain duration may be expected in all cases; this may extend from six months to possibly permanent cure. (3) That recurrence will take place in less than two years in more than half the cases subjected to vaginal hysterectomy, and in the greater part of the remainder within five years. (4) That possibly 10 per cent. of cases will survive at the end of six years.

As regards the operations of Ries, Clark, and Werder, further experience is required. The principle seems surgically sound, but we must not expect very striking alterations in the recurrence-rate in view of the large number of cases in which this occurs in the scar, or peritoneum; its benefit is only likely to be gained by lessening the number of cases in which recurrence takes place in the glands, or by extension through and from cellular tissues already partly infected.

Finally, the possibility of this disease being present should never be lost sight of by the practitioner in any case where irregular hemorrhages, apart from the puerperal state, ovarian or fibroid tumours, are present, especially after the menopause, and all women should be kept informed of the importance of early diagnosis and the necessity for physical examination when suspicious symptoms are present. Out of the last fifty cases seen by me, only five were fit for radical operation; in two

[1] *Am. J. Obst.*, 1898, xxxvii. 289.

others an operation was possible, but not likely to give rise
to other than the most temporary benefit.   This seems to show
an appalling state of ignorance, not on the part of the profession, since in all cases the disease had been already recognised, but on the part of the patients, on whom definite and
distinct symptoms had not appeared to impress the necessity
for seeking advice.   WALTER C. SWAYNE.

Reviews of Books.

Lippincott's Medical Dictionary. Prepared by RYLAND W.
   GREENE, with the collaboration of JOHN ASHHURST, Jr.,
   M.D., GEORGE A. PIERSOL, M.D., and JOSEPH P.
   REMINGTON. Pp. xii., 1154. London: J. B. Lippincott
   Company. 1897.

There seems to be no end to the enterprise of publishers of
medical works, for they publish enormous dictionaries which, we
fear, can never give an adequate return for the trouble and
expense incurred.   The one before us is one of the most complete we have seen, and must have involved a great amount of
labour in its compilation.   We can strongly recommend it to
all in need of a good medical dictionary.   It is especially strong
in the departments of chemistry and materia medica, in this
respect excelling most of those with which we are familiar.

English Sanitary Institutions.   By Sir JOHN SIMON, K.C.B.
   Second Edition.   Pp. xix., 516.   London: Smith, Elder,
   & Co. 1897.

We gladly renew acquaintance in this second edition of Sir
John Simon's *English Sanitary Institutions* with this fascinating
and instructive history of human sanitary endeavour.   The
successful writer on matters of universal history must be a man
of wide knowledge and of broad mind, able to sift and choose,
to prune and criticise, and to weave the disconnected threads of
record and tradition into one continuous whole. Sir John Simon
has the necessary qualities for the work, and it is fitting that
from the pen of so delightful a writer such a volume should
appear after a long life of usefulness, happily not yet completed.
   The introduction takes us back to "that nebula of times
which human records do not pretend to reach," and presupposes
that at a very early period when communities began to exist,
a desire must have originated "to amend, in the circumstances common to them, the conditions which they found
dangerous to their lives."   Hence through succeeding phases of

civilisation, from the evidence found amid the ruins of Nineveh, from the records relating to Greece, and through the more pretentious evidences such as the aqueducts and cloacæ of Rome, and the establishment in Rome of a public medical service for the poor, we pass through the darker centuries, the crusades, and the spread of leprosy, and the widespread and disastrous epidemics of the Middle Ages. The efforts of medieval philanthropy to relieve emergencies of distress threatening the poor are duly recognised, and the early and tentative efforts to cope with disease are in turn pointed out. Then it is shown that through the Tudor and Stuart reigns the changes developing later into the beginnings of modern medicine had been tending to define themselves in embryo; and medical science, previously "exercised from the widely different standpoints of the ecclesiastic, the barber, and the grocer," was able to "come into self-conscious existence."

In "New Momenta" we trace the beginnings of modern medicine, accompanying and following the revival of learning in Europe, starting from the fifteenth century, at first vaguely, more definite· in the sixteenth century when alchemy made progress in experiments and Vesalius achieved his daring dissections; through the more eventful quickening of the art of medicine in the seventeenth century, signalised in its earlier half by Harvey's discovery of the circulation of the blood, and later by Sydenham's careful and exact observations; leading to the far higher position of the practice of medicine in the eighteenth century, and its still more illustrious development in the present. Briefly, but with due appreciation, are sketched the work of Mead, whose *Short Discourse concerning Pestilential Contagion* gave advice wonderfully in advance of his age, and might even now repay study; Pringle and Lind's work on the Diseases of the Soldier and Sailor; Gilbert Blane's work in banishing scurvy from the navy; George Baker's work on the Cider Colic in Devonshire; and Jenner's imperishable triumph, whose "services to mankind, in respect of the saving of life, have been such that no other man in the history of the world has ever been within measurable distance of him."

And so we pass in chapters of unabated charm through the history of "The Growth of Humanity in British Politics," wherein John Howard's memorable work on *Gaols* is not forgotten; touch on the early experiences of Asiatic cholera in Europe, and reach the commencement of the present reign. Here Sir John Simon is thoroughly at home. Stimulating as it was to trace with him the inception, early beginnings, and gradual growth of preventive medicine, it is still more deeply interesting and instructive to follow under the guidance of his master-hand, and with the sidelight of his ripe experience, the actual growth of the great revival in the care of health which commenced with the reign of Queen Victoria and has progressed steadily, with occasional relapses, but in the main ever making for improvement and for progress. The volume must be read and studied to fully appreciate all the author's conclusions; but it may be stated that, in his belief, "the educational onward impulse" towards development of our sanitary institutions and their administration must come, as it has largely come in the past, from the medical profession. He looks forward with hopefulness, gladdened by "the immense development of altruism," by the "kindliness of man to man," and sees the human race "more and more, as the cycles are trodden," rising "to the religion of mutual helpfulness."

Sir Benjamin Collins Brodie. By TIMOTHY HOLMES. Pp. 256. London: T. Fisher Unwin. 1898.

Mr. Holmes has produced one of the most interesting books yet issued in the "Masters of Medicine" series. It does not perhaps quite equal in interest the *Life of John Hunter*, but it does not fall far short of it. Mr. Holmes thinks that Brodie is to be placed next to Hunter among the celebrated surgeons of the past, and his well-known books, *Diseases of the Urinary Organs* and *Diseases of the Joints* are sufficient to justify this estimate of his work.

We cannot attempt in this short review to give even a brief outline of the events which make this volume so well worthy of perusal. Brodie's character as a man deserves very careful study; and the insight which the book gives us into the condition of the profession and the state of society at the time when he lived is by no means its least instructive part.

Brodie had many interests outside his profession, and his views on various questions of psychology are given by Mr. Holmes. Perhaps the keynote of Brodie's life and work may be found in his statement that "there is no greater happiness in life than that of surmounting difficulties; and nothing will conduce more than this to improve your intellectual faculties, or to make you satisfied with the situation which you have attained in life, whatever it may be." The book will therefore interest the general reader.

The frontispiece is a very beautiful reproduction of a photograph of the portrait of Brodie, painted by Watts in 1860. The photograph was taken by his grandson, the present Sir Benjamin Brodie, to whom the reader is also indebted for much of the information relating to the home-life of the distinguished surgeon.

Justus von Liebig: his Life and Work (1803–1873). By W. A. SHENSTONE. Pp. 219. London: Cassell and Company, Limited. 1895.

Mr. Shenstone deals in popular style with the life-work of one who made no less important contributions to science as a means of education than to the advancement of his special province—chemistry. Liebig's name will be associated in most minds with the relations of the chemical composition of the soil to the growth of plants; but his establishment of a teaching laboratory, and the dissemination of the results of the researches of master and pupils, have probably had an even more important influence on modern scientific progress.

This biography, which is issued in "The Century Science Series," will be read with the greatest interest by all who are concerned with the foundations of our present knowledge of chemistry in its relation to life, and Mr. Shenstone is to be congratulated on the success with which he has depicted the main scenes in a memorable career.

On Certain Problems of Vertebrate Embryology. By JOHN BEARD, D.Sc. Pp. vii., 77. Jena: Gustav Fischer. 1896.
The Span of Gestation and the Cause of Birth. By JOHN BEARD, D.Sc. Pp. ix., 132. Jena: Gustav Fischer. 1897.

The author, in these two essays, puts forward a theory to explain certain phenomena which occur in the process of development of vertebrates. The theory is, that there is a hidden alternation of generations—an asexual larval form, succeeded by a sexual one. To the first belong such structures as a yolk-sac, transient nervous system and notochord, which in all vertebrate groups are found to disappear together and at a period when the embryo is just beginning to assume the body form characteristic of the adult. He calls this time the " critical period," and the interval from fertilisation of the ovum to this a " critical unit."

Monotremes alone of mammals have a well-filled yolk-sac, which is empty in all higher mammals. The cause of this disappearance of the yolk is probably to be found in the development of mammæ so that the young can be born in an early stage, the "critical" one, *i.e.* as soon as they are able to suck. This actually occurs in marsupials, and in such forms no allantoic placenta is ever formed. Most mammals, however, have a longer gestation-period, which becomes possible owing to the development of an allantoic placenta, and in such forms the gestation period is found to be a multiple of the "critical unit;" *e.g.* in the rabbit it is two, in the cow five, and in man six. The development of allantoic placenta renders the development of a marsupial pouch unnecessary.

In the case of some mammals, *e.g.* rabbit, the adult female is always with young, parturition is followed immediately by fertilisation; ovulation succeeds immediately on parturition. In other mammals, *e.g.* pig, lactation abolishes ovulation during its continuance.

The menstrual flow is not equivalent to the period of heat in lower animals, does not correspond with ovulation ; but is to be regarded as the shedding and abortion of a decidua prepared for an egg given off at the close of the preceding menstruation, but which was not fertilised. The ovulation-cycle is equal in length to the menstrual cycle; but the time of ovulation does not correspond with that of the catamenial flow.

The length of the " critical unit " in man is found to be from 45—47 days, *i.e.* twice the ovulation period. Abortions are particularly liable to occur at the end of the first " critical unit," which, according to the theory, represents an important change in the life-history of the individual, that in which the alternation of generations takes place, and at which the allantoic placenta is first formed, nourishment previously to this being obtained through the ecto-placenta derived from the yolk-sac.

The cause of birth is to be sought in a coming ovulation, *i.e.* is due reflexly to the ovary, and the formation of a corpus luteum is to be regarded as a means whereby ovulation is prevented during gestation.

The theory, of which the above is the slightest possible sketch, thus furnishes a clue to many normal and abnormal phenomena of the development of the embryo, and to the various periods at which they do or may occur. Whether it will be substantiated by future research remains to be seen.

Atlas of Methods of Clinical Investigation, with an Epitome of Clinical Diagnosis and of Special Pathology and Treatment of Internal Diseases. By Dr. CHRISTFRIED JAKOB. Edited by AUGUSTUS A. ESHNER, M.D. London : The Rebman Publishing Co. (Ltd.). 1898.

The earlier part of this book consists of 68 coloured plates, containing 182 illustrations, dealing respectively with clinical microscopy, chemical colour-reactions, the normal projection of the viscera upon the surface of the body, and their topography as determined by percussion, together with diagrammatic representations of diseases of the chest and abdomen. The plates are accompanied by descriptive letter-press, the object being to represent in a graphic manner the results of the clinical investigation of diseases by all the above methods. The number of the plates is so large that the microscopy of the blood, urine, sputum, gastric and intestinal contents is fully illustrated ; and they are uniformly good, so that, besides being useful to the practitioner for reference, they will doubtless greatly aid the student. The representations of the colour-reactions of the various chemical tests in clinical use will also be helpful. The diagrammatic pictures of abdominal and thoracic affections are taken from typical cases, of which a short abstract faces each plate.

The next portion of the book describes the method to be followed for the complete examination of a patient, and is followed by a detailed account of the clinical investigation of the systems of the body; of the blood and secretions, and of the chief bacteriological methods of use for direct clinical purposes, together with a short description of the normal state of each system and the chief pathological deviations from it.

Lastly, there is an epitome of special pathology and treatment. This is not so satisfactory as the rest of the book, as it attempts the impossible task of describing satisfactorily in brief abstract the symptoms and signs of disease. This is, however, a small part of the book, which for the rest is excellent, and we can recommend it as a very useful clinical manual of convenient size, and remarkable for the abundance and practical usefulness and beauty of its illustrations.

Psilosis or "Sprue." By George Thin, M.D. Second Edition. Pp. xii., 270. London: J. & A. Churchill. 1897.

Dr. Thin in this book gives a full account of this disease, for the differentiation of which from other forms of tropical diarrhœa and chronic dysentery we have mainly to thank his clinical acumen. His observations seem to establish the existence of psilosis as a distinct disease. The further question whether some varieties of so-called hill-diarrhœa and of diarrhœa alba met with in India are identical with psilosis is still uncertain, but now that the symptoms of psilosis have been differentiated this point should soon be decided. The exciting cause of the disease has still to be discovered. There is an interesting review of the literature, a chapter on the pathology of the disease, and a full description of the treatment—first advocated by the author,—which has been attended by successful results. A number of cases are reported in an Appendix. The book is written in a clear and interesting style, and gives the reader full information on the subject, which is of practical importance, as any medical man may be called upon to treat such a case in a patient who has lived in tropical countries. Three coloured plates of the appearance of the tongue will be found useful, as an early and characteristic sign of psilosis is the alteration of this organ.

A Manual of Surgery. By William Rose, M.B., and Albert Carless. Pp. 1162. London: Baillière, Tindall and Cox. 1898.

We have reviewed this book with much pleasure. It is an excellent work, of the type of small condensed surgical books now prevalent. The descriptions of surgical diseases and operations are well up to date and leave little room for criticism, which would be invidious upon a good book by experienced surgeons. Although we question the propriety of the regular administration of surgical knowledge in concentrated form, this

book may be safely recommended. The illustrations are largely
borrowed from Tillmanns. The printing and paper are good,
and there is evidence of very careful proof-reading.

Genito-Urinary Surgery and Venereal Diseases. By J. WILLIAM
WHITE, M.D., and EDWARD MARTIN, M.D. Pp. xix., 1061.
Philadelphia : J. B. Lippincott Company. 1898.

The need is often felt of a book which gives more information
than an ordinary text-book, and discusses more fully various
methods of treatment. Such a need, so far as genito-urinary
surgery and venereal diseases are concerned, will be supplied in
this book. It is a work of much value, written by two well-
known American surgeons. Indeed, Professor White is perhaps
as well known in this country in connection with the treatment of
hypertrophied prostate by castration as any American surgeon.

The anatomy of the various genito-urinary organs is given
before their injuries and diseases are described ; and this we
are inclined to think a very useful and convenient arrangement.
As an illustration of how fully the subjects are considered, we
may refer to a table giving the differential diagnosis of the
various parts of the urethra affected in gonorrhœa. The attempt
to give the reader an idea of the appearance of gonorrhœal
conjunctivitis by means of an uncoloured photograph, we must
say, is a complete failure. The coloured photographs of venereal
sores and syphilitic skin eruptions, also completely fail to represent the disease. Even coloured plates of venereal sores give
a very imperfect idea of them. But the other illustrations in the
book are very good, and some pictures of hypertrophied prostates
from Watson are particularly fine.

No less than 240 pages are devoted to syphilis. We are
glad to see syphilitic epididymitis mentioned, though it is not
very clearly described ; but attention is called to the similarity
of this disease to tuberculous conditions, a subject seldom
referred to in books. We are interested in the strong view expressed in favour of litholapaxy in boys, and the encouraging
statistics which are given. The important subject of cystoscopy
receives adequate consideration, and some very needful cautions
are given as to the mistakes which may be made in the interpretation of the appearances presented. We notice a reproduction
of a very clear skiagram of a stone in the kidney, and consider
that the subject of renal surgery receives careful and comprehensive treatment. Diseases of the seminal vesicles, about
which our knowledge is getting more precise, are here well
described, and it is perhaps needless to say that we can hardly
expect a better account of the treatment of prostatic hypertrophy
by castration and vasectomy than we have in this volume, no
doubt from the pen of Professor White. In the treatment of
rupture of the urethra we are not told to cut down on the rupture
if we can get a catheter into the bladder, nor is any mention

made of the fact that some eminent surgeons now recommend this proceeding in all cases in which the laceration is at all extensive, as a safeguard against urinary infiltration. But various views are as a rule very fully given, and in the pages devoted to the treatment of extroversion of the bladder the different methods are instructively discussed.

We strongly recommend the book as a modern guide to this branch of surgery.

Renal Growths. By T. N. KELYNACK, M.D. Pp. xiii., 269. Edinburgh: Young J. Pentland. 1898.

It is just time that this book should appear. A vast amount of periodical literature has now accumulated on the subject, and Dr. Kelynack has given us a careful digest of it, together with his own observations, which, as he is pathologist to the Manchester Infirmary, are likely to be as numerous as those of most men. But the book is not by any means limited to the pathological aspect of the subject; though this naturally occupies the greater part of the book, the clinical aspect is fully considered, and even the operative treatment exhaustively discussed.

At the present time there is a good deal of confusion about the classification of renal tumours—so many varieties are now recognised—and the reader must not expect to gain a perfectly clear knowledge of the subject by the careful perusal of this work. The fact is, the subject has not got beyond the stage of early enquiry; tumours of different forms are gaining recognition as distinct varieties. But the knowledge on the subject which we at present possess is well and clearly given by Dr. Kelynack. The illustrations, both of the naked-eye appearance and of the histology of these renal growths, are remarkably good, and the bibliography is very fully given. We heartily congratulate Dr. Kelynack on the result of the labour which he has obviously bestowed on the production of this work.

A Handbook of Medical Climatology. By S. EDWIN SOLLY, M.D. Pp. 470. Philadelphia: Lea Brothers & Co. 1897.

This book is intended for the use of three classes of persons: "the present generation of physicians who prescribe travel, the travelers themselves, and the rising generation of medical students should be taught to recognize the principles of medical climatology and its proper relation to general therapeutics." The author rightly summarises much of the mass of literature on the subject as a "desert of rubbish," in which commonly each writer claims for his own resort "the ability to cure all diseases, and the only invalids warned against coming are those in whom disease is far advanced." We may fairly class this book as one of the "bright oases of truth and reason" to which the author alludes. There are three sections: the first deals broadly with general principles of medical climatology,

the second treats of climate in relation to disease, and the third
is devoted to special climates in selected resorts.

The question has been asked,[1] "What constitutes a good
climate for the healthy?" The reply is, that one with constant
moderate variations calls forth the energy of the different organs
and functions, their power of adaptation and resistance, and
keeps them in a working condition. Such are the climates of
England all the year round: and they belong to the most health-
giving in the world; for here we see the finest trees, the finest
animals, the finest men—and they are most conducive to long-
evity, although not always the most agreeable or exhilarating.
The climates for invalids are those with an abundant supply of
pure air and water, the possibility of spending a great part of
the day in the open air, good hygienic and dietetic arrangements, and the presence of a good local physician. Our own
country—"Le pays ou il fait froid toujours, ou le soleil resemble
à la lune et la lune à un fromage à la crême" (Dumas)—is not,
however, the one where Dr. Solly derives his principal experience; and we naturally associate his name with the treatment of
phthisis at the elevated health-resorts of Colorado.

As to the nature of the influence of altitude, he shows that
the diminished barometric pressure is the principal factor; and
after giving interesting information on the hæmatogenic effects
of high altitude, more especially in consumptives, he quotes
the experiments of Egger, made at Arosa in 1891, showing a
marked increase of 16 per cent. in the number of the red blood
cells. From an analysis of eight thousand cases he deduces
the statement that there is a steady rise in the percentage of
improvement as we go upwards: "That the majority of consumptives do better, other things being equal, the further they are
removed from the sea, and that they do better in high than in
low altitudes, wherever situated" (p. 137). "Le fait est donc
pour nous indubitable, on ne devient pas phthisique à Quito"
(p. 101). Gardiner's researches on the immunity found at high
altitudes were commented on by us in the June number of 1898
(p. 127). We look upon the seventy-three pages on phthisis
and climate as the most valuable part of the work. Dr. Solly
has had a large experience and can speak with authority. His
résumé of the indications and contra-indications in the climatic
treatment of phthisis should be read by all on whom the responsibility rests of choosing a health-resort for those patients.
Section III. gives an excellent outline of the different climates
of all parts of the globe.

The Mineral Waters and Health Resorts of Europe. By HERMANN
WEBER, M.D., and F. PARKES WEBER, M.D. Pp. xiii., 524.
London: Smith, Elder, & Co. 1898.

Known in its original issue as *The Spas and Mineral Waters of
Europe*, this classical work has undergone much alteration and

[1] Clifford Allbutt's *System of Medicine*, 1896, vol. i. p. 284.

addition. The two entirely new chapters are amongst the most useful, inasmuch as they deal with the popular inland climatic health resorts, and the various special methods of treatment and sanatoria for phthisis. These resorts are classified in accordance with their elevation above sea level: those of high elevation being from 3500 feet and upwards, the medium class above 1500 and below 3500 feet, and those of slight elevation comprising places below 1500 feet. The localities of high elevation are described as "eminently stimulating and exhilarating and tonic. They promote the expansion of the chest and lungs, and the ventilation of the latter; they improve the appetite, the digestion, the nutrition and the oxygenation and quality of the blood. Under the diminished atmospheric pressure of high altitudes the number of red corpuscles in the blood rapidly increases, as also the percentage of hæmoglobin, though the latter does so more slowly." Accumulating evidence tends to show that we should not be content with any but the localities of high elevation if we wish to give a phthisical patient the chance of a radical cure, and if he is well enough and financially able to attempt it. After describing the dietetic cures and the various sanatoria for special treatment, the author adds the remark that "more sanatoria are undoubtedly needed, both institutions for the treatment of incipient and hopeful cases, and infirmaries for very advanced and very unfavourable cases, where patients who have no private means can be maintained, if necessary for the rest of their lives." Climatic treatment is usually expensive, as is the treatment of phthisis generally; and those who most need it are often those who can the least afford such luxuries as are to them necessities for the maintenance of life.

We are glad to observe that the authors do not encourage the practice of sending severe and advanced cases of diabetes to spas for treatment; they remark that "no complete and permanent cure of established diabetes is known to us from spa treatment"; and, further, "if the term 'diabetes' be accepted in this [Lauder Brunton's] sense, then one must say that only cases of 'glycosuria' are suited to spa treatment." We hold strongly to the belief that the ordinary glycosuria of middle life · is most amenable to spa treatment; but that the advanced diabetic should remain at home, and carry on there such dietetic and other treatment as may be possible.

The volume is one which may safely be consulted with the expectation of finding in it sound advice grounded on good judgment and experience.

A Manual of General Pathology. By WALTER SYDNEY LAZARUS-BARLOW, M.D. Pp. xi., 795. London: J. & A. Churchill. 1898.

Pathological anatomy is not touched in this book, which deals solely with experimental and general pathology. There is no doubt that the English text-books on pathology have in the past confined themselves too exclusively to pathological anatomy, and the sections devoted to general pathology have been comparatively brief and unsatisfactory. They have, therefore, failed to keep pace with the advances made in experimental pathology during recent years, and thus to give a satisfactory account of a subject which has made great strides. To deal with the whole of pathology, general and anatomical, and at the same time to give an adequate account of those researches and conflicting views, which cannot be omitted without endangering the usefulness of the work, is however no longer possible in a text-book of anything like moderate dimensions, and there is therefore much to be said in favour of the author's contention that it is more convenient to consider general pathology in a separate treatise. Thus this volume comes naturally from the aspect from which it views pathology to occupy a place not hitherto satisfactorily filled by other text-books, and in this way performs a distinctly useful function, and seems likely to have a successful future before it. The manner in which the author has fulfilled his task deserves success, for the book is well written, and gives a very good account of all the most important advances in our knowledge of general pathology, and is brought thoroughly up to the level of the most recent researches. From the author's own investigations into the pathology of the blood-plasma, œdema, and absorption, it would be expected that the chapter on this difficult and at present much-debated subject would be a particularly good one, and there is an extremely able account of it, fully representative of present knowledge, and forming a distinctive feature of the work. The book is one to be recommended as a trustworthy one for students, and will also be found very valuable to practitioners who desire to keep their knowledge of general pathology not only up to date, but to extend it.

Beiträge zur Pathologie und pathologischen Anatomie des Centralnervensystems. Von Dr. ARNOLD PICK. Pp. viii., 324. Berlin: S. Karger. 1898.

This book is made up of a number of essays on neurological subjects and reports of cases interesting either from the clinical or pathological side, and mostly from both. The cases, which are fully and clearly reported, are important as tending, many of them, to elucidate obscure or unsettled points in our knowledge of the pathology of the nervous system. In each instance there is a full critical commentary of the features of interest, and the references to the literature of the subject are unusually complete. In the first twelve papers, which, comprising about half the volume, deal with various kinds of aphasia, almost entirely sensory aphasia, will be found recorded many important cases, and special mention may be made of the studies of subcortical sensory aphasia, of the significance in localisation of quadrant hemianopsia, and of Wernicke's conduction-aphasia. A series of five papers describe various arrests of formation and malformations of the spinal cord; these are very copiously and well illustrated. Three other chapters are devoted to a case of disease of the interolivary layer, and to the consideration of degenerations of the comma-shaped tract in the posterior columns of the spinal cord, and of von Bechterew's "Olivenbündel." Two cases of tumour of the corpus callosum lead to a discussion on the diagnosis of tumours in this situation, and there are also essays on the return of the knee-jerk in some cases of disease of the posterior columns, and on the clinical features of tabes dorsalis when it occurs in young subjects.

The numerous and well-executed figures of the pathological changes form quite a feature of the book, and add to its value, which largely consists in the number of original observations on cases which have been carefully studied, and which form an important contribution to neurological literature.

A Short Practice of Midwifery. By HENRY JELLETT, M.D. Pp. xx., 323. London: J. & A. Churchill. 1897.

In this excellent compendium of the essentials of midwifery practice, the author commences with a well-written and precise chapter on aseptic principles and their practical application to midwifery. With reference to the principles laid down criticism is needless; the details concerning which some will disagree with the author are not important so long as the general principles underlying their application are correctly understood and carried out.

The chapter on abdominal palpation contains many very valuable hints on this important subject. The careful and precise explanation of manipulations gives no excuse for misunderstanding or mistake.

One or two practical points will meet with adverse criticism. In the treatment of accidental hemorrhage the author recommends plugging the vagina tightly; he brings good reason and authority for this method, which is not universally accepted as correct, but a view which is backed by the high authority of the Rotunda school must be received with a certain amount of deference. Had he added plugging the cervix to plugging the vagina, there would have been general agreement with him.

Dr. Jellett states that in the indications for the application of forceps, the head remaining four hours above the brim in the second stage is not of necessity an indication. We have known extensive sloughing follow less delay; with weak pains no doubt delay is harmless, but with strong pains danger is its early result. In the treatment of eclampsia he disapproves of the chloral and chloroform treatment, and prefers the hypodermic administration of morphia: here again he is supported by his school, and although we should object to the adoption of any hard and fast rule in the treatment of these cases, this opinion, enforced as it is by favourable experience, should be accepted with due regard.

The tables at the end referring to the work of the Rotunda during several years are very interesting and well worth study.

A Text-Book of Diseases of Women. By CHARLES B. PENROSE, M.D. Second Edition. Pp. 529. London: The Rebman Publishing Co. (Ltd.). Philadelphia: W. B. Saunders. 1898.

This is an excellent work which goes straight to the mark, untrammelled by needless anatomical, pathological, and histological details. The recommendation of one plan of treatment for each disease is useful for didactic purposes, but is not without its drawbacks when we consider the various clinical modifications of disease. For example, the operation for vesico-vaginal fistula described on pp. 400—402, though sufficient for the majority of cases, is inapplicable in many others in which the sloughing has been very extensive. In this connection, however, we are glad to see that the author condemns kolpokleisis. Dr. Penrose's style is clear and incisive, and the book may be taken as a trustworthy exposition of modern gynæcology.

Conservative Gynecology and Electro-Therapeutics. By G. BETTON MASSEY, M.D. Third Edition. Pp. xv., 394. Philadelphia: The F. A. Davis Company. 1898.

So much new work has been added in this edition of Dr. Massey's book, that it may practically be considered a new work. The author sounds a useful note in stating that every uterine malformation is not a pathological entity requiring treatment; but we must insist that in some pelvic and abdominal cases, and these generally the most grave ones, there will be with the most "conservative" and experienced surgeons an absolute necessity of abdominal section for diagnosis. As a means of diagnosis, the rectal examination of virgins is very properly insisted upon, as it is quite possible to make a complete pelvic examination by this method.

The chapters on the use of electricity in gynæcology are very good, and will repay a careful study; but we cannot agree with the author in all his statements as to the benefits to be derived from this mode of treatment, nor do we consider it safe to employ electricity in certain diseases of the Fallopian tubes or in extra-uterine gestation. The benefit of electricity in fibroid tumours of the uterus is proved most completely, and the various hints given as to the use of the battery, &c., will be of great service to those wishing to practise in this special department.

A striking feature of the volume is the excellence of its illustrations, which include half-tone reproductions of photographs of a professional model, whose services were called into requisition for the delineation of the typical methods of applying electric currents, and also for verifying the motor points of the nerves and muscles.

Guide to the Clinical Examination and Treatment of Sick Children. By JOHN THOMSON, M.D. Pp. xvi., 336. Edinburgh : William F. Clay. 1898.

Dr. Thomson's work is a useful manual for students, but, as he says, it is only supplementary to larger works on the same subject. While he was engaged in the work it seems a pity a more complete guide to clinical examination of children was not produced, as at present some parts might well have been amplified with advantage, more particularly where any help is intended to be given on treatment. The illustrations are anything but a success, and we very much doubt whether anyone could gain much from Fig. 8 or 9, or several others. Diagnosis at sight may be a useful faculty to possess, but it is a dangerous one on which to rely. We hope in a future edition to see these photographs left out, or very materially improved.

Medical Diseases of Infancy and Childhood. By DAWSON WILLIAMS, M.D. Pp. xvi., 634. London : Cassell and Company, Limited. 1898.

Of the many books on the diseases of children that have appeared lately, none strikes our fancy more than that by Dr. Dawson Williams. It is a handy volume, written in clear language and not over-burdened with statistics and tables on the composition of milk. As a practical treatise in a compact form, it is without a rival, and we can confidently recommend it to those who wish to improve their knowledge on this too often neglected subject. It will not of course compare with the larger volumes that come to us across the Atlantic, but they are too large and diffuse for the ordinary reader. The illustrations are few but excellent, being mostly reproductions of photographs. The only fault we have to find is, the small amount of space given to the treatment of skin diseases. They form a large part of the cases we see in the out-patient department of hospitals for children, and from the rapidity with which they improve and get well when the proper methods of dressing are impressed on the parents, we conclude that a little more knowledge on the part of the practitioner in the poorer parts of. our towns might be of use. It is, however, one thing to write and instruct, and another to learn and apply.

Tests and Studies of the Ocular Muscles. By Ernest E. Maddox,
 M.D. Pp. xv., 427. Bristol: John Wright and Co. 1898.

Those who are familiar with the work of Dr. Maddox on
ophthalmological prisms will anticipate in this volume a useful
and interesting book; and they will not be disappointed. The
problems dealt with are admittedly difficult and complex, but the
author's clearness and precision render them comparatively
simple; his happy and well-chosen expressions, his ingenious
methods and luminous suggestions, convert a somewhat dry
and tedious subject into a most interesting study.

We know of no book where so good a description of Tenon's
capsule is given; but what will probably be found the most
useful portions of the book are the chapters on ocular paralysis.
These are so admirably clear, so carefully led up to, and so
copiously illustrated, that if they are consulted a mistake in
diagnosis is scarcely possible. Numerous clever contrivances
and ingenious applications of already existing methods and
apparatus are described. The author's "torsion calculator,"
which anyone can construct for himself, illustrates very prettily
how, in certain cases of ocular paralysis, torsion of the false
image is brought about; and new uses for the "tangent scale"
are explained. The difficult and hitherto much neglected subject
of "latent torsion" of the eyeball deserves special mention as
indicating an advance in ophthalmology, and an attempt to
discover a cause and possibly a remedy for certain cases of
eye-strain.

Every chapter, every page almost, bears the stamp of the
author's originality, and the diagrams and general get-up of the
book leave nothing to be desired.

Nasal Obstruction. By W. J. Walsham, M.B. Pp. viii., 256.
 London: Baillière, Tindall and Cox. 1898.

The author of this work has proceeded on somewhat unusual
lines. He begins by working from the known conditions of the
parts, such as redness, hardness, swelling, &c., to the unknown
disease of which they are signs and symptoms, instead of first
describing the disease and then discussing how it may be
diagnosed from similar affections. He thus goes through all
the diseases which give rise to nasal obstruction, and then finally
he gives the treatment necessary for each variety in separate
chapters at the end of the book. This method of teaching is
frequently made use of in clinical lectures or in oral instruction
during clinical practice, but it has many disadvantages when
used in text-books. Thus it necessitates a great deal of repetition, it is wearying to the reader, and it separates the remarks
on treatment from their natural position immediately after the
diagnosis and symptoms and places them by themselves in
another part of the book. To these objections with the author's

methods we would add unstinting praise for his matter. The descriptions of the conditions giving rise to nasal obstruction are most lucid and admirable. They are clearly defined and well differentiated. The treatment advised is eminently cautious and conservative, and does not partake of that meddlesomeness so common in the present day. All "spoke-shaving" of turbinal bodies is deprecated, and we do not find any mention of that bogey "necrosing ethmoiditis." The author states that, although he has performed a large number of intra-nasal operations, he has never known them to be followed by any septic sequelæ. The most rigid precautions are always taken to work with absolutely aseptic instruments and hands, but the nose having been shown to be practically an aseptic cavity, he never employs antiseptics in the form of washes or douches before operating, and having taken care not to introduce any septic material from without, he leaves the cavity after the operation rigorously alone. When this is done, an aseptic blood-clot forms, and no better antiseptic dressing or preventive for the injured tissue can be found.

Lectures on the Theory and Practice of Vaccination. By ROBERT CORY, M.D. Pp. 122. London: Baillière, Tindall and Cox. 1898.

This book contains the substance of the lectures which Dr. Cory periodically delivers to vaccination students. The opening chapter is devoted to the discussion of the necessity for compulsory vaccination; and then follow chapters on the histology of the vaccine and small-pox vesicles, the difference between a primary and secondary vaccination, the eruptions that occasionally follow vaccination, the practical details of vaccination, and the relation of cow-pox to small-pox. The coloured plates and numerous statistical tables give an additional value to a work which undoubtedly should prove of service to the student. Unfortunately the work was written before the final report of the Royal Commission on Vaccination was issued, and consequently no reference is made to those changes in both the medical and lay minds which have led to the recent modification of our vaccination law, and to the adoption of glycerinated lymph. Indeed we find no reference to the bacteriological researches of Pfeiffer, Copeman, and Klein in connection with vaccinia; nor is mention made of the storage of lymph with glycerine, with a view to eliminating extraneous organisms. We should have wished that greater emphasis was laid upon the necessity for rendering the skin aseptic, sterilising the instruments, and the after-treatment of the arm on aseptic principles.

Dr. Cory regards generalised vaccinia as due to wholesale auto-vaccination, and that this is sometimes the case there can be no doubt. At the same time the experiments of Straus,

Chambon, Ménard, and Chauveau all point to the fact that a genuine general infection may follow vaccination—this quite distinct from auto-inoculation. Dr. Cory's book may be found suitable for elementary teaching purposes, but it cannot be regarded as embodying modern ideas in respect to the theory and practice of vaccination; and there is no excuse for the absence of an index.

Elements of Histology. By E. KLEIN, M.D., F.R.S., and J. S. EDKINS, M.B. Revised Edition. Pp. xii., 500. London: Cassell and Company, Limited. 1898.—Although it is not so stated on the title-page, this is the third edition of this useful manual, and between its first appearance in 1883 and the present issue there have been ten reprints. It is quite modern; for many additions have been made, especially in the sections treating of the cell and the nervous system. The improved methods of staining introduced by Golgi and others have made it necessary to introduce numerous fresh illustrations and diagrams. Only eighteen pages are given to the cell, but a great deal of new matter has been introduced, and the chapter may be taken as a fair *résumé* of the present knowledge of the subject. The somewhat puzzling terms that have been manufactured of late to express the different parts of the cell-structure and the changes in the nucleus, etc., are clearly used; but there is some redundancy—*e.g.* mitoma, intra-nuclear network, and chromosomes, all meaning the same. A noticeable feature is the photo-micrographs which appear in this edition. Some are useful; but many are very poor, especially those on pages 57, 205, 301, and 332. These are so indistinct as to be almost worthless. On the other hand, most of the illustrations and diagrams are decidedly good, and the account of the histology of the various organs is concise and clear; so that an average student can gain an excellent knowledge of minute structure from this work, which is sure to be popular.

Practical Organic Chemistry. By S. RIDEAL, D.Sc. Second Edition. Pp. x., 172. London: H. K. Lewis. 1898.—The second edition of this text-book has afforded the author an opportunity of including some additions to the lists of substances, a practical acquaintance with which is required of candidates for certain of the higher examinations. The properties and reactions of the more common organic bodies are concisely and accurately described, and the information is conveyed in a manner which will render it easily assimilable by those to whom it is especially addressed.

Notes on Malaria in connection with Meteorological Conditions at Sierra Leone. By Surgeon-Major E. M. WILSON. Second Edition. Pp. 16. London: H. K. Lewis. 1898.—We reviewed the first edition of this booklet some time ago, and pointed out the salient features of the opinions of the author. We have not yet heard that the Government have made the alteration in diet Major Wilson recommends. But then permanent officials move slowly.

Materia Medica, Pharmacy, Pharmacology, and Therapeutics. By W. HALE WHITE, M.D. Third Edition. Pp. xvi., 621. London: J. & A. Churchill. 1898.—Except to record that this third edition of Dr. Hale White's work is fully brought up to date and includes all the changes in the recent edition of the *British Pharmacopœia*, it is not necessary to enter into any detailed criticism upon it. It remains, as before, admirably concise, containing all that it is absolutely essential for a student to know about pharmacology and the therapeutical uses of drugs. Although treating mainly of substances included in the *British Pharmacopœia*, the book is not exclusively restricted thereto, for many useful but non-official remedies, such as exalgine, are noticed in their proper places. We heartily commend the work.

Notes on Pharmacy and Dispensing for Nurses. By C. J. S. THOMPSON. Pp. 101. London: The Scientific Press, Limited. 1898.—Nurses will find this small work of use in learning how to dispense medicines. The author has put what he wants them to learn clearly and as briefly as possible, but he has sometimes rather outstepped the range of what a dispenser has to do.

Baby Feeding. By A Doctor. Pp. 62. Bristol: John Wright & Co. 1898.—The information given by the author, who modestly appears as M.B., B.Ch. (Univ. Dub.), is of a thoroughly sound nature, clearly and forcibly expressed. We are afraid, however, there are a few "nots" in Chapter VI. that are seldom attended to, and, moreover, never will be as long as the world goes round. For all that, the advice is good and cannot be too often repeated. Drops of water wear the rock, and we wish every success to the author's drops on the rocks of superstition and ignorance.

Health Loss and Gain. No. 1. By M. A. CHREIMAN. Pp. 226. London: The Rebman Publishing Company, Limited. 1898.—The author proposes "that there should be instituted, as a custom, a system of periodical examination, to which all persons should submit themselves, and to which they should submit their children." We fear that his method would be an excellent means for the multiplication of the nervous hypochondriac, and we hold that if apparent health is working duly without friction it is best to leave it so. The writer has views on many things, and the volume is well worthy of perusal; but one cannot fail to observe that there is an absence of the medical instinct usually associated with the medical mind.

Dwelling Houses: their Sanitary Construction and Arrangements. By W. H. CORFIELD, M.D. Fourth Edition. Pp. xiv., 125. London: H. K. Lewis. 1898.—This edition has been carefully revised throughout by the author, and within its scope forms a good guide for the lay reader.

Association Française de Chirurgie. Onzième Congrès. Procès-verbaux, Mémoires et Discussions. Paris: Félix Alcan. 1897.— A large field is covered in these transactions; but especial attention should be directed to the papers and discussions on contusions of the abdomen, and the operative treatment of cancer of the rectum. The book is suitably illustrated in various parts, and reflects the highest credit on the work of French surgeons.

Recherches cliniques et thérapeutiques sur l'Épilepsie, l'Hystérie, et l'Idiotie. Vol. XVIII. Paris: Félix Alcan. 1898.—In the Bicêtre Asylum, of which this is the annual report there is excellent work being done. Records of many interesting cases of idiocy are given, amongst which are several of importance from a pathological point of view, and of great interest as regards the lesions of the brain. Dr. Bourneville finds in one case a further confirmation of his views as to false and true porencephaly, and it would certainly be well if the present vague use of this term was given up for a more restricted signification. A case in which there were lesions of both frontal lobes is also worthy of study. We must call especial attention to the beautiful reproductions of photographs of the brains of the most important cases, which are given in a series of fine plates, eighteen in number. We regard this volume as an important contribution to the pathology of the brain conditions underlying some forms of idiocy, and the cases recorded in it are worthy of careful perusal.

King's College Hospital Reports. Vol. IV. London: Adlard and Son. 1898.—This volume contains a continuation of John Curnow's historical sketch, and has an interesting account of the enthusiasm and the work of Robert Bentley Todd. The original papers are not numerous: Dr. Nestor Tirard gives an interesting account of albuminuria in children; Mr. Albert Carless advocates early operation in cases of appendicitis; Dr. Arthur Whitfield, writing on the diagnosis and management of syphilis, advocates the view "that iodide may be used to help in the improvement of some symptoms, but on mercury must we rely wherewith to combat the disease"; Dr. Raymond Crawfurd prefers a combination of belladonna and nux vomica to various barbarities which have been reputed to be of use for the enuresis of childhood; Dr. Hugh Playfair considers it to be absolutely essential to combine local application with constitutional treatment for most cases of leucorrhœa; and Dr. J. Curtis Webb gives some interesting reminiscences of gynæcology in Berlin. The statistical reports and records of cases of interest follow, and the account of what old King's men are doing is of especial interest to those whose names are found there.

Saint Bartholomew's Hospital Reports. Vol. XXXIII. London: Smith, Elder, & Co. 1898.—The volume of reports begins this year, as it has unfortunately done rather often of late, with an obituary notice of a member of the hospital staff. In the present volume Dr. Church gives a very interesting account of the life of Dr. James Andrew, who retired from work at the hospital some few years ago, and died in April, 1898. Such accounts are of sad but special interest to all old Bartholomew's students, and the graphic description of Dr. Andrew in his ward work is one which will recall many scenes connected with their study of clinical medicine. There are many papers of great value in the reports this year. As we might expect, many record interesting cases which have been in the hospital, and both the clinical and pathological sides of the work have yielded important results. There is perhaps no record of clinical work which gives so accurate an account of the difficulties and mistakes in diagnosis, and the failures in treatment, as the report of all cases of interest occurring in a large hospital during the year, and these we find admirably given in this volume. Instead of the publication of the successful cases only, to which we are all tempted, we have here many examples of failure both in diagnosis and treatment, which are really often more instructive than the successful ones.

The American Year-Book of Medicine and Surgery. London: The Rebman Publishing Co. (Ltd.). Philadelphia: W. B. Saunders. 1899.—*The American Year-Book*, a digest collected and arranged by a large staff under the general editorial charge of Dr. George M. Gould, has now become an established perennial in its fourth year. The volume covers a large scope, including all the special branches of medicine and surgery, pharmacology, anatomy, physiology, legal medicine, public hygiene and preventive medicine. Sixteen of the twenty-eight contributors are well-known specialists and teachers of Philadelphia; New York city claims four, Chicago three, Cleveland two; and Baltimore, Boston, and Montreal can each claim one. The staff may well be complimented on "that expertness of intelligence in gleaning and ripeness of judgment in deciding as to values which can only be gained by experience and knowledge." The book may be opened at any page, and the reader will find something interesting, novel, and well presented in excellent type. The omission of the name of Dr. William Pepper from the list of contributors is mentioned by the editor, and the whole world of medicine is the poorer by the death of that distinguished man.

Annual and Analytical Cyclopædia of Practical Medicine. Vol. II. The F. A. Davis Company. 1899.—The second volume of this great work has now arrived. It commences with bromide of ethyl and concludes with diphtheria. The volume contains exceptionally valuable articles on a number of exacting subjects, viz.: "Cerebral Hæmorrhage," by Dr. William Browning, of Brooklyn; "Cirrhosis of the Liver," by Professor Adami, of Montreal; "Cholera," by Professor Rubino, of Naples; "Cholelithiasis," by Professor Graham, of Toronto; "Diabetes," by Professor Lépine, of Lyons; "Diphtheria," by Drs. Northrup and Bovaird, of New York; "Constipation," by Professor Nathan S. Davis, of Chicago; "Dilatation of the Heart," by Dr. Vickery, of Boston. These and many other articles deserve the reader's special attention and study. The volume is beyond all praise or criticism, and Dr. Sajous deserves the hearty thanks of all engaged in the practice of medicine.

The Medical Annual. Bristol: John Wright & Co. 1899.— The amount of useful information given to the busy man·in this volume is remarkable. Most of the contributors to it are not mere abstractors, but are experienced in various branches of medicine and surgery, and so are able to select from and to criticise the great mass of newly-published work which they lay under contribution. The book is, as has hitherto been the case, well printed and illustrated, and we cordially recommend it to our readers. We think that many provincial societies deserve a place in the list of "Medical and Scientific Societies."

The Edinburgh Medical Journal. New Series, Vol. IV. Edinburgh: Young J. Pentland. 1898.—The half-yearly volume contains a collection of excellent papers worthy of careful study by those who have not received the monthly parts. Many of the papers read at, and a general summary of the proceedings of, the British Medical Association at Edinburgh are included. Dr. Finlayson has an interesting paper on "Medical Bibliography and Medical Education," in which he advocates the more general teaching of medicine by clinical work, and cites the instance of Johns Hopkins University, which has abolished systematic lectures on medicine. The reviews of British and foreign literature, and the reports on recent advances in medical science, are done with much care and by authorities in the various departments. We congratulate the editor on the result of his efforts.

Ἰατρικὴ Πρόοδος. *La Grèce Médicale.* Syra: Impr. Renieri Brindesi.—Medical journalism in Greece has had apparently rather a chequered career, one or two journals which we have seen in past years being now extinct. Ἰατρικὴ Πρόοδος is, however, in the fourth year of its existence, and has hitherto appeared in the Greek language only. In order, however, that the active advance of medicine in Greece may become more generally known among other nations, with the monthly issue of the Greek journal there is now published an appendix in French, *La Grèce Médicale.* Of both sections we desire to speak with much commendation; the subject-matter and occasional illustrations are thoroughly praiseworthy, and we wish this addition to our exchange-list long life, and its editor, Dr. Foustanos, a full measure of success.

Archives provinciales de Médecine. Paris: Institut international de Bibliographie scientifique.—We are glad to welcome on our exchange-list this new monthly journal, which, following somewhat on the lines of the *Archives provinciales de Chirurgie*, has started a career in the direction of decentralisation in medicine. With a large staff of supporters scattered throughout the principal cities of France, it may be expected to have a very successful and useful course, and we wish Dr. Marcel Baudouin, the editor, all possible recognition of this new effort which he is making, in addition to those many others which have so considerably benefited the profession.

The British Food Journal. Vol. I., No. 1. January, 1899. London: Baillière, Tindall & Cox.—This is one of the most remarkable—we had almost said impudent—pseudo-scientific publications that has ever appeared in print. The responsibility for its existence rests upon the shoulders of an "editorial staff" including some names which it is to be hoped decorate the cover without the knowledge of their owners. After drawing attention to certain excellent recommendations by the Censors of the Institute of Chemistry on the question of unprofessional conduct, with special reference to advertising and the issue of trade puffs, the "editorial staff" proceed to traverse the more important ones by offering themselves to the manufacturing world as testimonial-mongers on the co-operative system, on the principle, it is to be supposed, of the unkickability of the corporate body. The fact that this proposal is enshrined in a quantity of doubtful information collected apparently from the columns of the daily papers does not alter its character; and it is much to be desired that the Institute may use its influence to check a movement that can only tend to discredit one of the youngest, but not least useful, of the professions.

The Philadelphia Monthly Medical Journal.—Dr. Gould's excellent weekly journal is now to have a monthly supplement, which is to consist of original contributions only. For very good reasons no doubt, No. 3 is the first to be issued. It contains the prize essays in connection with the weekly journal. The first prize in the department of medicine was awarded to a paper by Dr. Henry Wald Bettman, of Cincinnati. It describes the shape, position and displacements of the stomach, and gives an excellent account of the diagnosis, prophylaxis, and treatment of gastroptosis and gastro-enteroptosis. A very complete bibliography is appended, and an analysis of the most important recent papers on the subject: on the authority of Meinert[1] we are informed that "every dress fastened about the waist worn by a girl before her fifteenth year leads inevitably to gastroptosis"; there is, therefore, no need to wonder why it is that 90 per cent. of adult women have gastroptosis, whereas it is present in only about 5 per cent. of men. The other papers

---

[1] *Centralbl. f. innere Med.*, 1896, xvii. 297, 321.

are worthy of careful consideration, and this new departure of Dr. Gould's deserves to be heartily supported.

The Polyclinic. Vol. I. No 1. May, 1899. London: H. K. Lewis.—Our Exchange-list has received the addition of this Journal of the new Medical Graduates' College. Sir W. H. Broadbent writes on "The Necessity for a Medical Graduates' College;" Mr. Jonathan Hutchinson gives "Some Account of the Formation and Aims of the College;" and Dr. Wm. Miller Ord, in considering "The Medical Practitioner as a Student," says: "The scheme of Post-Graduation Teaching now established will be found to offer large opportunities of self-improvement along many lines of work. The whole plan is framed to insure practical instruction in all departments. Those who will occupy the position of teachers, and those who come for instruction, will work side by side assuredly to the benefit of both. . . . The proverb 'Docendo discimus' is as true as ever." The list of officers and Council is one which will command success.

Notes on Preparations for the Sick.

Diastol.—THE STANDARD MALT EXTRACT CO. LIMITED, London.—The manufacture of this digestive is carried on at Clayton-le-Moors, Lancashire, by a special process, which gives excellent results. The diastasic power is high, and its use in many forms of dyspepsia gives good results, enabling cases of phthisis and other diseases of mal-nutrition to assimilate farinaceous foods in greater quantity than without it. In many cases of chronic dyspepsia we have found this preparation to be of real service. "If the starchy elements of the food were eliminated from the diet in a case of amyldyspepsia the alimentary troubles would soon cease," and so would the normal nutrition of the tissues unless the patient cared to run the greater risk of uric acid and urate poisoning. We think that the digestion, *even if artificial,* of the starchy foods is better than their elimination from the dietary.

Varalettes: Citrate of Lithia; Citrate of Piperazine; Glycerophosphate of Lime; Urotropine; Potass. Citrate, Lithia Citrate; Soda Salicylate, Antipyrine, Caffeine pure; Vichy Salts.—ALFRED BISHOP & SONS LTD., London.—These are the newer forms of Bishop's well-known preparations. The powder is compressed into what are called varalettes, which are said to have all the advantages of the tabloid combined with a greater solubility.

Meta - Cresol - Anytol.—GUSTAV HERMANNI, Jr., London.— This is specially prepared for the local treatment of diphtheria. It may be used as a three per cent. aqueous solution, either by inhalation or spray: the maker claims that it is non-irritating, is fatal to the cocci, and has a neutralising alterant action on the diphtheria toxin.

Public Vaccinator's Bag.—FERRIS & Co., Bristol.—In country districts it would be found convenient to carry such an assortment as is contained in this very complete and portable bag.

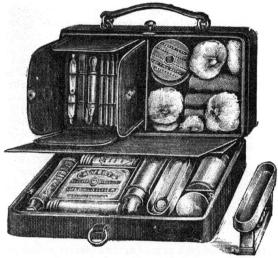

For use [in towns the pocket case included in the bag will generally be found sufficient. To those who over a long number of years have vaccinated thousands of children with excellent results these cumbrous paraphernalia seem quite unnecessary. Their introduction very much resembles the employment of a steam-hammer for cracking a walnut. The people who are charged with the administration of vaccination laws and practice are very nearly succeeding in making the whole thing ridiculous. In the *British Medical Journal* for February 25th there is an excellent illustrated satire on the new methods.

MEETINGS OF SOCIETIES.

Bristol Medico-Chirurgical Society.

March 8th, 1899.

Dr. R. ROXBURGH, President, in the Chair.

Dr. H. WALDO showed (1) a boy, aged 11 years, with Adenoma sebaceum of the face, which had existed for about a year. He said that this disease was characterised by the appearance of neoplasms papular in character, of congenital origin, but appearing at or before

12

puberty. There is a distinct outline to each lesion, and coalescence is unusual. A large proportion of the subjects are epileptics or imbeciles, and it was at one time supposed that bromides produced the eruption. Adehoid changes are found in the sebaceous glands. The papillary vessels are conspicuous, and there is an increase in the connective tissue. There is, in fact, a replacement of large numbers of hair-follicles and sebaceous glands by fibrous tissue, of which the little tumours are largely composed. There is extensive interpapillary hypertrophy. The lesions may be flat-topped, others rounded, convex or acuminate, while some may be warty-looking, and may be pedunculated, though the customary papule is sessile. Involution may occur, but the tendency is to persistence, the lesions recurring in spite of removal and even *in situ*. (2) A young woman with tuberculosis of the skin. The patient received a wound of the right leg six months ago. She says that shortly after this a rash extended all over her. When first seen there was a broad streak of lupus erythematosus extending down the left arm and forearm, with a circular patch the size of a half-crown on the right forearm, and also a well-marked bat's wing arrangement on the face and nose, with a slight implication of the left ear; in fact, the disease was becoming generalised. This condition had been present for four months. She thought she had lost flesh. There was no cough. He prescribed an emollient and slightly-astringent lotion during the day, and an ointment of sulphur and carbolic acid to be rubbed in at night. She was to take cod-liver oil and quinine; to keep her bedroom window well open at night, and to be in the open air as much as possible in the day. The patient was now nearly well.

Dr. J. E. SHAW showed (1) a case of acute anterior poliomyelitis, which had existed six months, involving the whole of the muscles of both legs, including the glutei; the case is remarkable in that not the slightest degree of recovery has taken place. (2) A case of spastic diplegia which began to develop at 9 months of age. Patient now has the usual cross-kneed progression, but the legs are permanently bent upon the thighs; the feet are long, flat, not in a position of talipes equinus, and are everted. (3) Two cases of pseudo-hypertrophic muscular paralysis occurring in brothers. The younger, aged 6, exhibits the usual phenomena of an early stage, being able to stand and walk alone and rise from the floor unaided; the knee-jerk is present. The elder, aged 12, cannot stand or walk alone, and cannot rise from the ground beyond getting on to his knees. He stands, when sustained artificially, upon his toes and toe-balls, the heel never coming down upon the ground owing to the contraction of the calf muscles maintaining the feet in the position of talipes equinus. The calf muscles are not very large, but are very hard; the knee-jerk is absent on both sides.

Dr. MICHELL CLARKE showed (1) a case of syringomyelia in a young man of 17. The illness began in July, 1898, with weakness and wasting of the muscles of the left hand. There had been no pain throughout. The symptoms present now are: atrophy of the small muscles of the left hand and of extensors of the left forearm, with paralysis of the left upper extremity; wasting to a less degree of the left deltoid, biceps, pectoralis major, and of the small muscles of the right hand; loss of sensation to pain, and to heat and cold, but not to touch, over left arm and left side of chest. There were also spastic rigidity of the legs, double ankle-clonus, left rectus-clonus, and exaggerated right knee-jerk. (2) A case of disseminated sclerosis in a sailor, aged 39, who had not had syphilis, and had enjoyed very good health. He attributed his illness to privation and exposure.

There were well-marked intention tremor of both arms, most in the right; scanning speech, exaggerated knee-jerks, weakness of arms and legs, attacks of vertigo, with defect of associated movement of the eyeballs to the left. (3) A case of progressive muscular atrophy with absent knee-jerks, and remarkably extensive distribution of the muscular atrophy for the presumably early stage of the disease.—Dr. WALDO asked Dr. Clarke if the retinæ had been examined ophthalmoscopically, as he considered that atrophy of the papilla was very often found in cases of disseminated sclerosis, and might assist in the diagnosis of an obscure case.—Dr. CLARKE, in reply, said that the optic discs were pale.

Dr. E. C. WILLIAMS showed a case of hemiplegia, with wasting of the muscles of the leg, of six years' duration in a child aged 11 years. The onset was sudden—pain over the left temporal region, followed by a convulsion. After the convulsion, there was loss of speech and paralysis of right side of face, right arm, and right leg. She gradually recovered from the aphasia and facial paralysis in about fourteen months. There was no history of rheumatism, chorea, or any infectious disease. She is of slow intellect and very forgetful. On admission to the Children's Hospital, under Dr. Lees, her right arm was in a spastic condition—elbow and wrist more or less flexed, fingers flexed or extended and rigid, movements being slow and usually tremulous. The right arm measures more than the left, the increase being probably due to the constant choreiform movements. Electrical reactions, normal; heart and lungs, healthy. Right leg measures 1 inch less than left. There is pes cavus. Some of the leg muscles give the reaction of degeneration; knee-jerks, glib. The seat of the lesion appears to be in the upper motor segment, for the following reasons: 1, The lesion is a hemiplegia; 2, aphasia and facial paralysis at onset; 3, no reaction of degeneration in upper limb; 4, reflexes present. The lesion is double; i.e., there is an anterior poliomyelitis as well as an upper segment lesion (polio-encephalitis). It would appear the two lesions are the result of the same poison, which more commonly affects the anterior horns, but also affects the ganglion cells of the cortex. The disease is often epidemic, many cases being reported in the *Journal of the American Medical Association*, xxvi., 1896, in which the characteristic symptom was paralysis in young children. It was attributed to insanitary surroundings. An elder brother of this child had a similar attack seventeen years ago, but made a fair recovery.

Mr. MUNRO SMITH showed a boy on whom erasion of the knee-joint had been performed, a year ago, for extensive disease of the synovial membrane and cartilage. The bone was slightly affected. Two operations were performed before the disease was eradicated. The boy can now walk easily and well, and there is very slight shortening.

Mr. C. A. MORTON showed a woman, aged 59, from whom, in November last, he had excised the cæcum for a carcinomatous growth. The ileum was joined to the ascending colon with a Murphy button. The growth had been so movable that it simulated movable kidney. Not only could it be pushed into the loin, but also as far inwards as the umbilicus. The patient had gained 2 stone in weight since the operation.—Mr. ROGER WILLIAMS said cancer of cæcum was such a comparatively rare disease that but few examples of its successful removal have been reported. He could at that moment recall only two cases in which an operation of this kind had been done. One was by Homans, in which he successfully excised a sarcoma of the cæcum from a girl of 5. In another case Abbe excised the cæcum and several feet of intestine from a youth of 16, uniting the divided ends of gut by a Murphy button. The patient died shortly after operation. It was interesting that in Mr. Morton's case there were no symptoms of obstruction, as this had been noted in several cases of cæcal cancer, wherein it differed so markedly from other cancers of large intestine. Of 100 consecutive cases of cancer of the large intestine, Mr. Williams found that ·5 per cent. were cæcal and ·5 per cent. of ileo-cæcal valve, whereas Fagge found 4 per cent. were cæcal.—Dr. Lacy Firth remarked that one of the difficulties in the operation of removal of the cæcum was due to the difference in size of the two portions of bowel which had to be united. He had heard of one successful case, in which the end of the colon was partially closed by sutures and the small intestine then fixed to the portion remaining open by means of a Murphy button. He had on one occasion removed the cæcum for malignant disease, and had attempted to overcome the difficulty mentioned by closing up the end of the colon and then fixing the end of the ileum to its side with a Murphy button, but the patient unfortunately died on the seventh day. He asked if Mr. Morton had found any difficulty in his case in approximating the ileum to the colon by reason of the difference in calibre.—In reply to Mr. Roger Williams and Dr. Firth, Mr. Morton said he had not yet had time to look up the literature of the subject, but would refer to it when he published the case. There was considerable difficulty in getting the cut edge of the ascending colon into the grip of the button, which was the one used for the junction of small intestine.

Mr. T. Carwardine showed two patients after excision of the rectum for malignant disease by a method which he had devised and described in the *British Medical Journal*, 1898. Each patient has a partially renewed and bifid coccyx and intact sphincter, and perfect control over fæces, and the case operated on six months ago has control of flatus also. Defæcation is performed voluntarily once or twice a day, and rectal sense is perfect.—Mr. C. A. Morton asked if Mr. Carwardine left a segment of the lower end of the rectum in his two operations. He thought that if the growth extended far up the rectum the peritoneum must of necessity be opened in the removal of the growth, as in the ordinary Kraske's operation.—Mr. Carwardine, in reply, said the amount of anal mucous membrane left may vary with the case. The facility with which the peritoneum can be deflected from the presacral glands and tissue in this method of operation avoids the necessity, as in Kraske's operation, of frequently opening the peritoneum.

Dr. E. H. E. Stack showed a case of precocious menstruation. The girl was 5½ years, and mentally a little deficient. Periods began at 18 months, and have been nearly regular ever since, lasting three days and requiring seven diapers. The breasts began to develop about the same time, and have progressed since; now the diameter is 3 inches, and depth at nipple 1¼ inches. The pelvis has a grown-up appearance, and, comparing its measurements with about twenty others of ages from 5 upwards, it conforms to the average of those of 12 years. The external genitals are not much abnormally developed; there is a little downy hair over them about ¼ inch long. She has been twice seen menstruating, and blood had the appearance of a normal period. There have been thirty to forty cases reported, and about twenty of these seem genuine and do not include cases beginning at 7 or 8 years or the bleeding once of new-born babes. They are very much alike. Average beginning was 2 years; most, but not all, had distinct growth of hair on pubes, but not in axilla. All had well-developed breasts;

most were otherwise normal children; some seemed older than their years. Longest record is a child of 11, who began at 16 months. Only one case of very early puberty in a boy was found. No cause appears in the way of family history, climate, etc.—Dr. AUST LAWRENCE said that he would have liked to have had some information on the condition of the pelvic viscera as ascertained under chloroform or by rectal examination.—Mr. ROGER WILLIAMS regarded the condition as not so rare as was generally believed, and he had collected notes of over fifty cases. Nothing was more remarkable in the history of the development of the body than the great punctuaity with which the different developmental events came off, although in exceptional cases a wide range of variability in this respect was not incompatible with health. Developmental anomalies with regard to time were quite as interesting and important as structural anomalies; and they were met with in respect to dentition and other conditions, besides sexual development. He thought many cases of this kind might be ascribed to reversion. Very few animals arrived at sexual maturity at such a late age as man; and among savages—where the waste of life was great—sexual maturity and reproduction ensued at much earlier periods than in modern communities. In this connection it was interesting to note that among the Hindoos—who were a branch of the same stock as ourselves—sexual maturity usually set in at an earlier age than with us, girls often attaining puberty at 8 years or even earlier. Premature sexual development was met with in boys as well as in girls, although most of the recorded cases were of the female sex. It might supervene at any time from birth to the normal age of puberty. A curious feature in many cases was that this precocity only manifested itself in respect to some of the constituent phenomena that go to make up sexual maturity. Thus in some cases the only evidence of it was mammary overgrowth; in others, menstruation; in others, undue development of the genitalia, etc. In most cases, however, the *ensemble* of the phenomena of sexual maturity was affected. Mr. Williams thought it might be inferred from the foregoing that the various phenomena which together constitute sexual maturity had been gradually integrated and co-ordinated, rather than that they had suddenly sprung into existence as a physiological unity. The internal sexual organs were often affected, as well as the external ones; for in necropsies on cases of this kind maturing Graafian follicles, corpora lutea, and recent ovarian cicatrices had been found with the pubescent uterus, ovaries, tubes, and pelvis; in short, there could be no doubt but that in these cases we had to do really with puberty. In support of this, he referred to cases of early pregnancy, at from 8¾ to 12 years, these young mothers having manifested signs of sexual precocity from earliest infancy. In one case of this kind the mother, aged 12, was impregnated by a boy of 14, and in due course she was delivered of a healthy child. Many cases of premature sexual development had been met with in children having intra-abdominal tumours, such as ovarian cystomata, sarcomata, etc., and adrenal tumours. In these cases the condition seemed to be caused, and the local congestion determined, by the presence of the tumour. In this connection it was interesting to recall the cases in which lactation had been excited—in young children and others—by repeated suction of the nipples, etc. Thus it seemed that sexual precocity might result from extrinsic as well as from intrinsic causes. —Dr. C. ELLIOTT stated that all cases of so-called premature menstruation should be carefully examined, as the discharge of blood from the vagina was not always from the uterus. Some years ago a young girl was brought to the Children's Hospital who had been seen by more than one medical man, and the mother was told by them that it was a case of premature menstruation. Not being satisfied with this diagnosis, he admitted the child into the Hospital and had the bladder examined. A hairpin was found with one point protruding through the urethra, and a phosphatic calculus had formed around it. His colleague, Mr. Norton, broke down the calculus, and removed the hairpin with some difficulty.

Dr. F. H. EDGEWORTH read a paper on the treatment of bronchitis, which will appear in a subsequent number of this *Journal*.

Mr. ARTHUR PRICHARD read notes on a case of hæmatometra in which, by strict antisepticism and slow draining of the tumour through the imperforate hymen, a cure resulted. The case was that of a girl aged 18, who first noticed a swelling in the lower part of the abdomen seven months before coming under observation. There was no pain at regular intervals. She had never menstruated. The vagina was occluded by a tense membrane, slightly bulging, to which an impulse could be communicated by pressure on the abdominal swelling. It was drained into sterilised wool pads by a small tube, and the catheter used when required. In three days the tumour, which before reached to 1 inch above the umbilicus, was almost gone. The discharge lasted for fifteen days. The vagina was subsequently dilated. The upper part was capacious, and had constituted part of the abdominal tumour. The os uteri would admit the tip of one's forefinger.—Dr. AUST LAWRENCE mentioned three cases of hæmatometra which he had seen. 1. Imperforate hymen, vagina and uterus distended, with retained menstrual blood. Treated by slowly draining through cannula and tubing into a bottle containing carbolic lotion. Perfect success. 2. Occluded os uteri, the result of *post-partum* sloughing of cervix uteri, the retained fluid caused uterine enlargement equal to a six months' pregnancy. Treated by slow draining through an opening made in position of normal os uteri, as case 1. Complete success. 3. Imperforate os uteri in one half of a bifid uterus, the other half menstruating normally. Treated as No. 2, but patient died from septic peritonitis, due to escape of menstrual blood into the abdomen, owing to rupture of the adherent and distended tube on that side. The symptoms of this were very indefinite.

April 12th, 1899.

Dr. J. E. SHAW in the Chair.

The CHAIRMAN showed a patient with peroneal type of muscular atrophy, which will be described in a later number of this *Journal*. —In connection with this case Dr. MICHELL CLARKE showed photographs of the hands of a patient, aged 10, under his care eight or nine years ago. There was wasting of the small muscles of the hands and of the muscles of the forearms, and the fingers were contracted in flexion. The disease came on after one of the acute specific fevers. The wasting appeared to be stationary, and the patient after attending at the Hospital for some time was lost sight of. Her case was one of neuritic atrophy.—Dr. E. J. CAVE mentioned the interesting pathological question raised by the fact that what appeared to be a primarily neuritic affection should be liable to occur in members of the same family, especially in regard to the part played by measles in the etiology of the condition. Such family groups were more familiar in primary muscular or spinal affections.

Dr. H. WALDO showed a patient with tubercular peritonitis treated by operation. He was brought to the Infirmary with a tubercular temperature, a tender and swollen abdomen, depending in the first instance upon tympanites and shortly afterwards on ascites. He was acutely ill, and Dr. Waldo thought an abdominal incision would give him the best chance. The most satisfactory results from this treatment occur in the ascitic variety.—Mr. W. H. HARSANT said that when the boy came under his care he seemed so ill and hectic, and was so rapidly losing weight and strength, that it was obvious he would not recover unless something were done. A small incision was made and 4½ pints of fluid were evacuated. The peritoneal cavity was then freely washed out with sterilised water, and the wound closed without drainage. Recovery was rapid and most satisfactory; and though it was too early yet to speak of a cure, it seemed as if this boy would probably remain well. It had been laid down by some observers that a cure could not be said to be assured until five years had elapsed. The cases most favourable for operation were those occurring in young patients with an acute history and where there is a free exudation of fluid, and all these circumstances were combined in the present case.— Dr. WALTER SWAYNE stated that he himself, some years ago, suffered from an affection which was diagnosed as tubercular peritonitis, with symptoms of abdominal distension, general wasting, slight ascites, and for a short time some evening rise of temperature. He recovered without operation, and was pleased to hear Mr. Harsant's statement that after five years the patient might be considered safe.—Mr. C. A. MORTON alluded to three cases under his own care in which ascites from tubercular peritonitis had been present, operation had been postponed, and in all the cases recovery had taken place without. He thought that surgeons had brought forward theories which, as Dr. Waldo had stated, were most unsatisfactory explanations of the improvement after laparotomy, because they had failed to recognise the fact that probably a large number of the cases operated on would have recovered without. Hawkins [1] had shown that 59 out of 100 cases of tubercular peritonitis, treated in the wards of St. Thomas's Hospital, got well without operation. But he thought that when it was necessary to evacuate the fluid on account of the pressure which it exerted, it was far safer to do so by incision than by tapping. A short time ago he had seen a lady suffering from ascites from tubercular peritonitis who had a few hours before been tapped, and only fæces had escaped. The area tapped had been quite dull, no doubt because the adherent bowel was at the time empty of gas. He thought the chance of adhesion of bowel to the anterior abdominal wall was so great in these cases that a free and careful incision was a much safer method of evacuating the fluid.—Dr. SHINGLETON SMITH mentioned an interesting history which had come to his knowledge. A patient in early life was supposed to be dying of tubercular peritonitis: she recovered, but some ten years later had spinal disease which caused considerable angular curvature: ten years later again she had hæmoptysis and indications of tubercular disease of lungs, together with a tubercular intercostal abscess. Death occurred some twenty-two years after the first indications of abdominal tuberculosis, but there was no return of the peritoneal symptoms.— Dr. J. O. SYMES said that in other collections of tubercular fluid it was noteworthy that evacuation was followed by rapid disappearance of tubercle bacilli. Thus pus aspirated from a tubercular hip-joint might be found crowded with bacilli, but if the discharge were examined twenty-four hours after opening the abscess the discovery of the bacilli

[1] St. Thomas's Hosp. Rep., 1892, xx. 25.

would be a matter of great difficulty.—Mr. PAUL BUSH mentioned that in operating on these patients he endeavoured to admit as much air as possible into the peritoneal cavity, and that he had observed that the mere evacuation of fluid was often not sufficient to obtain a cure.—Dr. E. H. E. STACK remembered a case at St. Bartholomew's Hospital in a young man who, without ascites, had chronic intestinal obstruction which no medical treatment relieved. An incision was made through the abdominal wall, and the intestines were so matted that nothing further was done; but within a few days the obstruction was relieved, and in a few weeks the boy seemed quite well, and he was still well a year afterwards.—Dr. F. H. EDGEWORTH called attention to the statement of Fagge to the effect that the majority of cases of ascitic tubercular peritonitis are cured by the application of linimentum hydrargyri on lint to the skin of the abdomen.—Dr. MICHELL CLARKE said that he agreed with Mr. Morton that the majority of these patients got well from the immediate attack. Operation was unnecessary unless there was ascitic fluid, and then a certain time should be allowed for medical treatment to be carried out before operation was undertaken. If, however, an extreme amount of fluid was present so as to cause pain from distension, the abdomen should be opened without waiting. He mentioned a case in which a large quantity of ascitic fluid was absorbed as the result of extensive blistering of the abdominal wall, occurring from the application of a carbolic pad as a preliminary to operation. Tuberculous disease of the lungs, or persistent diarrhœa indicating intestinal ulceration, as a rule, contra-indicated operation. In these cases, as in a patient lately under his care, death might take place from obstruction of the intestine through adhesions or bands. Though the immediate prognosis of an attack of tuberculous peritonitis was good, the ultimate issue of the case was doubtful; three instances had occurred to him in the last three years in which the lungs became affected.—Mr. J. EWENS spoke in favour of blistering the abdomen with mercurial dressing in all cases of fluid in the abdomen; he had seen very good results. In some cases of ascitic fluid, when digitalis, squill, and other direct diuretics failed to reduce the swelling, small doses of mercury, given to the extent of affecting the gums, produced immediate diminution of the fluid.—Dr. R. C. LEONARD asked whether it was possible to exclude tubercular lesions of the intestine in cases of tubercular peritonitis, and whether if it was suspected operation was contra-indicated. He quoted Dr. Whitla's results with cod-liver oil in these cases.—Dr. C. ELLIOTT mentioned that in cases of tubercular peritonitis the secretion of urine was usually considerably diminished, and this fact he had found useful for diagnosis in obscure abdominal cases. For instance, he had once ventured on this ground to question the accuracy of his surgical colleagues in the case of a young woman who had been admitted for a supposed ovarian cyst. When operated upon, as he expected, simple peritoneal fluid was let out, and the patient made an excellent recovery. His treatment accordingly aimed at increasing the urinary excretion, and for this purpose he usually employed infusion of broom, combining it with iron, and the results were satisfactory.—Dr. WALDO, in reply, said that in cases where operation was not considered advisable he used lin. hydrargyri and a dry diet.

Dr. WALTER SWAYNE showed a specimen of diffuse sarcoma of the uterus with complete inversion. The patient, a nullipara, aged 17, was admitted to the Royal Infirmary with what looked like a piece of placenta protruding from an intact vaginal orifice. This was found to be immovable and to consist of part of the fundus covered with a placenta-like growth, a section from which showed that it was composed of mixed spindle- and round-celled sarcoma. The growth covered the whole of the body of the uterus, which was completely inverted and rreducible. A large vesico-vaginal fistula was present, the opening being about the size of a shilling. As the growth appeared to have infiltrated the surrounding parts, it was dealt with by removal of the growth from the fundus by scissors and curette. The patient improved markedly in health after this; but was readmitted three months later with recurrence of the growth, and again treated in the same way. Improvement again followed the removal; but four months later the patient was readmitted, and died on the third day after arrival of asthenia. While sarcoma of the uterus was rare, and inversion also rare, diffuse sarcoma of the fundus uteri was specially apt to cause inversion.—Dr. W. H. C. NEWNHAM said that inversion so complete as shown in this specimen must be extremely rare. He had only met with *five* cases of complete inversion : four were produced by the midwife pulling upon the cord; these were admitted into the Hospital, replaced, and all recovered. The other was produced by the dragging down of a large fibroid tumour, which was sloughing and projecting from the vulva. He passed the wire of an ecraseur round what he believed to be the neck of the tumour and removed it. On looking at the specimen, he found he had also removed the upper half of the uterus with the Fallopian tubes in addition to the tumour He did not take any further operative steps, and strangely enough the patient recovered absolutely without a single bad symptom or rise of temperature.

Dr. E. H. E. STACK showed a specimen of retro-pharyngeal abscess. The child was 2½ years, and had been ill a fortnight before admission. He came in under Dr. Shaw and seemed to be a case of diphtheritic laryngitis. The fauces looked natural. There was so much recession that tracheotomy was decided on almost at once, but on the first stroke of the knife he cried with such a good voice that it seemed evident there was no laryngitis. Exploring with the finger, a retro-pharyngeal abscess was felt and opened from behind the sterno-mastoid, several ounces of pus were evacuated, and very soon the breathing was relieved and he could swallow; but in a day or two he died, not having been able to recover the serious dose of septic infection he had received. The specimen shows no evidence of tubercle of the spine or other evidence of the cause of the abscess.

Dr. BERTRAM ROGERS read a paper on a case of thrombosis of the portal vein (*see* page 107 of the current number).

Mr. PAUL BUSH read a·paper on some peculiar operation cases in lunatics, which will be published in a subsequent number.

May 10th, 1899.

Dr. A. J. HARRISON in the Chair.

Mr. PAUL BUSH showed a boy with a marked displacement of the right scapula, which was raised about 3½ inches and rotated, the lower angle of the bone being situated over the spine of the vertebræ; there was no winged condition of the scapula. He considered the case was one of spasm of the trapezius muscle. A clear skiagram showed that the upper vertebræ were drawn over to the affected side.

Mr. J. LACY FIRTH showed a case of cervical ribs present on both sides, but more conspicuous on the left side. There were some signs of pressure on the brachial plexus and the subclavian artery on the left side.—Mr. ROGER WILLIAMS said a few years ago Prof. Debierre read a paper at the International Medical Congress on " The Human Thorax: is it regressing?"[1] In support of his views, he referred to man's lost cervical and abdominal ribs, regarding specimens such as that shown this evening as due to reversion. The first and the two last ribs were normally of stunted and imperfect formation, indicative of tendency to disappear; and sometimes the first rib had no connection with the sternum, or it was represented only by a fibrous band. The chest muscles, especially the intercostals and those over the ribs, presented signs of regression in the great abundance of their tendinous structures. Similarly the thoracic (dorsal) nerves were seldom complete, for certain of them were wanting in 81 out of 100 cases; and nerve roots were defective in many cases. Mr. Williams had been specially interested in this subject, because his studies in polymastia had independently led him to a similar conclusion, he having shown that man had lost six pairs of mammary glands from the front of the thorax, three from above and three from below the normal pair, and traces of these lost mammæ occasionally reappeared owing to reversion. From the great thickening of the abnormal rib structure in the case exhibited, and from the fact that pressure-symptoms had been noticeable of late, he thought the redundant rib was growing in a very irregular manner; and in many cases irregular osseous growths, like exostoses, had resulted from the abnormal evolution of these formations.

Dr. W. H. C. NEWNHAM showed two specimens from the same patient —a large ovarian cyst, which was pressing on the bladder and rectum (being wedged down in the pouch of Douglas), and a fibroid uterus. The patient, aged 40, had one child thirteen years ago, and was sent by Dr. E. Walker for complete obstruction to micturition and partial obstruction to defecation. The ovarian tumour was distinctly felt in the pouch of Douglas. On April 20th he removed the cyst, also the fibroid uterus, by the operation of intra-peritoneal hysterectomy. The right ovary he left behind, it being apparently healthy. The woman recovered without a bad symptom, and was walking about the ward eighteen days after the operation.—Mr. C. A. MORTON said that evidently the ovarian cyst, which he understood had been supposed to be a myoma before operation, was the cause of the pressure-symptoms, and he did not think any need had been shown for performing hysterectomy. He thought that the mere fact that the abdomen had been opened was not sufficient reason, for the great majority of myomata never caused any trouble at all, and unless they grew very large, or caused pressure-symptoms or serious hemorrhage, there was no need to interfere with them. He quoted from Mr. Bland Sutton's recent papers advising removal of every myoma just as we remove every ovarian cyst, and he contended that a surgeon who did this would be likely to have a run of simple cases, and that his results by the intra-peritoneal method could not be compared with those of surgeons who only operated on very large tumours or those causing pressure-symptoms or serious hemorrhage by the extra-peritoneal method; and he referred to the mortality of one such operator who had had a more successful run of cases by the extra-peritoneal method than Mr. Bland Sutton by the intra-peritoneal. He also pointed out that the mortality in Bland Sutton's twenty-eight cases was 7 per cent., and that this was a high mortality for ovariotomy at the present time, and that therefore the mortality of the intra-peritoneal method

---

[1] *Atti d. xi. Cong. med. internaz.*, 1894, ii. Anat., 12.

could not be said to be the same as that of ovariotomy. Mr. Morton also referred to the dreadful picture of the results of the extra-peritoneal method drawn by Dr. Newnham in his recent paper in the *Journal*,[1] and said he ventured to think it was altogether an exaggeration. He asked, what evidence was there that dragging on a pedicle had ever caused peritonitis? and denied that fetid pus was discharged from the pedicle, or that there was a danger of pus leaking into the peritoneal cavity and causing peritonitis. He asked if there was no possible risk of peritonitis by the intra-peritoneal method from septic infection from the interior of the uterus, and if one could ignore the risk of injury to the ureters in the ligation of the uterine arteries? He did not wish to plead for the extra-peritoneal method in all cases, but mentioned some conditions in which it might be an advantage, and referred to one of his own cases treated by that method, with success, in which the tumour was very large—reaching up to the costal margin,—and in which the operation was rendered difficult by intimate adhesions to the bladder, and an expansion of the broad ligaments so that he was glad to use the serre-nœud.—Dr. JAMES SWAIN said that it was an easy matter to criticise another man's work when the specimen appeared on a plate, but the operator could best determine the right course of action to pursue, for at the time of operation we might consider it desirable to do that which might afterwards appear to others to be unnecessary. Speaking of the removal of fibroid tumours of the uterus in the abstract, he thought that the surgeon who performed hysterectomy in such cases should always be able to give a good reason for his action apart from the mere presence of a tumour. With reference to the battle which was being waged between the extra-peritoneal and the intra-peritoneal treatment of the pedicle in hystero-myomectomy, he felt that statistics were not altogether trust-worthy, especially as such men as Bland Sutton apparently favoured the removal of all myo-fibromata, apart from their size or symptoms. He thought that of more value than statistics was the significant fact that most operators all over the world were now adopting the intra-peritoneal, or rather the retro-peritoneal, method. Thanks to the use of antiseptics, the employment of the clamp in extra-peritoneal hysterectomy had not been attended with such disastrous results as had accompanied the use of the clamp in the early days of ovariotomy. The extra-peritoneal method had been most successful, and he had not seen any of the unpleasant accompaniments which had been said to follow this mode of treatment. Each method appeared to be attended with good results, and he thought that the balance in favour of the intra-peritoneal method was to be looked for not so much in a diminished mortality as in greater precision in operating, a more speedy convalescence, and a lessened tendency to ventral hernia. He had recently adopted the retro-peritoneal method, and would continue to use it in suitable cases, for he regarded it as the operation of the future. At the same time, he had had such successful results with the clamp that he did not think it should be entirely discarded, for he thought there were cases where this method might advantageously be adopted, though not as routine treatment. The question was in a transition stage, and he declined to pin the whole of his faith to a pedicle clamp with the "extra-peritonealists," or to cast it free in the abdomen with the "intra-peritonealists." Our duty was to get the patient well by the best means at our command, and all would prefer to do a successful operation by what might be considered an incomplete technique, rather than to perform a surgically

[1] 1899 xvii. 8.

perfect operation resulting in the death of the patient.—Dr. WALTER SWAYNE was of opinion that it was impossible to say from seeing pathological specimens after operation whether operation was indicated in a particular case or not. It is a matter of experience that the most serious symptoms are not always produced by the largest tumours. He had now under his care a patient suffering from a fibroid which reached nearly to the ensiform cartilage, and was accompanied by profuse hemorrhage; by treatment and natural processes (the menopause) the hemorrhage and general symptoms soon ceased and the tumour retrogressed. The patient refused operation, perhaps wisely. At the same time small tumours produce occasionally very severe symptoms, and in any case when pain produces such disturbance that the patient is prevented from earning her living and her life is made a burden to her, then operative removal is imperative. He thought that if Dr. Newnham had not removed the uterus and the patient's symptoms had been unrelieved, his position as regards the patient would not have been a pleasant one. It appeared to him that the question of what was to be done at the operation must be left to the operator, and could not be settled by the inspection of a specimen previously removed by those unacquainted with the particular symptoms present. —Mr. T. CARWARDINE spoke in favour of the intra-peritoneal method of treatment of the pedicle in hysterectomy. With regard, however, to the extra-peritoneal treatment of the stump, any moisture and suppuration in the stump are usually due to faulty procedure and after-treatment. — Mr. ROGER WILLIAMS thought the term " hysterectomy " ought to be restricted to total extirpation of the uterus. The application of this term to all sorts of other operations comprising partial removal of the uterus tended to produce confusion. Dr. Newnham's case was one of amputation of the myomatous corpus. The small size of the tumours, the fact that the largest of them was connected with the fundus by but a slender pedicle, and that the other two tumours were of sub-peritoneal evolution, led him to ask the author why he had preferred amputation of the uterus to myomectomy, the procedure which Mr. Williams would have preferred, as it would have left the uterus intact, and was safe and efficient. Mr. Williams said it was misleading to compare statistics as to mortality, unless like things were compared with like things. The class of cases a surgeon had to deal with who undertook to remove every myoma, as soon as its presence could be recognised, was totally different from the class of cases that had to be dealt with by those who only operated when urgent symptoms arose. The former had to deal only with small tumours without extensive adhesions, and the mortality from such operations was from 5 to 10 per cent. In these early cases the condition of the uterus and its adnexa differed but little from the normal. In the other class of cases, however, the tumours were often of great size, very vascular, extensively adherent, inflamed and otherwise complicated, so that equally good results could not fairly be anticipated. In most of the former class of cases Mr. Williams thought operation unnecessary and unjustifiable. Hysterectomy, as a conservative operation, was a remedy worse than the disease it was meant to cure.—Dr. NEWNHAM, in reply, said it was a matter of opinion as to whether this was the right operation for this patient. She was complaining, in addition to her other troubles, that she had to keep her bed for ten days every month on account of the uterine hemorrhage. Supposing he had left these fibroid tumours, would she not rightly have returned complaining he had not cured her of her ailments. He did not think it possible that the ovarian cyst was the cause of the hemorrhage. In all probability the myomata would grow to a large size in a woman whose age is only 40. He did not say that it is necessary to remove every myoma, for he had dozens of women attending as out-patients, and not one of them did he propose to operate on, because they had no serious symptoms. Neither did he say that every case that is undertaken must be done by the intra-peritoneal method, each case should be decided on its own merits; but he did think that intra-peritoneal hysterectomy is the operation of the future. He thought that if he had attempted to enucleate these fibroids from the uterus, as Mr. Williams suggested, the hemorrhage would have been more profuse, and, in his opinion, the danger of the operation would be greater than that of intra-peritoneal hysterectomy.

Dr. T. FISHER showed the following specimens:—(1) A pancreas containing several calculi from a man, aged 58, who died in the Bristol Royal Infirmary of senile gangrene. Apparently the calculi had given rise to no symptoms. (2) One of fibroid myocarditis, from a young man, aged 18, who had died suddenly while at work. There was disease of the aortic valves, but no affection of the coronary arteries. The chief points of interest were—firstly, that the fibroid disease was with very little doubt due to rheumatism; and, secondly, that, as so commonly occurs in cases of fibroid disease in later life, the patient died suddenly. (3) A specimen of broncho-pneumonia breaking down into cavities. Dr. Fisher thought that many cases of so-called dilated bronchial tubes are really the sequence of actual lung-destruction consequent upon broncho-pneumonia. (4) Specimens of sarcoma of the cæcum and of the ileum.—Mr. ROGER WILLIAMS said much interest attached to examples of malignant disease of the cæcum and small intestine, on account of their variety. Of 1,066 primary sarcomata tabulated by him, there was not a single instance of sarcoma of the small intestine. In 1892 Madelung reported three cases, and gave references to eleven others. Mermet, in 1896, reported a case of sarcoma of the jejunum in a woman, aged 32, who died the day after resection of the diseased bowel. She suffered from pain and diarrhœa, but not from obstruction. Twenty-three other cases were cited. Since then a few others had been reported. Several cases had been met with in quite young infants. In Stern's patient—an infant only a few days old—the disease presented as polypoid angio-sarcoma of the ileum, which caused death by intestinal obstruction. He thought these polypoid sarcomata generally arose from congenital adenomata of the intestinal mucosa.— Dr. P. WATSON WILLIAMS remarked that dilatation of the bronchial tubes, due to paresis of the muscular coat, was usual in bronchitis of the smaller tubes and broncho-pneumonia, and almost invariably found in fatal cases, and in this way the great majority of dilatations of bronchial tubes originated. In a comparatively few cases, as in the specimen shown by Dr. Fisher, the dilatation was due to the action of various micro-organisms leading to erosion or destruction of the bronchial wall and the neighbouring pulmonary tissue.

Dr. BERTRAM ROGERS showed two microscopic sections of the liver of a child. The patient had been for about eight weeks in the Hospital, when she developed a high temperature and died. The only symptoms were fever, an enlarged liver and slight jaundice. The liver *post mortem* presented a very mottled appearance, parts being fatty and parts very deeply congested, and in places a deep red from hemorrhages. Under the microscope, there were large patches where the liver substance seemed to have disappeared, leaving only a fine reticulum of connective tissue. There were extensive small hemorrhages into the substance of the liver.—Dr. T. FISHER, in connection with this case, showed a drawing he had made of a very similar condition he had found in a case of heart disease.

Dr. E. H. E. Stack showed the following kidney specimens:—Two showed abscesses following bladder disease, one acute, the patient having only lived nine days after he broke his back. Two cases show hemorrhage in the pelvis of the kidney, the first from a case of purpura, under Mr. Munro Smith, in which the source could not be discovered. The patient was a man who had epistaxis, melæna and hæmaturia, as well as exten-sive hemorrhages in skin and muscles. Microscopically, the blood was normal. The second is from a case presented to the Infirmary by St. Bartholomew's Hospital—it is a kidney from bubonic plague. The two specimens are very much alike, the pelvis and ureter being filled with blood-clot. Two cases show adenoma of the kidney—one a single one, and the other multiple small ones. Two cases show hydro-nephrosis—one from stone impacted in the ureter, the other much larger, and for which, although the ureter was found by operation to be quite occluded, no cause could be discovered. Two cases show dilata-tion of the ureters, both from babies. No cause can be assigned for this, as there is no obstruction to the flow of fluid from ureter to bladder. One case of small multiple sarcomata from a child who died of diarrhœa, no other growth found. The last case is one of throm-bosis of the renal vein. The child died of infantile diarrhœa. It is interesting in the light of recent bacteriological research on the streptococcus nature of this variety of diarrhœa. Dr. Symes grew from the clot many colonies of streptococci.

Dr. W. H. C. Newnham read a paper on " Removal of one Ovary—with Cases." The record of the following cases may be of interest, as they include some women who have been under treatment for long periods (occasionally extending to years) by pessaries and various intra-uterine medication without relief. He simply included cases of painful pro-lapsed or inflamed ovary on one side. The operation for the removal of the diseased organ is simple, takes a very short time, and in the cases given below appears to have relieved all the symptoms and changed the patient from a chronic invalid to a worker.

(1) S. J., aged 26, laundry-maid, single. Has suffered with pelvic discomfort for eleven years,—much worse the last six, especially during catamenia. The pain was always on the left side. She had been previously treated with a pessary after some intra-uterine application. On April 7th, 1892, he removed the ovary, enlarged and deeply grooved apparently by the edge of the Hodge's pessary. She left the Hospital well on May 17th, and continues in good health.

(2) K. T., aged 25, unmarried, was admitted complaining of intense pain on the right side and down the right groin. He removed a large cystic and prolapsed ovary of the right side on August 10th, 1892, and the patient left the Hospital well on September 12th.

(3) A. B., aged 28, unmarried, came with a history of gonorrhœa some six years previously. She complained of intense pain in the right ovarian region. He removed a large inflamed right ovary on March 19th, 1898. She left the Hospital well on April 27th, 1898.

(4) F. O., aged 26, married. Had been ill for three years, com-plaining of dyspareunia and menorrhagia. Has had no children. He removed an intensely painful prolapsed ovary on the right side on April 21st, 1898, and patient left the Hospital on May 28th, 1898, quite well. She is now six months pregnant.

(5) M. L., aged 32, waitress, unmarried, with a history of gonorrhœa. Nine years ago she had first child. For the last eight years has been constantly in bed with some inflammatory attacks in the lower

part of the abdomen. *Per vaginam* on right side was felt a swelling, about the size of a small orange, which was acutely painful. He removed the right ovary on December 20th, 1898; it was very large and congested, and the tube itself was much swollen. For the first three days after the operation patient was very sick, in great pain, and distended to an uncomfortable degree. This all subsided under appropriate treatment, and patient left the Hospital quite well on January 17th. She now appears to be in perfect health.

(6) A. J., aged 32, married ten years, has had one child. Has had pain in left groin for twelve years. He removed a large tender and prolapsed ovary on the left side on February 20th, 1899, and she left the Hospital quite well on March 24th, 1899.

(7) M. R., aged 25, single, came with a history of localised peritonitis. On examination he found a large inflamed and apparently adherent ovary on left side This he removed August 20th, 1898, with some difficulty, as the adhesions were very dense all around. Patient, however, recovered without a bad symptom, and left the Hospital on September 28th, 1898, quite well.

(8) J. I., aged 28, had suffered from abdominal pain and discomfort for four years in the region of the left ovary. She is a married woman and has had three children. He removed a cystic ovary from the left side on April 12th, 1899, and patient is now well.

Dr. WALTER SWAYNE considered that there were many useful points. to be noticed in connection with the series of cases. The first case illustrated very well the importance of a correct use of pessaries; it should be an axiom that a pessary should never be used if it pressed on solid visceral structures, *e.g.* uterus or ovary; intra-uterine applications also should be avoided, except after free dilatation and provision for drainage. In any case where symptoms of one-sided tenderness. on pressure, backache, dysmenorrhœa, sterility, and dyspareunia were present, the condition of the ovary, if felt to be enlarged, should be investigated by operation, unless the symptoms were alleviated by rest and local treatment; in a large number of these cases, even when temporary alleviation took place, operation was ultimately necessary. He mentioned a case in which he removed the left ovary from a patient suffering from the above symptoms. On bringing the ovary into the wound it was seen to be cystic: the cysts were punctured, and the fluid contents evacuated; but as the diseased portion proved more than one-half of the ovarian substance, instead of removing the cystic portion from the ovary and returning the remains of the latter after suture, he removed the entire ovary. The patient was able to go home on the twenty-first day after operation, perfectly well. The ovary at present might be seen in the museum.

J. PAUL BUSH, *Hon. Sec.*

Devon and Exeter Medico-Chirurgical Society.

November 18th, 1898.

Dr. P. M. DEAS, President, in the Chair.

The PRESIDENT read a paper on " Sleep-producers and Sedatives." He called attention to the large number of drugs that were on the market, and to the fact that every doctor had his favourite one. Often the drug acted in the way of hypnotic suggestion. The doctor told the patient that he was go ng to give him something that would send him to sleep, and consequently the patient slept. The subject of the treatment of insomnia was most important, as the condition was on the increase. The following varieties of insomnia were distinguished: (1) Psychical or emotional insomnia, due to grief, &c.; (2) insomnia in connection with bodily disorder, such as pain, fever, diseases of the heart or urinary system, eczema, with errors of diet, such as abuse of tea, coffee, or alcohol; (3) insomnia which precedes or follows insanity. These cases are apt not to get treatment sufficiently early. *Physiology of sleep.*—According to the latest theory, the cortical cells or "neurons," and their processes "dendrons," are not in organic connection with the nerves which bring up afferent stimuli and carry away efferent orders. This is important with regard to the views held as to sleep, dreaming, and somnambulism. The essence of sleep is that the neurons are out of action. The telephonic exchange ceases to exist during sleep, and the lower nerve centres in the brain and spinal cord are depressed, together with a general lowering of the vital processes. As to the proximate cause of sleep, there are various theories; namely, that it depends on periodicity, fatigue of brain cells, or increased supply of blood to the brain. The last is certainly not true. There is diminished supply and pressure of blood in the brain due to contraction of vessels. The inhibiting action of the highest centres is in abeyance. Dr. Deas believed that sleep was due to the absorption by neurons from the blood of some material circulating in the blood, and that when a certain amount has accumulated sleep is produced. The conditions which tend to insomnia are—1, excitement and over-action; 2, depression (a) central or mental, (b) peripheral or bodily. In these conditions there is a state of vascular excitement, and the neurons are over-stimulated. The circulation is kept at such a state of tension that the neurons cannot be withdrawn from the irritation of the nerves, and their inhibiting action is still maintained. A drug may act as a sedative, and produce sleep, by putting the body into a more favourable condition for sleep. Unfortunately, nearly all sedatives are heart depressants. A sleep-producer acts directly on the neurons. He then called attention to some of the drugs available. *Bromides* had a remarkable effect in diminishing reflex irritation. Bromide of sodium, gr. 20, with tincture of lupuline ʒ i., was a good combination (at bedtime). In more urgent cases bromides must be given several times a day. In sleeplessness in connection with a rapid neurotic heart, digitalis may be combined with bromides. Bromide of potassium is the most depressing, and so is useful in cases of sexual excitement (with liq. extract of salix nigra). It is very useful in acute mania. *Chloral.*—Dr. Deas did not recommend this drug strongly. Chloral is better as a sleep-producer than as a sedative. It is uncertain and very depressing; occasionally useful when combined with bromides. He laid stress on the importance of only giving sleep-producers at bedtime, and when the conditions are favourable for the production of sleep. *Trional* is a good sleep-producer, and there is very little risk in its use. Grains 25 may be given for 2—3 nights running, and then a smaller dose. *Sulphonal* wants very careful watching. It is a treacherous drug, and is not to be depended upon. It is a powerful sedative, and does best for violent cases of acute mania. It is very useful if given at regular intervals and with proper precautions. It tends to interfere with the secretions, and has a cumulative action. It paralyses the peristaltic action of the bowels. It has a very depressing effect on the nerve-centres, causing ataxia, &c. Aperients are necessary during its use. In conditions of excited circulation with weakness, causing insomnia, do not hesitate to give stimulants with the sedative. In conditions of depression, causing insomnia—such as grief, melancholia, stupor, hypochondriasis, where there are vague feelings of discomfort, and mental pain—the neurons are in a state of irritation, very different from the feeling of comfort and well-being which precedes natural sleep. Here insomnia is well marked, and the depression is much worse during the sleepless hours. *Paraldehyde* is an ideal sleep-producer; it first stimulates the neurons, and then natural sleep is produced with no depression. In cases of melancholia with stupor, paraldehyde has sometimes a remarkable effect. After taking the drug the patient wakes up and talks for about ten minutes, and then falls fast asleep. The dose of paraldehyde is 3 i.; in exceptional cases 3 iij. to 3 iv. may be given, with liquid extract of liquorice to disguise the unpleasant taste. Dr. Deas did not advise drugs in all cases of insomnia. In cases of acute excitement ordinary means may act as well as drugs. The want of sleep is not so important in excited cases as in depressed cases. It may be necessary to prevent struggling, which would otherwise exhaust the patient. In general paralysis some authorities keep their patients during the stage of excitement in a condition of sulphonal intoxication, and so steer them into the haven of dementia. He did not advise the use of morphia or opium for insomnia without pain. These are narcotics, and not sleep-producers. In giving sleep-producers, give a sufficient dose that you think will produce sleep, and only at bedtime, and diminish the dose afterwards. In giving sedatives, begin with a small dose and go on increasing it. It is often more necessary to stimulate than to depress. Sleep is wanted, and not a condition of unconsciousness.

R. V. SOLLY, *Hon. Sec.*

The Library of the Bristol Medico=Chirurgical Society.

The following donations have been received since the publication of the list in March :

May 31st, 1899.

American Dermatological Association (1) ... ... 10 volumes.

Dundee Medical Library (2) ... ... 1 volume.

L. M. Griffiths (3) ... ... 7 volumes.

Editor of *Illustrirte Rundschau der medicinisch-chirur-gischen Technik* (4) ... ... 1 volume.

G. T. Jackson, M.D. (5) ... ... 1 ,,

E. D. Mapother, M.D. (6) ... ... 1 ,,

R. Shingleton Smith, M.D. (7) .. .. 1 ,,

E. H. E. Stack, M.B. (8) ... ... 1 ,,

Surgeon-General, United States Army (9) ... ... 29 volumes.

B. W. Walker, M.D. (10) ... ... 18 ,,

John Wright and Co. (11) ... ... 1 volume.

Unbound periodicals have been received from Mr. L. M. Griffiths. A framed picture has been presented by Mrs. Greig Smith; and unframed pictures have been given by Mr. H. Kerslake, Herr J. F. Lehmann, and Dr. William Warren Potter.

THIRTY-SECOND LIST OF BOOKS.

The titles of books mentioned in previous lists are not repeated.

The figures in brackets refer to the figures after the names of the donors, and show by whom the volumes were presented. The books to which no such figures are attached have either been bought from the Library Fund or received through the *Journal*.

Adams, J. H. ...	*Life of D. Hayes Agnew*	1892
Adams, R.	*Illustrations of Rheumatic Gout* ... ... (8)	1857
Allbutt, T. C. [Ed.]	*A System of Medicine.* Vol. VI.	1899.
Bailey, J. B. ...	*The Diary of a Resurrectionist, 1811–12*	1896
Barbour, A. H. F.	*The Anatomy of Labour* ... ...▲ 2nd Ed.	1899
Bettany, G. T. ...	*Eminent Doctors.* 2 vols. ... . 2nd Ed.	[1885]
Bramwell, B. ...	*Anæmia and Diseases of the Blood-Forming Organs and Ductless Glands*	1899.
Brockbank, E. M.	*The Murmurs of Mitral Disease*	1899
Brown, A. M. ...	*Elements of Alkaloidal Ætiology*	1899.
Bruce, J. M. ...	*Materia Medica and Therapeutics* ... ... [5th Ed.]	1896
Bryce, J.	*On the Inoculation of Cowpox* ... ... 2nd Ed.	1809
Burghard, W. W. Cheyne and F. F. *A Manual of Surgical Treatment.* Part I.		1899
Cheyne and F. F. Burghard, W. W. *A Manual of Surgical Treatment.* Part I.		1899
Crile, G. W. ...	*Surgical Shock* ... ... [1899]	
De Foe, D.	*A Journal of the Plague Year* ... ... [N.D.]	
Evans, A. H. ...	*Golden Rules of Medical Practice* ... ... [1899]	
Feltoe, Rev. C. L.	*Memorials of John Flint South* ... ... (7)	1884
Fernie, W. T. ...	*Animal Simples*	1899.
Floderus, B. ..	*Om Medfödda Uretermissbildningar ur Kirurgisk Synpunkt*	1899
Freeman, E. C. ...	*The Sanitation of British Troops in India*	1899
Hawthorne, C. O.	*Some Aspects of the Mental Discipline Associated with the Study of Medicine*	1899.
Helferich, H. ...	*On Fractures and Dislocations.* (Tr. from 3rd Ed. by J. Hutchinson, jun.)	1899
Herschell, G. ...	*Constipation*	1899
Hime, M. C. ...	*Schoolboys' Special Immorality*	• 1899
Hurst, A. M. Marshall and C. H. *Practical Zoology.* 5th Ed. (Revised by F. W. Gamble)		1899.
Jackson, G. T. ...	*A Dermatological Bibliography* ... ... (5)	1891
Katalog over det Norske Medicinske Selskabs Bibliotek—Tillægs No. 1		1899
Kirkes, [W. S.] ...	*Hand-Book of Physiology.* 15th Ed. (Ed. by W. D. Halliburton)	1899
Leeuwenhoek, A. à	*Opera Omnia.* 4 vols. ... ... Editio Novissima 1719–22	
Mapother, E. D. ...	*Papers on Dermatology, &c.* ... ... (6) 2nd Ed.	1899
Marshall and C. H. Hurst, A. M. *Practical Zoology.* 5th Ed. (Revised by F. W. Gamble)		1899

Moure, E. J. ...	*De la Réunion immédiate du Pavillon de l'Oreille après la Cure radicale de l'Otorrhée*	1899
, ...	*Sur un Cas d'Ostéo-Myélite Aiguë du Temporal consécutive à l'Influenza*	1899
Newsholme, A. ...	*Vital Statistics* ... ... 3rd Ed.	1899
Ogle, J. W. ...	*The Harveian Oration, 1880*	1881
Osler, W.	*The Principles and Practice of Medicine* ... ... 3rd Ed.	1898
Park, R.	*An Epitome of the History of Medicine* ... ... 2nd Ed.	1899
Parke, T. H. ...	*Experiences in Equatorial Africa*	1891
Pedley, R. D. ...	*The Hygiene of the Mouth* ... ... [N.D.]	
Prichard, J. C. ...	*The Natural History of Man.* (Ed. by E. Norris) 2 vols. ... ... 4th Ed.	1855
,, ...	*Celtic Nations.* (Ed. by R. G. Latham)	1857
Ratzel, F.	*The History of Mankind.* (Tr. from 2nd German Ed. by A. J. Butler) 3 vols.	1896-98
Raynalde, T. ...	*The Byrth of Mankinde*	1604
Roberts, C.... ...	*Eastbourne as a Health Resort*...	1899
Rolleston, H. D.	*The Diseases and Primary Tumours of the Thymus Gland* [N.D.]	
Rosenberg, A. ...	*Die Krankheiten der Mundhöhle, des Rachens und des Kehlkopfes* ... ... Zweite Auflage	1899
Sandefjord Svovl- og Sobad i Norge		1899
Savill, T. D. ...	*Neurasthenia*	1899
Schools, A Code of Rules for the Prevention of Infectious and Contagious Diseases in ... ... 4th Ed.		1899
Simpson, J. Y. ...	*Syphilis in Scotland in the 15th and 16th Centuries* ... [1862]	
Sisley, R.	*The London Water Supply*	1899
Smith, E. N. ...	*Growing Children: Their Clothes—and Deformity* ...	1899
Smith, F. W. ...	*The Natural Waters of Harrogate*	1899
Spitta, E. J. ...	*Photo-Micrography*	1899
Therapeutics of Tuberculosis, Bronchitis, and Scrofula ... ... [N.D.]		
Thompson, C. J. S.	*The Mystery and Romance of Alchemy and Pharmacy* ...	1897
,, ...	*Poison Romance and Poison Mysteries*	1899
Tillmanns, H. ...	*A Text-Book of Surgery.* Vols. I. (Tr. from 3rd German Ed. by J. Rogers and B. T. Tilton. Ed. by L. A. Stimson), II., III. (Tr. from 4th German Ed. by B. T. Tilton. Ed. by L. A. Stimson)	1898-99
Tuchmann, M. ...	*The Exploration of the Urethra and Bladder*...	1899
Turner, R.	*Lord Lister and Surgery*	1899
Verworn, M. ...	*General Physiology.* (Tr. from 2nd German Ed. and Ed. by F. S. Lee)	1899
Whitelegge, B. A.	*Hygiene and Public Health* ... ... [8th Ed.]	1899
Williams, C. J. B.	*Memoirs of Life and Work*	1884

TRANSACTIONS, REPORTS, JOURNALS, &c.

Alienist and Neurologist, The... ... ... Vol. XIX. 1898
American Dermatological Association, Transactions of the (1) 1878, 1879, 1886, 1889-93, 1896-98
American Gynæcological and Obstetrical Journal, The Vols. XI., 1897, XIII., 1898

American Journal of Obstetrics, The ... ...   Vol. XXXVIII.   1898
American Journal of Ophthalmology, The ... ...   Vol. XV.   1898
American Ophthalmological Society, Transactions of the...   Vol. VIII.,
                                                            Part 2   1898
American Pediatric Society, Transactions of the   ... ...   Vol. X.   1898
American Practitioner and News, The... ... ...   Vols. XXV., XXVI.   1898
American Year-Book of Medicine and Surgery, The...   1899
Annales de la Société Belge de Chirurgie ... ...   Tome VI.   1898
Annali di Ostetricia e Ginecologia...   1898
Annual and Analytical Cyclopædia of Practical Medicine   ... Vol. III.   1899
Archiv für Verdauungs-Krankheiten ... ...   Band IV.   1898
Archives of Surgery ... ... Vol IX.   1898
Archives provinciales de Chirurgie   ... ...   Tome VII.   1898
Australasian Medical Gazette, The   ... ...   Vol. XVII.   1898
Bristol and Clifton Directory ... ... (11)   1899
Bristol Medico-Chirurgical Journal, The   ... ...   Vol. XVI.   1898
Buffalo Medical and Surgical Journal, The... (9) Vols. XX.—XXVI.   1881-87
Bulletin de l'Académie de Médecine   3e Sér., Tomes XXXIX., XL.   1898
Bulletin de l'Académie royale de Médecine de Belgique ...   Tome XII.   1898
Canadian Practitioner, The ... ...   Vol. XXIII.   1898
Centralblatt für Chirurgie   1888,   1898
Centralblatt für Gynäkologie   1877-92,   1898
Centralblatt für innere Medicin   1898
Cincinnati Lancet and Clinic, The   ... ... (9) Vols. XL.—LI.   1878-84
Cincinnati Lancet-Clinic, The   ... ... Vol. LXXX.   1898
College of Physicians of Philadelphia, Transactions of the   3rd Ser.,
                                                            Vol. XX.   1898
Dublin Journal of Medical Science, The   (3) Vols. LXIX., 1880, LXXI.   1881
Écho médical du Nord, L'   1898
Food Journal, The ... ...   (3) Vols. I.—IV.   1871-74
France médicale, La   1898
Gazette des Hôpitaux de Toulouse   1897,   1898
Gazette hebdomadaire des Sciences médicales de Bordeaux   Tome XIX.   1898
Gazzetta Medica Lombarda   1898
General Medical Council, Minutes of the   ... ... Vol. XXXV.   1899
Hospitals—
     Middlesex Hospital, The—Registrars' Reports for 1897   1898
Illustrirte Rundschau der medicinisch-chirurgischen Technik   ... (4)   1898
Intercolonial Medical Journal of Australasia   ... ... Vol. III.   1898
International Medical Magazine ... ...   Vol. VII.   1898
Journal d'Hygiène ... ...   Vol. XXIII.   1898
Journal of Laryngology, Rhinology, and Otology, The   ...   Vol. XIII.   1898
Journal of Mental Science, The   Vols. (10) XIX.—XXII., 1874-77;
                          (2) XXV., 1880; (10) XXVI.—XXXVII.,
                                1881-91, XXXIX., 1893, XLI.,   1895
Journal of the American Medical Association, The ... ...   Vol. XXXI.   1898
Laryngoscope, The ... ...   Vols. IV., V.   1898
Library, The   ... ...   Vol. X.   1898
Liverpool Medico-Chirurgical Journal, The   ... ...   Vol. XVIII.   1898
Medical Age, The   ... ...   Vol. XVI.   1898

Medical Annual, The 1899
Medical Chronicle, The ... ... N.S., Vol. X. 1898-99
Medical Defence, A Year's Work in (1898)... ... ... [1899]
Medical Officer of the Privy Council, 11th Report of the... ... ... (3) 1869
Montreal Medical Journal, The ... ... Vol. XXVII. [1898]
Newquay Urban District Council—Annual Report of the Medical
  Officer of Health 1898
New York Journal of Gynæcology and Obstetrics, The Vols. I., II. 1891-92
New York Medical Journal, The (9) Vols. V., 1867, IX.—XII., 1869-70,
    XIV., 1871, XIX.—XXII., 1874-75; LXVIII., 1898
Nord médical, Le ... ... Tome IV. 1898
Northumberland and Durham Medical Journal, The 1898
Nursing Directory, Burdett's Official 1899
Occidental Medical Times ... ... Vol. XII. 1898
Post-Graduate, The ... ... Vol. XIII. [1898]
Preparations, Annual Report on New Medicinal, 1898 1899
Progrès médical, Le ... ... 3° Sér., Tome VIII. 1898
Revue de Thérapeutique médico-chirurgicale 1896, 1898
Revue générale d'Ophtalmologie ... ... Tome XVII. 1898
Revue hebdomadaire de Laryngologie, d'Otologie, et de Rhinologie
            Tome XVIII. 1898
Revue médicale, La 1898
Revue médico-chirurgicale des Maladies des Femmes ... Tome XIX. 1897
Sanitary Record, The ... ... · ... ... Vol. XXII. 1898
Society of Medical Officers of Health, Transactions of the 1885-87
Therapeutic Gazette, The ... ... Vol. XXII. 1898
Treatment ... ... Vol. II. 1899
Wiener klinische Wochenschrift 1898
Zeitschrift für Krankenpflege 1898

Local Medical Notes.

ABERGAVENNY.

MONMOUTHSHIRE ASYLUM.—During the year 1897 this asylum increased the number of its patients by 37, and on the last day of the year it contained 1,012. Of the year's admissions 18 owed their insanity to moral causes, 21 to intemperance in drink, 45 to hereditary influence, and 42 to previous attacks. Courses of lectures on nursing are given by the medical officers, and eighteen of the staff entered for the examination of the Medico-Psychological Association, and seventeen of them obtained the nursing certificate. The committee express their "high appreciation of the services of Dr. Glendinning and his able assistants, Dr. Nelis and Dr. Black." At the meeting of the Monmouthshire County Council, held on May 3rd, it was decided to purchase at an approximate cost of £8,000 a farm adjacent to the county asylum for purposes of further development.

BARNSTAPLE.

PUBLIC HEALTH.—Mr. M. R. Gooding has been re-appointed Medical Officer to the Port Sanitary Authority.

. . ... BATH.

ROYAL UNITED HOSPITAL.—At the Guildhall, Bath, under the presidency of the Mayor, the annual meeting of the Governors and others interested in the Bath Royal United Hospital was held. According to the report the number of in-patients that had been treated was 1,190, whilst in 1897 the number was 1,264. The out-patients numbered 8,209, whilst during the previous year the number was 8,988. An increase of subscriptions from factories and workshops was shown; but there had been a falling off in subscriptions and donations during the past year. Several improvements have been effected, the operating theatre and the new chapel having been refurnished and kitchens constructed.

EYE INFIRMARY.—At the annual meeting of the Governors of the Bath Eye Infirmary, the report showed that against 262 in-patients treated during 1897, 208 were admitted during the past year. £245, the amount of legacies received, and the balance in hand, which was a good one, had been carried to the capital account.

ROYAL MINERAL WATER HOSPITAL.—The annual meeting of this institution was held on May 1st, under the presidency of General Mainwaring. The report showed that during the past year 1350 patients had been admitted, the largest number in the history of the hospital; the average number in the hospital was 150, and the average stay of each was 40 days. The expenditure amounted to £5,514 and exceeded the income by £142. The balance in hand was £527. Colonel Vaughan was elected president for the ensuing year.

BRISTOL.

HOSPITAL SUNDAY FUND.—In our last number we stated that the collection this year on behalf of the Medical Charities would exceed that of 1898, and we are pleased to say that about £500 more was obtained. This must be very gratifying to the organisers, who certainly worked very hard to make the fund a success. In only the second year of its existence, that the collections in the numerous places of worship in our city should contribute £1500 is good, but when compared with what is accomplished in other towns it is evident that much remains to be done to stimulate interest in our medical charities and their impoverished condition. Comparing the lists of last year and of this, it is a curious fact, and one of which no explanation has yet been given, that while the money received from Church of England churches is less than previously, that from Nonconformists has increased. It may be that the Nonconformist conscience has been awakened; if so, we hope that the Established conscience will be awakened next year.

ANNUAL REPORTS OF MEDICAL CHARITIES.—Since March all the Medical Charities have published their annual reports, and in all of them there is the same cry for more subscribers to carry on the work. The ever increasing debt of these institutions is a very serious matter, and must be faced. Several of them have employed legacies to pay current expenses—a proceeding which does not meet with the approval of every-one; but when the income year by year fails to meet the expenditure, something of this kind must be done.

THE PREVENTION OF CONSUMPTION.—The Committee mentioned in our last number have been at work, but not much progress has been made beyond a most excellent report on the condition of the city from a medical and legal point of view presented by Dr. Davies. We believe that this will be printed in the Medical Officer's annual report, so that at least every medical man as well as town councillor will have an opportunity of seeing how much consumption there is in Bristol now as compared with forty years ago; and how we are still in a very impotent state as regards the inspection of meat or dairies. We regret that so little interest has been shown outside our profession in the matter, but it may be aroused later.

THE JUBILEE CONVALESCENT HOME will be opened, according to present arrangements, by the Queen in November. The Committee has got so far as to elect a Medical Officer, and out of a large number of candidates chose Mr. John S. Griffiths for the post. The interior is still undergoing alterations.

OBITUARY.—It is with deep regret that we learn that the plague in India has caused the death of Dr. Fenton Evans, who was some years ago a very able Medical Tutor at the School, and afterwards House Physician at the Royal Infirmary.

BURNHAM.

PUBLIC HEALTH. — Dr. F. C. Berry has been re-appointed Medical Officer of Health.

CARDIFF.

PUBLIC HEALTH.—Dr. E. M. Spencer has been appointed Medical Officer to the Penarth Sanitary District. Dr. R. Mathias has been appointed Medical Officer for the Pentyrch Sanitary District.

THE INFIRMARY.—At a meeting of the Cardiff Infirmary, held on April 12th, under the presidency of Dr. Edwards, it was decided that a sub-committee should report upon the proposed reception of paying patients in the institution. . A recommendation of the medical board that no member of the honorary staff should hold office longer than twenty years was deferred for future consideration. It was decided that the supply of milk to the infirmary should be only from cows certified to be free from tuberculosis. Legacies to the amount of £2,100 have been recently received by the institution, and the reverse balance is now reduced to £2,900. A resolution was proposed at a special meeting of the governors that a deputation should approach the Mayor and County Council of Cardiff with a view to obtaining a grant of not less than £500 a year from the Council to the Infirmary towards maintenance expenses; but the resolution was rejected by a majority of ten.

PROPOSED SEAMEN'S HOSPITAL.—The Mayor of Cardiff has embarked upon a useful and praiseworthy scheme; namely, that of building and organising a Seamen's Hospital for the town. Already the sum of £16,500, including a generous donation of £10,000 from Lord Bute, has been raised, but £5,500 more are required before the work can be proceeded with. Cardiff is a wealthy town, and there is every probability that this sum will soon be forthcoming. Moreover, the object is so good a one that there can be no excuse for those able to do so from withholding their liberal support. The important shipping centre which the town has now become makes the needs of a Seamen's Hospital almost imperative, and hence the activity and enthusiasm displayed by the townspeople in the Mayor's enterprise. It is proposed to hold a bazaar in aid of the building fund in December next. We wish the new charity every success.

CONVALESCENT HOME.—The annual meeting of those interested in this institution was held at the Cardiff Town Hall on April 24th, under the presidency of the Mayor, Alderman T. Morel. The report showed that the receipts in 1898 were £1,453, and the expenditure amounted to £1,109. There still remains a deficit balance of £2,500 on the extension fund. There were 738 patients admitted, the average period for which each remained in the Home being seventeen days. The cost of maintenance was 1s. 5d. per head per day. It was decided that a special committee should be appointed to devise means for raising funds to remove the debt upon the building.

DISTRICT NURSING.—The ninth annual report of the Cardiff Branch of Queen Victoria's Jubilee Institute for Nurses has been issued. The Honorary Treasurer, Dr. Sheen, reports that the total cost of this excellent work was £888 9s. 6d., which was raised by various methods.

CARMARTHEN.

PUBLIC HEALTH.—The decision at the last quarterly meeting of the Carmarthenshire County Council to set up a Sanitary Committee, to whom is delegated the question of securing the appointment of a County Medical Officer of Health, is a long delayed step which will eventually bring this County Authority in line with its compeers throughout the country in matters of public health.

OBITUARY.—The death of Mr. James Rowlands in his eighty-fifth year occurred on April 10th. He received his medical training at St, George's Hospital, London, and was believed to be the oldest St. George's man living. For forty years he was surgeon to the prison at Carmarthen, and for many years also surgeon to the local infirmary. He was Coroner for a long period, and an Alderman and J.P. He was deeply respected and beloved by all classes of the community, and remained in practice until illness compelled him to retire about six months ago. He married in 1835, and celebrated his diamond wedding in January, 1895.

CHELTENHAM.

PUBLIC ABATTOIRS.—The Medical Officer of Health for Cheltenham, Dr. J. H. Garrett, refers to the abattoirs question in his report for 1898. He asserts that it is not only nor chiefly to avoid a nuisance from filth and general insanitary conditions, such as may be prevented to a great extent by by-laws, that private slaughter-houses should give way to public abattoirs, but rather in order that the very necessary inspection of animals intended for slaughter, and of their organs and carcasses after slaughter, and of their mode of slaughter, should be rendered possible, and the seizure or setting aside of the flesh and parts of diseased animals. be facilitated.

TUBERCULOSIS.—Dr. Garrett points out that it would be misleading to the public to grant a Corporation certificate, which would be taken as a guarantee of the freedom of the products of a dairy from the germs of tuberculosis, whilst in reality our knowledge of the subject does not at present admit of the possibility of any such guarantee. This has prevented him hitherto advising the use of certificates in his district.

DEVIZES.

PUBLIC HEALTH.—Dr. Leonard Raby has been appointed Medical Officer of Health, vice Mr. E. N. Carless, deceased. Mr. J. T. Thomas. has been appointed Medical Officer of Health for Wiltshire.

DEVONPORT.

PUBLIC HEALTH.—Mr. H. Gard has been appointed Medical Officer for the Northern Sanitary District.

ROYAL ALBERT HOSPITAL.—A scheme has been prepared for extending and improving the Royal Albert Hospital at an estimated cost of £4,000.

ISOLATION HOSPITAL.—The Devonport Town Council at their meeting on April 13th decided to endeavour to purchase seven acres of land adjoining the Infectious Diseases Hospital, which was built in 1882, and is in need of enlargement.

EXETER.

DEVON AND EXETER HOSPITAL.—The special meeting of Governors of the Devon and Exeter Hospital dealt with a large number of questions of vital interest to all institutions of the kind. The Devon and Exeter Hospital has experienced a large amount of criticism recently, and a complete inquiry into its financial condition has taken place. At the meeting it was proposed to close one large ward, to decrease the yearly deficit. Discussion brought out the fact that the capital of the Hospital equalled upwards of £100,000, from which a yearly income of £3,000 was derived. In the face of this fact, a resolution in favour of resorting to other means of diminishing the adverse balance was passed, and it was also decided that a reinvestment of the capital should be considered. A proposal to open a paying ward did not receive much attention, and another suggestion for the more satisfactory admission of patients met with no definite result. Nevertheless, the meeting showed that amongst the governing body a distinct advancement has been made in realising the measures which tend generally towards progress and judicious administration.

WEST OF ENGLAND EYE INFIRMARY.—The foundation stone of the new West of England Eye Infirmary was laid by Mr. Franklin on April 11th, after a short service by the Bishop of Crediton. This infirmary was founded in 1808, and was the second in the United Kingdom devoted exclusively to diseases of the eye. In 1895 it was decided to entirely rebuild the institution, and property adjoining the infirmary was purchased for that purpose. The section now commenced will cost about £8,500, towards which £7,500 has been raised.

THE PREVENTION OF CONSUMPTION.—A useful leaflet, entitled *Advice on the Prevention of Consumption*, has just been issued for circulation among the people by the Health Department of Exeter, of which Dr. John Woodman is the Medical Officer of Health, and Drs. Edward A. Brash, George T. Clapp, and John Mackeith the Assistant Medical Officers.

EXMOUTH.

DISPENSARY. — Dr. J. Shapland has been appointed Medical Officer, *vice* Mr. Reginald Martyn, resigned.

FALMOUTH.

PUBLIC HEALTH.—Dr. W. K. Bullmore has been re-appointed Medical Officer of Health to the Falmouth and Truro Port Sanitary Authority.

GLOUCESTER.

PUBLIC HEALTH.—The report of the Medical Officer of Health (Dr. Campbell) of the Gloucester Urban Sanitary Authority for 1898 has just been issued. Dr. Campbell estimates the total population of the city at 41,450, an increase of 284 in the year. The births numbered 1315—688 males and 627 females—compared with 1336 in the previous year. The rate is 31·7 per 1000, compared with 32·6 per 1000. There were 694 deaths as compared with 726, a rate of 16·7 as compared with 17·6 in the previous year. Dealing with the water supply, the report states that the three sources of supply now available are capable of providing twenty gallons per head per day for double the population now supplied. On the whole, the supply generally will, it is stated, compare favourably with that of the best supplied towns; and the only fault that can be found is that the Witcombe and Robinshood Hill supplies are not sand filtered as well as decanted, and that the Newent supply is not chemically softened.

GLOUCESTER GENERAL INFIRMARY AND GLOUCESTER EYE INSTI-
TUTION.—At a quarterly meeting of this institution, held on March 30th,
under the presidency of Colonel Curtis Hayward, the Chairman stated
that during the past ten years the expenditure of the Infirmary had
increased by £1,000 a year, while the income had only increased by
£200.

DISTRICT NURSING.—The annual meeting of the Gloucester District
Nursing Society has been held, under the presidency of the Dean.
There was a good attendance, and the novelty of the proceedings
was an address on the subject of "District Nursing" by Mrs. Clare
Goslett. The Chairman, in addressing the meeting, remarked that
general approval was sometimes not so profitable as a little wholesome
abuse. Everyone approved of this most needful and helpful institution,
but at the present moment they were from £30 to £40 to the bad. It
has been decided to buy a house for the use of the nurses. The
hon. secretary's report also contained a strenuous appeal for a larger
income. The committee deplore the loss, by death, of Dr. Ancrum,
vice-president of the Society since its institution, and of Miss Taynton,
an energetic colleague.

ISLES OF SCILLY.

MEDICAL MAGISTRATE.—Dr. T. Thornton Macklin, Medical Officer of
Health for Scilly, has been appointed to the Commission of the Peace for
the Isles of Scilly in the County of Cornwall.

KEYNSHAM.

PUBLIC HEALTH.—Mr. F. W. S. Stone has been appointed Medical
Officer for the Sanitary District of Kelston and Northstoke.

LOOE.

PUBLIC HEALTH.—Dr. J. E. Webb has been re-appointed Medical
Officer of Health.

MAESTEG.

ACTION FOR LIBEL.—At the Glamorganshire Assizes, held on
March 21st, before Mr. Justice Darling, a libel action was brought
against Dr. John Davies, of Maesteg, by Dr. W. H. Thomas, J.P., of
the same place. The cause of the action was the publication of a
letter to the Bridgend Board of Guardians and also to a local newspaper, in which defendant complained of the absence of professional
etiquette on the part of the plaintiff. The plaintiff claimed £1,000
damages. Eventually the defendant withdrew absolutely the statement which he had made against Dr. Thomas. In the result a juror
was withdrawn.

We regret to record the sudden death of Dr. Thomas on April 13th.

MERTHYR-TYDVIL.

PUBLIC HEALTH.—The Medical Officer of Health (Mr. Dyke) reports
that during 1898 there were 2495 births registered, giving a rate of 34·7;
of these 73, equivalent to a rate of 2·92, were illegitimate. Vaccinations
were performed in 1870 instances by public vaccinators. There were
1409 deaths, compared with 1598 in 1897, equal to a rate of 19·5 per
1000, which is the lowest rate ever recorded in the district. The present
population is 71,903, with 12,912 occupied houses.

MIDSOMER NORTON.

PUBLIC HEALTH.—Mr. A. H. Whicher has been re-appointed
Medical Officer of Health.

NEWPORT.

PUBLIC HEALTH.—The Sanitary Committee of the Corporation has decided to continue for another term of five years the old system of dealing with street and trade refuse; viz., by tipping it on scavenging heaps instead of purchasing and erecting refuse destructors. Inquiries as to the taking of further land for cemetery purposes have brought in a valuation of ten acres of land belonging to Lord Tredegar at £8,750, in addition to the cost which would be imposed for drainage.

NEWTON ABBOT.

PUBLIC HEALTH.—Mr. H. Goodwyn has been re-appointed Medical Officer for the Islington Sanitary District. Mr. R. H. Grimbly has been re-appointed Medical Officer for the Ipplepen Sanitary District. Mr. A. E. Hayward has been appointed Medical Officer for the Teignmouth Sanitary District.

PENZANCE.

VACCINATION.—At the meeting of the Penzance Board of Guardians, held on April 13th, it was stated that £102 would be paid for vaccination fees in the western district of the union, as compared with £15 paid for the whole union in the corresponding quarter of last year. One of the members thought that the names of persons vaccinated by the public vaccinator should be published.

PLYMOUTH.

BOROUGH ASYLUM.—At a meeting of the Plymouth Town Council, held on May 8th, the report for 1898 of the Visiting Committee of the Plymouth Borough Asylum at Blackadown was presented. This stated that the result of the recent controversy between the Guardians and the Council with regard to the weekly rate charged for pauper patients from Plymouth was that the Council in future would pay £1000 a year extra and the Guardians £1000 per annum less than formerly. The weekly maintenance rate of patients had been reduced from 12s. 1d. to 11s. 2d.

PROPOSED HOME FOR INCURABLES.—At an influential meeting, held at Plymouth on March 29th, it was decided to establish a Home for Incurable Patients at Plymouth, and a committee was appointed to prepare a scheme for the purpose to be submitted to a public meeting to be held shortly.

PONTYPRIDD.

PUBLIC HEALTH.—Mr. D. N. Morgan has been appointed Medical Officer to the Tonyrefail and Gilfach Sanitary District.

PORTISHEAD.

SEWERAGE SCHEME.—These works have been completed, and the house connections are being rapidly proceeded with. The sewage, without treatment of any kind, is discharged into the river Severn at a point about a third of a mile from the shore. Valves are provided to keep the sea water out of the sewers; and the low-level sewers are distinct from the high-level, the sewage having to be lifted from the former to the latter. The total length of main sewers on the high and low levels is about eight miles. The whole works cost, approximately, £16,500.

SWANSEA.

SWANSEA HOSPITAL.—Mr. C. N. Chadborn has been appointed House Surgeon.

DIPHTHERIA EPIDEMIC.—In the recent diphtheria epidemic at Swansea a good effect was produced by closing the elementary schools.

TAUNTON.

TAUNTON AND SOMERSET HOSPITAL.—Dr. A. C. Anderson has been appointed Assistant House-Surgeon.

TAVISTOCK.

RESPIRATORY DISORDERS AMONG ARSENIC WORKERS.—Since the decline of the copper and tin mining industries in Cornwall, a number of arsenic works have been in operation on the sites of the old mines, and the attention of the Tavistock Board of Guardians has been directed to the large number of persons employed at these works who have been disabled and have come upon the parish for support. Dr. C. C. Brodrick, Medical Officer of Health for the Tavistock Rural District, and Dr. Albert Bowhay, Medical Officer of Health for the Calstock Rural District, at the request of the Board, have investigated the state of affairs in the parish of Calstock, and find that a large number of persons once employed at the arsenic works are in receipt of parish relief, and are suffering from respiratory diseases attributed to the effect of arsenic fumes. They have also discovered that out of 100 persons employed at these works who have died in the last three years, 83 have died of respiratory diseases. On visiting the works they observed that the furnace men used no protection at all, while the millers and grinders had the mouth and nostrils covered only with lint and a handkerchief. They recommend the use of a wire mask covered with gauze by all those employed at the works. The Board of Guardians have sent copies of this report to the managers of the works, and also to the Local Government Board. These two medical officers have for many years been familiar with the arsenic works, and are well acquainted with the medical history of the workers, so that their opinion is deserving of serious consideration. (For further information relating to this subject, see *British Medical Journal,* April 15th, 1899, p. 926.)

TOTNES.

NEW HOSPITAL.—At the meeting of the subscribers of the Totnes (Devon) Cottage Hospital, held on March 22nd, under the presidency of the Mayor (Dr. G. J. Gibson), the Duke of Somerset's offer of a site for a new hospital at Bridgetown was gratefully accepted, and it was decided to advertise for plans for the new building.

TROWBRIDGE.

PUBLIC HEALTH.—At a special meeting of the Urban Council held last week, consideration was given to the question of the proposed formation of an isolation hospital district for the urban district, the Melksham urban district, and the rural district of the Melksham union. A resolution against joining the hospital district was passed unanimously.

TRURO.

PUBLIC HEALTH.—At the meeting of the Sanitary Committee of the Cornwall County Council, held at Truro on April 13th, under the presidency of the Hon. John Boscawen, Mr. Martyn drew attention to the desirability of appointing a Medical Officer of Health for the County. The chairman agreed as to the necessity of such an appointment, and upon his motion a sub-committee was elected to act.

TUBERCULOSIS.—The Medical Officer of Health for Truro Union (Dr. Bonar), in his report to the Sanitary Committee, recently referred at length to tuberculosis in cows, and stated that one cow's milk with tubercle mixed with the milk of twenty healthy cows would contaminate the whole. He also referred to the importance of the tuberculin test, and said it would be an advantage to every milk purveyor to be able to say that his dairy was free from suspicion. Commenting on the report, Dr. Bonar said he thought that all dairies from which milk was brought to Truro should have their cows tested. Those who lived by milk-selling ought to be able to say they had had their animals tested, and that these were free from tubercle. Dr. Bonar said the time was coming when no one in Truro or anywhere else would buy milk from cows that had not passed the test.

CORNWALL NURSING ASSOCIATION.—The Earl of Mount Edgcumbe presided at the annual meeting of the Cornwall County Nursing Association, recently held at Truro. There was a large and influential attendance. The village nurses, trained by the Association free of cost to themselves, have been started with a view to meet the want of trained nursing in scattered rural districts, where it is impossible to raise the sum required to maintain a Queen's nurse. The minimum time required for training village nurses is six months, but the Executive Committee have decided in some instances to allow twelve months instead, so as to better qualify them for their work. These nurses are required to pass the examination of the London Obstetrical Society, and to obtain its certificates. Arrangements have been made to give the village nurses six months' additional training in the South Devon and East Cornwall Hospital, Plymouth, and the Royal Cornwall Infirmary, Truro, subject to certain conditions. The Association has now altogether expended £229 on the training of nurses, and has received a grant of £100 from the Cornwall Technical Education Committee.

WEYMOUTH.

PUBLIC HEALTH.—Mr. James Nimmo has been appointed Public Analyst to the Borough of Weymouth and Melcombe Regis.

A Memorial to Dr. Joseph O'Dwyer.

A representative committee has been formed for the purpose of doing honour to the memory of Dr. Joseph O'Dwyer. Dr. Geo. F. Shrady has been elected permanent Chairman, and Dr. Alfred Meyer permanent Secretary, and the following Committee on Scope and Plan was appointed: Dr. Dillon Brown, Chairman, and Drs. Robert Abbe, R. G. Freeman, L. Emmet Holt, and Louis Fischer. The memorial will probably take an educational form.

The "Index Medicus."

The announcement has just been made that with the current number the *Index Medicus* will cease to exist. The death of this periodical will be an irreparable loss, as during the twenty-one years of its able editorship it has become an indispensable necessity in the field of medicine. Some steps must be taken to continue it under under new conditions. We are not in a position to say how this can be done; but as the question is a cosmopolitan one, some scheme by which the great medical institutions and societies of all countries could become guarantors ought not to be an impossibility. Could not the Royal Colleges of the United Kingdom take the initiative in the matter?

SCRAPS

Clinical Records (27).—This excellent story has been recently revived :—
" A well-known Archbishop of Dublin was, towards the end of his life, at a dinner
given by the Lord-Lieutenant of Ireland. In the midst of the dinner the
company was startled by seeing the Archbishop rise from his seat, looking
pale and agitated, and crying, ' It has come—it has come ! ' ' What has come,
your Grace ? ' eagerly cried half-a-dozen voices from different parts of the
table. ' What I have been expecting for some years—a stroke of paralysis,'
solemnly answered the Archbishop. ' I have been pinching myself for the
last ten minutes, and find my leg entirely without sensation.' ' Pardon me
my dear Archbishop,' said the hostess, looking up to him with a quizzical
smile, ' pardon me for contradicting you, but it is my leg you have been
pinching ! ' "

Medical Satire.—A friend has kindly supplied me with the following :—
Wisdom ceases not to be wisdom when it pleases her to assume the cap
and bells of Folly ; hence much profit can be derived from a perusal of the
recently-issued " Comic Number " of the *Münchener medicinische Wochenschrift*, if
readers, to borrow an expression from Rabelais, are wise enough " rompre l'os.
et sugcer la substantifique moelle."
Amongst the advertisements are to be seen : " Iodosanin," a new remedy
for syphilis, wherein the iodine is so firmly secured no power on earth can
release it ; the organism is therefore protected against it ; it is guaranteed to
produce no iodism, *nor any other effect*.—Girls suffering from Dramatic
Neurosis are thoroughly cured at the establishment of Schmierfink [Oily-
tongue], Theatrical Manager, Vienna.—" Medical Assistant wanted for
Hospital ; " Salary £25 per annum, with board and lodging ; a deduction
of £22 15s. is made for attendance ; liable to dismissal at a month's notice,
but Assistant is otherwise bound for two years.—" Doctors required for a
Club." Salary about 10d. a day ; every other Good Friday a half-holiday ;
responsibility small, as every prescription is duly examined by the lay Committee, and if necessary corrected. Quacks and pot-house practitioners
excluded, as the expense for soap and water would be too great.—" Exoteric
Food for Invalids." This needs merely to be shown to the patients ; strongly
recommended, on the score of economy, to Hospitals and Infirmaries.—
" Artificial Assistants." These are of glass and iron, with electrical and steam
motive power ; the surgical ones are transparent, sterilisable, call out " Lint,"
" Sponge," and then use them.
There is an original article by Dr. Michael Squirt on " The Artificial
Production of Unsexual Generation in Man." Struck with Tolstoi's suggestion in the *Kreutzersonate*, that the actual method of generation, so crude, so
coarse, is quite unworthy of our modern refinement and culture, the writer
tries a lymph prepared by him from Protozoa that propagate by self-division.
He experiments, by subcutaneous injection near the shoulder-blade, upon a
wealthy banker, married, childless, eagerly desirous of an heir. Two heads
soon form and complete themselves ; but as each now claims to be the
original banker and denounces the other for a scoundrel who is seeking to get
possession of immense wealth and a handsome wife not his own, the dialogue
grows animated. Finally two complete men are formed, to the utter
bewilderment of the ever-watchful mother-in-law. Not to be outwitted, she
too resolves on sub-division, and is injected accordingly. Division into four
perfect individuals ensues. These now enter the bankers' mansion arm-in-arm.
At the sight of the common enemy, the bankers blench with terror and
collapse in a death-like swoon.—Dr. Pantschenberger's article, " A New
Method of Feeding Infants," is admirable satire. The writer starts by
condemning natural milk in every form, mother's milk included ; maintains
that modern Chemistry can in this matter excel Nature herself ; and advances
elaborate arguments in support of his thesis. He accordingly opens an
experimental klinik with twenty-one infants, fourteen from three weeks to two

months old, and seven from four to ten months These are fed with the doctor's artificial food exclusively. Results: Twelve out of fourteen of the former perish of inveterate stomachic affections; there are hopes three of the latter seven may survive the year. Now, the Professor's sunny optimism is by no means overclouded by these results, apparently so unfavourable; on the contrary, inasmuch as the preparation contains every element that is needful for the reparation and growth of the infantile organism, Nature is manifestly in error. "Let us but hold fast to Theory," says he, "Experience must and will give way!"—The article, "A Triumph of Modern Surgery," by Professor Swindel of Mississippi College, is aimed at the extravagant hardihood of Quixotic operators. The case is as follows: A young German, engaged for two and a half years in a paint-factory in America, falls ill. Symptoms: Several times a day the stomach, after premonitory noises—rolling, gurgling, gulping,—discharges its fluid contents. Great thirst supervenes, but the drinking of fluids only aggravated the evil. As no treatment relieves, Dr. Swindel boldly determines to excise the stomach and substitute a swine's. The operation is performed. Then in the stomach is discovered the cover of a beer jug, swallowed in student days and long forgotten. Complete success. Healing *per primam*. In the exuberance of restored health, the young man shortly afterwards climbs a lamp-post, which snaps off and flings him to the ground, the lamp descending with terrific force upon his occiput and causing compound fracture of the skull Brought almost *in articulo mortis* into Dr. Swindel's klinik, a hasty examination reveals the skull-cavity all but empty, the brain-matter having been lost through the wound. As a desperate resort, a calf's brain is planted therein, with the happiest results. The patient recovers: every mental operation is soon normal. He quits the paint-business and turns art-critic with marked distinction. "This brilliant success," says the writer, "secures for brain-transplantation an enduring place in surgery."

New Books received:—

> Alois Strampfer. *The Most Common Forms of Injury arising from Cycling —to Foot-passengers.* Leipzig. 1898.
>
> G. Sorcier. *Acceleration of the Mental Development of New-born Infants by Inoculation with Extract from the Pituitary Gland.* Paris. 1898.
>
> John Grudger. *The Morbid Sensibility of the English—particularly in Reference to the Naval Advancement of Other Nations.* London. 1898.
>
> Paolo Firlefanzi. *The Voluntary Procreation of Twins.* Firenze. 1898.

Contributions in verse occupy about half the number. Of these, the best perhaps is the short epigram, "The Mistaken Examination," concerning a physician whose custom is to look for fever *per anum*.

At the sitting of the Medical Association in München, November 31, 1898, Dr. Masculine proposed certain addenda to the usual code of professional etiquette, which, legislating for men only, is now obsolete. Among them are these: The male consultant is on no account to assume airs of superiority over the Doctoress, nor presume to criticise the treatment followed. Children of a Doctor and Doctoress may choose by a bare majority which parent is to take medical charge of them. In case of illness occurring in the medical husband or wife, either may give medical aid to the other gratis. This rule extends to childbirth. But if the latter event is too often repeated, the husband's fees must be settled by mutual arrangement.

Medical Philology (XXX.).—The *Promptorium* has "DYDERYN' for colde. *Frigucio, rigeo*," and "DYDERYNGE, *Frigitus*." Mr. Way's note quotes "dadir" from the *Catholicon Anglicum*, and from Cotgrave "*Barboter de froid*, to chatter or didder for cold, to say an ape's Paternoster;" and adds, "Skinner gives this word as commonly used in Lincolnshire, '*a Belg.* sitteren, *pra frigore tremere*.' The Medulla renders '*frigucio*, romb for cold.' In the Avowynge of King Arther, edited by Mr. Robson, to 'dedur' has the sense of shaking, as one who is soundly beaten; and in the Towneley Mysteries, Noah's wife, hearing his relation of the approaching deluge, says,

> 'I dase and I dedir
> For ferd of that taylle.' p. 28.

Didder, to have a quivering of the chin through cold' FORBY."

Mr. Herrtage, in his edition of the *Catholicon*, has a note on "to dadir" (the Latin equivalent of which is *Frigucio*), saying: "*Dither* is still in use in the Northern Counties with the meaning of 'to shake with cold, to tremble': see Peacock's Gloss. of Manley & Corringham, Nodal's Glossary of Lancashire, &c. *Dithers* is the Linc. name for the shaking palsy, *paralysis agitans*. The Manip. Vocab. gives 'to dadder, *trepidare*.' Cotgrave has '*Claquer les dents*. To gnash the teeth, or to chatter, or didder, like an Ape, that's afraid of blowes. *Frisson*. A shivering, quaking, diddering, through cold or feare; a trembling or horror.' See also *Friller, Frissoner*, and *Grelotter*.

> Boyes, gyrles, and luskyth strong knaves,
> *Dydderyng* and *dadderyng* leaning on ten staves.'
> The Hye way to the Spyttel Hous, ed. Hazlitt, p. 28."

Didder and dither are fairly common in colloquial speech even now. The *New English Dictionary* quotes "ditthering, rippling hysteria," from Rudyard Kipling's *Soldiers Three*.

Mr. Herrtage, calling attention to its connection with "Dayse" (which in the *Catholicon* has the meaning "to be callde" with *frigere* as one of its Latin renderings), in his note has: "Icel. *dasdr*, faint, tired; *das*, a faint, exhaustion."

The *Catholicon* has "Calde of þe axes; *frigor*." This is interestingly illustrated by Mr. Herrtage, who says "Palsgrave gives 'Chyueryng as one dothe for colde. In an axes or otherwise, *frilleux*. Ague, axes, *fyeure*.' *Axis* or *Axes* is from Lat. *accessum*, through Fr. *accez*, and is in no way connected with A.S. *æce*. Originally meaning an approach or coming on of anything, it at an early period came to be specially applied to an approach or sudden fit of illness: thus Chaucer has, 'upon him he had an hote *accesse*.' *Black Knight*, l. 136, and Caxton, 'fyl into a sekenes of feures or *accesse*.' *Paris & Vienne*, p. 25." *The Complaint of the Black Knight* is not now considered to be Chaucer's work, but the word in this sense occurs in his undoubted *Troilus and Criseyde*:

> "A charme that was right now sent to thee,
> The whiche can thee hele of thyn accesse."   II. 1314-15.

> "What nedeth you to tellen al the chere
> That Deiphebus unto his brother made,
> Or his accesse, or his sikly manere."   II. 1541-43.

Under "Axes," which in the *Catholicon* has a reference to fevers, Mr. Herrtage has this note: "In the Paston Letters, iii. 426, we read—'I was falle seek with an *axez*.' It also occurs in *The King's Quhair*, ed. Chalmers, p. 54:

> 'But tho begun mine *axis* and torment,'

with the note—'*Axis* is still used by the country people, in Scotland, for the ague.' Skelton, Works, i. 25, speaks of

> 'Allectuary arrectyd to redres   These feverous *axys*.'

'Axis, Acksys, aches, pains.' Jamieson. 'I shake of the axes. *Je tremble des fieures*.' Palsgrave. 'The dwellers of hit [Ireland] be not vexede with the *axes* excepte the scharpe axes [incolæ nulla febris specie vexantur, excepta acuta, et hoc perraro]. Trevisa, i. 333. See *Allit. Poems*, C. 325, '*þacces* of anguych,' curiously explained in the glossary as blows, from A.S. *þaccian*." The *New English Dictionary* quotes from Andrew, who, in his 1527 translation of *Brunswyke's Distyll. Waters*, recommends a certain treatment "for the dayly axces or febres." Jamieson, in the passage here quoted from him, seems to have fallen into the error of interpretation against which Mr. Herrtage warns us in the note on "Calde of þe axes" given above. Concerning the different pronunciations of "ache" as a noun and a verb, I had a long note in the *Journal* for June, 1892. This is a word which we get from the Anglo-Saxon, *æce* or *ece*, a pain or unpleasant feeling.

"To say an ape's Paternoster," which occurs in Mr. Way's note above, was a proverbial expression for chattering with cold, and probably had some reference to the noise of the beads in the Rosary at every tenth of which a Paternoster was said. In addition to the instances in Cotgrave to which Mr. Way and Mr. Herrtage refer, Halliwell, in his *Dictionary of Archaic and Provincial Words*, gives Batre, Cressiner, and Dent. Under the first of these Cotgrave has "Batre le tambour avec les dents. *To chatter, didder, say an apes Paternoster*."

The Bristol
Medico-Chirurgical Journal.

SEPTEMBER, 1899.

THE ANTISEPTIC AND DISINFECTANT PROPERTIES OF SOAP.

BY

J. O. SYMES, M.D. Lond., D.P.H.,

Bacteriologist to the Bristol Royal Infirmary.

SOME months ago I was asked by an operating surgeon whether plain toilet soap might not be a medium in which germs could flourish, and whether therefore it would not be an advantage to use a disinfectant soap. The present investigation was undertaken with a view to answering these questions. I am indebted to Dr. J. M. H. Munro, of Bath, for much valuable assistance in carrying out the experiments and analytical work.

In all cases the organism with which the soaps were tested was the staphylococcus pyogenes aureus, the commonest and most resistant of the pus organisms. The soaps examined were those in use at the Bristol Royal Infirmary at the time, viz.:—
(1) Brown Windsor; (2) Izal, containing 4 per cent. izal oil; (3) Toilet carbolic soap; (4) Scrubbing carbolic soap, 10 per cent. carbolic acid; (5) Germicidal soap, Dr. C. T. McClintock's formula, made by Parke, Davis & Co., and containing 2 per cent. of biniodide of mercury; (6) A potash soft soap, containing 20 per cent. of lysol.

14

With regard to the first question, *viz.*—" Can germs live and multiply on soap ? " I may at once say that all soaps possess antiseptic properties in greater or less degree. The following experiments serve to illustrate this fact : (1) Fragments taken from the centre of a cake of soap by means of a sterile cork borer, and incubated in nutrient broth, were found in all cases to be sterile. (2) The hands were washed in hot tap water with each soap; the tablet was placed on a clean surface, and cultures made from the soap at the expiration of three minutes. Those from germicidal and from scrubbing carbolic soap were sterile, and those from izal, toilet carbolic, lysol, and brown Windsor soaps showed growth of various organisms. (3) Small slabs of each soap were moistened and then heavily inoculated with a culture of staphylococcus aureus, and kept in a moist hot chamber for two days. At the expiration of this time the surfaces of the brown Windsor, lysol, and germicidal soaps were sterile, but scrapings from the others all gave rise to growth of the organism first inoculated. On none of the surfaces was there any apparent increase of growth, nor have we found it possible to grow moulds or bacteria on surfaces of soap kept under ordinary conditions. We may conclude, then, that organisms which may get rubbed into a soap in the process of washing hands, clothes, or other surfaces, or which may settle upon soap from the air, are not capable of multiplication thereon. Of the soaps tested, this antiseptic property was most marked in that containing biniodide of mercury.

For practical purposes the second point—namely, the disinfectant value of the soaps—is the more important. To test this the following method was adopted :—A 1 per cent. solution of each soap was made (this representing what we judged to be the strength of the solution which comes into contact with the hands), and to 5 c.c. of this solution there was added a drop of a fresh broth-culture of staphylococcus. The tube was then shaken and allowed to stand for a stated period, and then 5 drops of the mixture were added to a broth tube which was incubated for 48 hours. Obviously, if the antiseptic property of the soap solution were sufficient to kill the organisms in the one drop of broth-culture added, then the tubes inoculated from the mixture should be sterile; whilst if the solution had no antiseptic power, or if the time allowed were insufficient, then growth would occur.

I do not purpose giving here the details of many experiments extending over several months, but simply to state the result arrived at, viz., that tested in this way it was found that; a 1 per cent. solution of germicidal soap killed staphylococcus aureus in one minute, whilst the same strength of izal, toilet carbolic, scrubbing carbolic, lysol, and brown Windsor soaps failed to do so in ten minutes, half an hour, an hour, or three hours. These solutions were, however, all sterile in from 12 to 14 hours; the exact time in which this result was attained was not observed, nor is it of much importance, for under no conditions would objects be as long as three hours in contact with the soap.

It is a matter of some importance to note that all organisms are not affected alike by soap solutions. Thus the cholera vibrio, the typhoid bacillus, the bacillus coli, and the streptococcus are killed much more quickly, or by very much more diluted solutions, than are the staphylococci. For instance, the bacillus coli is killed by a 2 per cent. solution of plain curd soap in from two to four hours. Our antiseptic precautions are, however, commonly directed against the more resistant organisms, the staphylococci, and, therefore, in testing the germicidal power of a soap it is preferable to work with these organisms. We have tested the germicidal soap with bacillus coli, bacillus typhosus, the cholera bacillus, streptococcus and staphylococcus albus, all of which were killed by admixture with a 1 per cent. solution (equal to biniodide of mercury 1 in 5,000) in one minute.

We conclude, then, from these experiments, that for practical purposes most of the so-called disinfectant soaps have no value, but that in the combination of biniodide of mercury with soap we have a useful means of disinfecting hands, instruments, surfaces, &c.

Although a large number of trials were made, we did not succeed in sterilising our hands by washing with the soap containing biniodide of mercury, although much better results were obtained with this than with any other variety. This points to the necessity of the operator first washing his hands and then soaking them in an antiseptic solution.

It has been thought that the germicidal action of soaps is due to their alkalinity, especially to the free alkali present. We do not think that this can be the case, for Dr. Munro, from a careful analysis of the samples, finds that the difference in the amount of *free* alkali is infinitesimal. Moreover, we obtained no better results with soaps with high *total* alkalinity than with the others.

Although the exact combinations formed are not known, there are many observations to prove that certain antiseptics when mixed with soap partly lose their power. This is certainly the case with carbolic acid, lysol, and izal. Rideal,[1] who has done much work on this subject, considers that for an antiseptic soap an olein base is the best. Superfatted soaps are in his opinion not so suitable vehicles for antiseptics as soaps with a moderate excess of alkali. The presence of free fat or oil strongly militates against germicidal action, witness Koch's discovery that carbolised oil has no antiseptic value. Acids and free halogens are incompatible, the one being neutralised and the other combining with the fat. Boracic acid is converted into sodium borate, and most mercury salts into insoluble mercuric oleate. Oleates do not generally mix well with soap; fluorides, sulphates, and oxides give better results. Rideal found the double iodide of mercury and potassium to mix well and form a good antiseptic with soap, compatible with strong alkalies and not precipitating albumin. In composition this resembles the soap with which we obtained the best results.

In conclusion, I would point out that the matter is one of considerable importance with regard to nurses, attendants upon sick persons, and the general public, who may be led to think that in using so-called antiseptic soaps they are ensuring efficient disinfection. There is also an economic side of the question, for most of the soaps impregnated with chemical disinfectants are very much more costly than plain soaps, though as disinfectants they are of no greater value.

[1] *San. Rec.*, 1898, xxii. 6.

ESTIMATION OF ALKALINITY.

By Dr. J. M. H. Munro.

Brown Windsor, total alkalinity equal to 9.5 % Soda (Na_2O)
Izal   ..   ,,   9.7 % ,,   ,,
Toilet Carbolic   ,,   9.6 % ,,   ,,
Scrubbing Carbolic   ,,   ,,   6.82 % ,,   ,,
Germicidal   ..   ,,   9.9 % ,,   ,,
Lysol   ,,   7.75 % ,,   ,, or
                             11.75 % Potash (K_2O).

These determinations were made with methyl orange as indicator, litmus being of no use with soaps.

The soaps were somewhat drier than when bought, consequently the alkali is higher than would be found in fresh cakes of soap.

Free alkali was greatest in the lysol and the scrubbing carbolic, but there was very little in any of the samples.

ON THE TREATMENT OF SUBACUTE BRONCHITIS.[1]

BY

F. H. Edgeworth, M.B., B.Sc., B.A. Cantab.,

Assistant-Physician to the Bristol Royal Infirmary.

The following notes deal with the treatment of ordinary subacute bronchitis, of such cases as come in numbers to the out-patient department of a hospital and are found so frequently in medical practice. They do not touch on questions of complications and sequelæ, or on the methods that may be adopted in severe cases of the disease.

[1] A paper read at a meeting of the Bristol Medico-Chirurgical Society, on February 8th, 1899.

As a result of the causes of bronchitis, upon the nature of which I do not intend to dwell, a hyperæmia and swelling of the mucous membrane lining the bronchial tubes take place. This is succeeded after a variable interval by a secretion of mucus from the epithelium and glands. The mucus, at first very thick and tenacious, becomes more watery and gradually diminishes in amount until health is restored. The course of an attack of bronchitis may be correspondingly divided into a first and second stage, the onset of secretion from the mucous membrane marking the division between them. The inflammation of the bronchial mucous membrane may be associated during all its stages with a greater or less degree of spasm of the underlying bronchial muscles.

The beginning of even a mild attack of bronchitis is generally accompanied by a slight elevation of temperature, the patient has a dry cough, feels "tight" or "raw" within his chest, the breathing is more rapid and is accompanied by a sense of oppression. Physical examination of the lungs in this stage reveals nothing, or perhaps a little sibilus and rhonchus.

Now one finds, from observation of the course of the disease, that, as soon as the mucous membrane begins to secrete, the increased rate of breathing and its accompanying difficulty disappear, and the patient feels better. Our efforts then should be directed towards two ends—the reduction of temperature and the speedy induction of secretion.

The patient should obviously be kept in bed until all fever is gone. Antipyretic drugs are certainly not required in the mild cases here dealt with. All that is needed is some sudorific —for instance, sweet spirit of nitre or acetate of ammonia. The latter is more suited for continuous administration, whereas the former if given in a sufficient dose acts more quickly. Two drachms of nitre, mixed with water immediately before administration, will generally produce perspiration in an adult, and can generally be taken by a child of say ten years; some children, however, vomit a dose greater than one drachm.

The induction of secretion by the inflamed mucous membrane can be most speedily brought about by the administration of alkalies. The results of clinical observation agree with physiological observation in showing that alkalies rapidly produce a secretion from the bronchial mucous membrane, or, if there be already a secretion going on, increase the proportion of water and so render the mucus thinner and more easy of expectoration. Direct antacids are to be avoided, as in large doses they may irritate the stomach. Of indirect antacids the best are citrate of potash and acetate of soda, of which the latter is perhaps the preferable, as sodium salts are less poisonous than potassium ones.

Ipecacuanha has an action on mucous secretions very similar to that of alkalies; but it has the defect that adults, unless cyanosed, are sometimes nauseated by even ten minims of the vinum; so that its use is best confined to children.

Antimony, if given in small doses, say seven and a half minims of the vinum, is a most useful drug at the commencement of an attack of bronchitis. If the patient be feverish it acts as a sudorific, and it diminishes the inflammatory hyperæmia of the bronchial mucous membrane. In large doses antimony has a depressing effect, so that even small ones are best withheld if there be any cardiac weakness. If there be any troublesome cough, 3 ss. to 3 j. of syrup of tolu is a useful addition to the above drugs. A mustard leaf, too, will quickly relieve "tightness" or "rawness" of the chest and the accompanying irritating cough.

The last point worthy of mention in the treatment of the first stage of bronchitis is the use of antispasmodics in cases where there is spasm of the bronchial muscles. The inconvenience of such drugs as nitro-glycerine and erythrol tetranitrate is that they are apt to produce headache, and of such drugs as nitrite of sodium that their effect is evanescent. But good results may be obtained by the administration of caffeine, the usefulness of which was advocated by Dr. Skerritt some time ago. The only bad effect I have found is that it occasionally prevents sleep.

The antispasmodics act very imperfectly in relieving spasm of the bronchial muscles due to inflammation of the mucous membrane, until secretion has set in. For instance, whilst a combination of alkalies and caffeine will be found to act very well, caffeine by itself will fail to relieve. This absence of effect may be due to the fact that in some cases narrowing of the calibre of the bronchial tubes is the result of the swelling of the mucous membrane; but I doubt if this be the full explanation of the fact.

At the commencement, then, of an attack of subacute bronchitis, good results will generally be found to follow from (1) the administration of a sudorific; (2) the administration of an indirect alkali, such as citrate of potash or acetate of soda, in 20 to 30 grain doses every three or four hours, combined with a small dose of antimony if circumstances permit; (3) the application of a mustard leaf if the chest feel "raw"; and (4) a caffeine pill, of say 5 grains, at night if there be any bronchial spasm. One finds that expectoration is soon established and the patient relieved of his symptoms. He passes on into the second stage more quickly than he does if left untreated, or treated, for instance, with carbonate of ammonia.

The further question then presents itself, whether it be possible to diminish the secretion of mucus from the bronchial mucous membrane more quickly than would take place if the patient were left untreated. Patients are often first seen in this stage, especially in hospital practice. In regard to this, I should first say that as long as expectoration is difficult, or if it become so during treatment, the administration of indirect alkalies is indicated.

In this second stage there may be a large or moderate amount of phlegm coughed up. If there be a large amount of secretion, accompanied with not more cough than is sufficient to get rid of it, no drug probably does so much good as ammonium chloride, in, say, 20-grain doses every four hours. It has, unfortunately, an unpleasant taste; but this may be partially corrected by spirit of chloroform and syrup. Sometimes a large amount of secretion coming up freely is accompanied by a troublesome tickling cough, and in such a case phosphate of codeine (which is freely soluble in water) in gr. $\frac{1}{4}$ to $\frac{1}{2}$ doses, every four hours, will be found most effectual.

But as a rule the amount of expectoration is moderate, and one needs drugs which will act as astringents, diminish and lessen the total secretion from the mucous membrane, whilst preserving the ratio of its constituents one to the other. Many drugs which are employed for this purpose are apt to have a greater effect on the water than on the mucus, the result of which is that the secretion, though less in amount, is more viscid and difficult of expectoration, and so a troublesome cough is set up. Senega and ammonium carbonate are valuable drugs in diminishing bronchial secretion, but occasionally they produce the above-mentioned untoward result. Tincture of Virginian prune, in ℥ss. to ℥j. doses, is useful; it reduces the amount of phlegm and also allays any irritating cough. This latter action is probably dependent on the fact that it contains a small amount of hydrocyanic acid. Its astringent effect, however, is not very great. Tincture of hydrastis is a more effectual astringent, in ℥ss. to ℥j. doses, and may often with advantage be combined with the former drug. Euphorbia pilulifera has a somewhat limited use. It is useful in diminishing secretion, and has also the advantage of allaying bronchial spasm. Like stramonium and lobelia, it is apt to cause nausea if given in too large a dose. I have used it in spasmodic asthma; but though its effects are often striking, they are liable to wear off in the course of a few weeks. But this is hardly a defect in the case of an attack of bronchitis. It may be given in the form of the tincture, in ♏ 10 to 30 doses.

Yerba santa—the sacred herb of California—has been used by Indians for many years in the treatment of coughs and colds. Though little known in England, experience in its use shows that it is extremely efficacious in the treatment of the second stage of bronchitis; it seems to diminish the watery and mucous constituents of the phlegm proportionately, so that this does not become more difficult of expectoration. The dose is ♏ 15 to 45 of the liquid extract. It forms a somewhat muddy mixture with water, owing to precipitation of the contained gum-resin; but the addition of a little alkali, ammonium carbonate or bicarbonate of soda, for instance, makes it clearer.

Bronchial spasm in the course of the second stage of bronchitis is best treated with caffeine or iodide of potassium.

The above-mentioned drugs, used for the varying conditions which may arise in the course of an attack, will be generally found to give excellent results in ordinary subacute bronchitis.

In the discussion which followed Dr. Edgeworth's paper, Dr. E. H. E. STACK wished to know if Dr. Edgeworth had tried large doses of vinum ipecacuanhæ in cases of bronchitis of the second stage with spasm, as he had found it very useful in doses of about a drachm every hour for a few hours, and then less frequently, without producing either vomiting or depression.—Dr. MARKHAM SKERRITT was glad that Dr. Edgeworth endorsed his recommendation of caffeine in certain conditions of bronchitis. Similarly to its effect in asthma, caffeine relieved the spasmodic element in bronchitis. In the latter disease, the narrowing of tubes, which caused a certain proportion of the dyspnœa and was expressed by the dry *râles* or rhonchi, was due to two factors: first, inflammatory swelling of the lining membrane and adherence of thick mucus to its surface; and, secondly, spasmodic contraction as in true asthma. In bronchitis, caffeine relieved the latter condition, but did not touch the former; and hence the apparent uncertainty of its effect.—Dr. G. PARKER agreed with Dr. Edgeworth as to the great value of vinum antimoniale in vigorous patients, especially children. The syrup of apomorphia and iodide of potassium were also drugs which he had found very useful. The latter, from its power of favouring exudation, had even been recommended for diagnostic purposes in early phthisis, since its use was followed in a day or two by moist sounds where none previously existed, though some lesion was suspected. He asked also for any experience as to the results of giving vinum ipecacuanhæ by a throat spray, instead of in a draught, which had been recently advised.—Dr. WATSON WILLIAMS desired to emphasise the utility of the old-fashioned poultice, not only for the comfort of the patient, but because there is very clear evidence that these applications of moist heat to the surface of the chest might actually shorten and favourably modify the general course of an attack of acute bronchitis. Simple acute bronchitis is almost invariably due to superficial chill, acting reflexly on the bronchi and producing the vascular engorgement, and it was only reasonable to suppose, as experience seemed to prove actually was the case, that the effect of the poulticing was, by reflex action, to lessen the vascular engorgement and relieve any associated bronchial spasm. The sooner this could be done the less pronounced would be all the further changes that ensued on this bronchial vascular engorgement.—Dr. R. ROXBURGH remarked on the great potency of potassium iodide in releasing bronchial spasm, but insisted on large doses as generally requisite. In spasmodic asthma he would give twenty grains, combined with a like quantity of tincture of belladonna and spirit of chloroform, and would repeat the dose in an hour if necessary; while in bronchitis with much spasm he gave rather smaller doses.

SOME GROUPS OF INTERESTING CASES OF ABDOMINAL SURGERY.

BY

Charles A. Morton, F.R.C.S. Eng.,

Professor of Surgery in University College, Bristol, and Surgeon to the Bristol General Hospital and to the Hospital for Sick Children and Women.

From the records of eighty-two abdominal operations [1] which I have performed, I have selected three groups of cases as of special interest and worthy of record.

Group A.—Cases of operation for obstruction of the bile ducts by calculi. This group does not include cases in which only cholecystotomy (or removal of stones from the gall-bladder) was performed, but only those in which the ducts were obstructed by stones.

Group B.—Ovarian cysts burrowing deeply into the broad ligament, and therefore without a pedicle.

Group C.—Cases in which collections of pus within the peritoneal cavity have been evacuated through that cavity, *i.e.*, cases in which the general cavity was not shut off by adhesions.

These are records of all the cases of the kind which have been under my care.[2]

GROUP A.

Cases of Operation for Obstruction of the Bile Ducts by Calculi.

Case I.—Stone impacted in the cystic duct, with distension of the gall-bladder. Incision of duct and removal of stone.

Mrs. H. was sent to me by Dr. J. Wilding, in July, 1897, with a swelling in the position of the gall-bladder, and a history of typical attacks of gall-stone colic during the preceding four years. The swelling had been first noticed during the last attack of colic, a month before I saw her. There was a smooth, hard swelling, 3 in. by 3 in.

[1] These do not include hernia, or operations on the kidney from the loin, or vaginal hysterectomy, but include all abscesses arising in connection with disease of the appendix.

[2] This paper was written in March. I have had several cases of this kind since then.

in size, exactly in the usual position of a distended gall-bladder. There was no jaundice.   I advised operation, but she was not able to come into the hospital until November 23rd.   In the interval she had had unusual freedom from attacks of colic, but she had one lasting twenty-four hours, and followed by jaundice.   The condition of the gall-bladder swelling was the same as in July.

I operated on November 26th.   The gall-bladder was greatly distended with mucus, and from it I removed three gall-stones, the size of marbles.   I then felt another stone just beyond the neck of the gall-bladder in the cystic duct, but neither by manipulation with one finger in the gall-bladder and one finger outside the duct, nor by efforts to drag the stone back into the gall-bladder by forceps, could I remove it.   I therefore made an incision an inch long into the cystic duct on to the stone and removed it, and then sewed up the opening with a double row of Lembert's stitches of fine silk, the second row invaginating the first.   Owing to the depth at which the duct lay the manipulation was difficult.   The parts were of course carefully isolated with sponges, but no bile was seen, and there appeared to be no extra-vasation of mucoid fluid from the opened duct.   I closed the incision in the gall-bladder except at one spot which I left open for a drainage tube.   One end of a strand of iodoform gauze was placed below the sutured duct, and the other end brought out at the lower angle of the wound, which was shut off by suturing the parietal peritoneum and abdominal aponeurosis across the wound.   In this way the opening in the abdominal wall was divided into a lower smaller one, through which the gauze protruded, and a larger upper one, and to the edges of this, the gall-bladder was united, with a small drainage tube passed into the interior.   The skin was then sutured across between the openings, and then the end of the drainage tube and the strand of gauze buried in a mass of cyanide gauze and wood wool.   The gauze plug was removed the day after the operation, but the gall-bladder drainage tube was retained some days longer.   On December 4th bile was found discharging through the opening into the gall-bladder where the drainage tube had been.   This rapidly closed, and the patient went out quite well.

After the cystic duct had become obstructed, and the gall-bladder distended with mucus, an attack of colic occurred and was followed by slight jaundice.   Where did the gall-stone come from which thus temporarily obstructed the common duct?   The gall-bladder was at that time shut off by the stone impacted in the cystic duct.   Possibly there was more than one stone impacted in the cystic duct, and one of them moved on down the common duct.

Case II.—Obstruction of cystic and common duct by calculi calculi removed from the gall-bladder, and a floating stone crushed in the common duct.

S.P., aged 39, was sent to me by Dr. J. Young, on January 25th, 1898.   For six months she had suffered from attacks of pain in the right hypochondrium every three weeks.   They usually lasted about twenty minutes, but she had been in constant pain in the same region for a fortnight before admission.   There had never been any vomiting.   On admission to the hospital she was very slightly jaundiced, and a small round swelling could be detected in the position of the gall-bladder.   The jaundice became much more marked directly after admission, but the pain disappeared until February 12th and then returned. The swelling in the position of the gall-bladder could not always be felt. I operated on February 17th and found the gall-bladder, the size of a hen's egg, full of mucus and containing ten small gall-stones, which I removed. I also discovered a stone which darted up and down in a dilated common duct. Owing to the great difficulty in reaching the duct in this case and the way in which the stone lay on the under surface of the lesser omentum, I was obliged to crush it between my thumb and finger rather than remove it by incision. I did not find any stone in the cystic duct. After the operation, bile discharged, from the gall-bladder drainage tube and the jaundice gradually passed off. The opening into the gall-bladder closed before her discharge, on March 21st. It re-opened, however, after her discharge from the hospital, and a little bile escaped daily. She was re-admitted at the end of April, and then the fistula closed in a week. I saw her again this month (February, 1899), and found that she had remained free from jaundice and abdominal pain, and the scar had remained sound. When she came round from the anæsthetic after the operation we found she had left hemiplegia. From this the leg slowly recovered, but the hand remains useless. Its cause was uncertain—possibly some cerebral hemorrhage during the condition of cerebral congestion caused by the ether. My dresser, Mr. Johnson, has discovered records of two other cases of hemiplegia coming on after administration of ether.

Case III.—Obstruction of common duct by floating gall-stones : anastomosis between gall-bladder and duodenum.

Miss P., aged 62, was seen, in consultation with Dr. Emily Eberle, in August last, with a view to performing cholecystenterostomy. In the previous autumn the patient began to suffer from attacks of gall-stone colic, and she had been subject to the febrile attacks resembling ague, which are often present with impaction of a calculus in one of the bile ducts. In the early autumn Dr. Eberle had discovered a gall-stone in the motions. Before the end of 1897 Dr. Eberle ceased to attend her, and in the spring of 1898 she got much worse, jaundice became very marked, and an operation was performed. Many adhesions were found around the gall-bladder, some stones were removed from its interior, but the cause of the obstruction in the common duct was not apparent, and as she was too ill for cholecystenterostomy to be performed, a biliary fistula was established, and the bile continued to discharge externally. When she had recovered from this operation, Dr. Eberle again became her medical attendant, and fearing that the continued loss of bile was preventing her complete restoration to health, asked me to see her with a view to making a communication between the gall-bladder and the intestine, and closing the external biliary fistula, from which ten to twelve ounces of bile discharged every twenty-four hours Diarrhœa and flatulence had been relieved by the administration of ox gall by the mouth. The patient was anxious to get rid of the annoyance of the fistula. I operated on August 17th, assisted by Dr. Eberle. The bile was so viscid I could not draw it off with the aspirating cannula passed into the fistula, and I therefore plugged the latter with iodoform gauze before making the incision. There were so many adhesions in the region of the gall-bladder and bile ducts, it took some time to reach them. On passing my finger deeply behind the duodenum, I felt in the region of the head of the pancreas a large round hard body the size of a marble. When palpating it, it slipped upwards in what was evidently a greatly dilated common duct. Dr. Eberle then grasped the duct below the stone, and I did the same above it, thus fixing it, and I was just about to incise the duct over it, when I thought it lay rather too much on the under surface of the lesser omentum, and I released my grip in order to shift it further round, when it disappeared, and I was never again able to find it; but in a prolonged search for it, I found another stone half the size, also close to the head of the pancreas. This one I could easily float upwards in the duct, and could readily have removed, but I considered it was not worth the risk of incising the duct unless the larger stone could also be found and removed. I discovered another calculus the size of a small shot, fixed, very high up near the liver. Failing to remove the cause of the obstruction, I detached the gall-bladder from the abdominal wall, and united it with a Murphy button to the duodenum. The button was not the ordinary one used for the purpose, for the half which lay in the duodenum was distinctly larger than the gall-bladder half, so that the button, when detached, could not pass into the gall-bladder instead of the duodenum. I drained the region of the anastomosis with a rubber tube and a strand of iodoform gauze, and united the incision in the abdominal wound around their protruding ends. There was only a moderate degree of prostration after the operation. She was fed by the rectum only for the first twenty-four hours, and the gauze drain was removed the day after the operation. Her progress was quite satisfactory until August 30th, when she had a severe attack of hæmatemesis, but no melæna. After this she slowly regained strength, and the drainage-tube opening was healed during the following month. The button was passed ten weeks after the operation. The old fistula-opening has discharged, every now and again, a few drops of watery fluid. She gained flesh and was able to walk a mile and a half, and has had none of the old attacks of colic or pyrexia until the beginning of this year, when she had some return of the old pain. Since the operation in August, she has only had a slight conjunctival tint of jaundice for a few days in January. But serious valvular disease of the heart has developed, and her condition in January was very critical.[1]

The fourth case of this series was published in the *Bristol Medico-Chirurgical Journal* for 1897.[2] I removed a large stone which was floating freely in the common duct, and had caused a very uncommon form of pyrexia. A very interesting series of operations on the bile-ducts has lately been published by Mr. Mayo Robson[3]; and as the surgery of the bile-ducts is considered in such an exhaustive manner in Mr. Mayo Robson's paper, I would refer the reader of these records to it for further information on the subject. The difficulty in dealing with the ducts, lying as they do at a considerable depth and amongst

[1] This patient died from heart disease on May 17th, and at the necropsy I found a stone the size of a small marble in an enormously-dilated common duct.

[2] xv. 317. [3] *Brit. M. J*, 1898, ii. 1404.

important structures, is often very great. I have not thought it safe to close the abdominal cavity without any drain, after incision and suture of the duct, and hence in Case I. the difficulty arose as to how the gall-bladder should be drained of mucus, and the peritoneal cavity in the neighbourhood of the duct drained at the same time through the same opening in the abdominal wall. I might have drained the gall-bladder through the abdominal wound, and the region of the sutured duct by means of Rutherford Morison's method of drainage through a lumbar incision. But I do not like to make this additional lumbar wound if it can be avoided, and the plan which I adopted answered very well.

The difficulty of finding floating stones in the common duct is well shown in the last case. The patient had been previously operated on by another surgeon, and no stone discovered; and after finding the largest stone, I lost it, and could not find it again. What happened must remain uncertain. I am inclined to think it darted up into some dilated and pouched portion of the hepatic duct, and there remained. I manipulated the common duct, as one would milk a cow, and had the patient's shoulder raised to a considerable extent to try and dislodge it.

GROUP B.

Cases of Ovarian Tumours burrowing deeply into the Broad Ligament.

Two of the cases may be called broad ligament cysts, for they lay wholly within the broad ligament; in the other case the cyst reached to the costal margin, and yet its base extended deeply into the broad ligament up to the side of the uterus. Parovarian cysts of course start in the broad ligament, but do not always burrow deeply between its layers. Paroöphoritic cysts—i.e., cysts starting in the hilum of the ovary, and often containing much watery growth—do commonly burrow between its layers. So also would cysts arising in the upper segment of the canal of Gärtner. The exact origin of the cysts in these cases which I record I do not know.

The removal of an ovarian cyst, large enough to ascend into the abdomen, with a distinct pedicle and with no very important or numerous adhesions, is about as simple and easy an abdominal operation as we could well have to perform. But when there is no pedicle, when the cyst lies deeply in the pelvis, and we have to open up the broad ligament and shell it out, with the danger of injury to the ureter lying just beneath, it becomes a much more difficult and anxious proceeding.

CASE I.—Mrs. S., aged 52, came under my care in the General Hospital in March, 1894, for a swelling in the lower abdomen, which she had noticed for three months. A definite swelling was visible in the centre of the lower abdomen, extending rather more to the right than the left, and from just above the pelvis to two inches from the umbilicus. It was dull all over, with resonant intestine around, softly fluctuating, and could be moved laterally with considerable freedom. Nothing abnormal could be felt *per vaginam* until the tumour was pressed down, and then it could be felt bulging at the right of the cervix.

I operated on April 2nd, and found a cyst the size of a young child's head, covered by a thin layer of peritoneum, which was reflected on the tumour from the iliac fossa, and the cyst also extended deeply into the right broad ligament, and the uterus was pushed by it over to the left side of the pelvis. It lay in contact with the right side of the uterus, and there was no pedicle. It was so soft I could not satisfactorily evacuate the clear watery fluid it contained with the ovariotomy trocar and cannula; but by pushing it well forwards against the anterior abdominal wall, I was able to guide the fluid out of the incision in the latter without any passing into the peritoneal cavity. Before the cyst was emptied, a large cyst within the one first opened had to be incised. I then found that the cyst extended very deeply into the broad ligament, and in enucleating it the ureter was exposed to view, running beneath the cyst. I divided the peritoneum over the cyst, and shelled it out, clamping and dividing strands of tissue here and there, and ligating the tissue between it and the fundus of the uterus in two places. The ovarian artery and a large vein passing into the tumour were recognised and tied separately. The uterine appendages on the left side were all buried in old adhesions. The cavity from which the cyst had been removed in the broad ligament was drained by a glass tube for several days. She made an uneventful recovery, and was discharged at the end of April. In this case, the bilocular nature of the cyst is of interest. Most cysts of the broad ligament, parovarian, and paroöphoritic cysts are unilocular.

CASE II.—E. H., aged 43, was sent to me in March, 1898, by Dr. L. B. Trotter, of Coleford, with a swelling in the abdomen, of nine months' duration She had a good deal of pain in the position of the swelling at times, and some frequency of micturition.

On admission, on March 20th, there was visible fulness in the right lower abdomen, and a very soft fluctuating swelling could be felt beneath the lower part of both recti, but projecting more to the right than the left. No definite outline could be made out, and the limits of the swelling could only be defined by the fluctuation wave. Nothing abnormal was made out on vaginal examination. I operated on April 5th, and found a very soft cyst in the right broad ligament. It raised the peritoneum from the right iliac fossa, so that the cyst lay over the iliac vessels and in contact with the bladder and the side of the uterus. The only place where it was free was on its posterior aspect. It was too soft to puncture with the ovariotomy trocar, so I wedged a sponge between the cyst and the abdominal wall, turned the patient over on her side, and evacuated straw-colored serous fluid from the cyst by incision. Through the opening thus made I was able to separate the cyst-wall from its capsule of peritoneum. At the upper part the cyst-wall was very thin, but shelled out with ease, after division of some strands of connective tissue containing vessels. At its lower part the cyst was much thicker, and it extended deeply, so that I felt there was considerable risk of wounding the ureter in its removal; but by clamping and dividing various strands of tissue, and peeling the cyst away where I could, I enucleated it from the broad ligament. The cyst was unilocular, and the size of a large cocoa-nut. There was no trace of the ovary attached to it. I drained the cavity left in the broad ligament for twenty-four hours. She made an uninterrupted convalescence, and went home early in May.

CASE III.—N. I., aged 40, was sent to me by Mr. J. C. Smyth, of Glastonbury, for ovariotomy, in January, 1899. Her friends had first noticed an increase in size of the abdomen early last summer, and Mr. Smyth had been called in to see her a fortnight before she came under my care, and had then discovered the abdominal tumour. She had had a good deal of abdominal pain at times. There was a fairly firm, smooth tumour, which extended from the pubes to the left costal margin. It occupied more of the right half of the abdomen than the left. There were no bosses on the surface, and no thrill on percussion, or distinct fluctuation on palpation.

I operated on January 28th. On plunging the ovariotomy trocar into the cyst, nothing came through it, but thick jelly-like material welled out round it. I dragged the cyst forwards with large forceps, and my assistant kept the cyst pushed well forward against the anterior abdominal wall. I then made a free incision into the cyst (after enlarging the incision in the abdominal wall) and drew out a large mass of this viscid material. After partly emptying the cyst in this way, I made the incision into it large enough to get my hand in, and bailed out more of the jelly from the large cyst, and numerous secondary cysts which I broke into with my fingers. In this way I was able to deliver the empty cyst, except at its base. I found it had no pedicle, but burrowed to some depth into the right broad ligament, and lay by the side of the uterus. There were no adhesions, but the peritoneum of the right iliac fossa was raised by it. I got a ligature around the reflection of peritoneum from the iliac fossa into the cyst, which contained the ovarian vessels, and another around the Fallopian tube just by the side of the uterus, and after dividing the peritoneum between these two points, enucleated the cyst out of the broad ligament, dividing strands of connective tissue here and there, and clamping and dividing some vessels. The iliac vessels were freely exposed, but I did not see or feel the ureter. A small cyst was also removed from the region of the left ovary. I washed out the abdomen with sterilised saline solution, but I do not think any of the colloid material had entered it. I drained the cavity left in the right broad

15

ligament for forty-eight hours. There was a good deal of sickness and
flatulent distension of the abdomen for some days after the operation,
and the urine had to be drawn off for some considerable time.

The contents of this cyst were more like those of an ovarian
adenoma; but the structure of the cyst was not like that form of
ovarian tumour.'

It is interesting to note that in none of these cases could
the cyst be evacuated by the ovariotomy trocar and cannula in
the ordinary manner, but the evacuation of their contents was
effected by incision without fouling the general peritoneal
cavity and setting up peritonitis. In the first two cases the
cysts were too soft, and in the third the contents were too
viscid, for their evacuation in the ordinary manner.

GROUP C.

Cases in which Collections of Pus within the Peritoneal Cavity have been Evacuated through that Cavity.

When the parietal peritoneum becomes firmly adherent to
the wall of an appendicitis abscess, and we can open straight
into the collection of pus without implicating the general
peritoneal cavity, the proceeding is not as a rule a difficult
one. There may be uncertainty as to whether we have an
adherent coil of bowel beneath the adherent peritoneum, and
therefore we have to work very cautiously, and work through
the thickened tissue mainly with the point of a blunt instrument such as a director; but when we have first to open up
the general peritoneal cavity and then evacuate offensive pus
through it, it becomes a more risky and difficult business.
And yet we are certainly not wise in leaving pus shut up
amongst adherent coils of bowel, even though adhesion may
not have fixed them to the peritoneum of the anterior
abdominal wall. Too often such collections of pus leak into
the general peritoneal cavity before these adhesions form,
and fatal peritonitis is set up. If we carefully pack around
the adherent coils forming the abscess-wall with iodoform
gauze, or sponges before we break down the adhesion of the
coils and liberate the pus, we shall effectually prevent contamination of the general cavity of the peritoneum at the

time of operation; and by the retention of a plug of gauze for twenty-four to forty-eight hours after, we can drain the abscess sac with equal safety. Some of the cases in this series show that even if pus has been freely discharged into the peritoneal cavity from the rupture of an intra-abdominal abscess, free flushing and drainage may prevent the onset of peritonitis.

In dealing with these abscesses, the method which I adopt is as follows. Directly the mass of adherent bowel around the pus is exposed, on opening the peritoneal cavity over it, it is very carefully isolated by packing around it with iodoform gauze or sponges. I then look for a spot on the surface of the mass where I think I can break through the adhesions between the coils and reach the interior; here I gently work with the end of a director and my finger-tip. Presently a little, usually offensive, pus escapes, and is quickly caught on a sponge. The opening is enlarged by the finger, the pus caught on sponges as it wells up, and then when it ceases to flow the cavity is plugged with a strand of iodoform gauze so that no pus can escape. The surrounding mass of gauze, or the sponges, are then removed, and the neighbouring coils examined, by inspection and gentle sponging, to see if any pus has found its way amongst them. In my own cases, the gauze packing has always prevented this. If a little pus had escaped amongst the coils of bowel, it would be sponged up; if anything like free escape of pus into the general peritoneal cavity had occurred, it would be flushed out with boiled saline solution. A fresh strand of gauze is then packed around the mass, and the end brought out of the incision in the abdominal wall. The piece of gauze within the abscess cavity is then replaced by a large glass drainage tube, in which lies a strand of iodoform gauze to act by capillary attraction. The general peritoneal cavity is thus shut off while the abscess sac is drained. Sometimes I have used the wick drain, introduced by Morris of New York, instead of the glass one. This consists of a strand of gauze, surrounded by green protective, just as the tobacco is surrounded by the paper in a cigarette. The gauze acts as a capillary drain, and the green protective prevents adhesio surrounding tissues. Usually an anæsthetic is required for a few minutes when the gauze is removed from around the suppurating mass, forty-eight hours after the operation. By this time, and probably sooner, protective adhesions will have shut off the general peritoneal cavity around the gauze-plugging. The adhesion of the gauze to the peritoneum is so firm that it often requires some force to dislodge it, and hence the need for an anæsthetic.

Only a certain number of the cases in this group have been cases of appendicitis. Two are cases of suppuration from perforation of the bowel, one in a malignant growth and one from a fish-bone. One is a very interesting case of abscess in the mesentery from localised necrosis. Fæcal matter, as well as pus, was flushed out of the general peritoneal cavity in one case, which recovered without peritonitis.

The cases in this group are too numerous to give their histories, and I have had to be content with a brief outline of the operations and results. In the first seven cases, the abscess probably arose in connection with disease of the appendix. In most of the cases, the discovery of the perforated appendix, or an appendix concretion in the pus, placed their origin beyond doubt, and the origin of the others from the appendix was extremely probable.

CASE I.—W., aged 22. There was a collection of pus shut in by adherent coils around a sloughing appendix. On opening the peritoneal cavity, a mass of adherent intestine was found lying just internal to, and slightly below, the cæcum, which was adherent to it, and overlapped it to a slight extent. There were no adhesions to the anterior abdominal wall. I carefully packed sponges around it in all directions. At first I did not see where I could break into the mass and evacuate the pus, but what looked like the junction of ileum and cæcum (so smooth was it) turned out, on further examination, to be only an adhesion, and by breaking it down I liberated a few drops of pus. The pus was at once sponged up, and I then gradually broke into the abscess cavity through the adhesions. The cavity was the size of a hen's egg, and I did not feel the appendix within it, but I avoided much manipulation for fear of breaking down adhesions on the under aspect of the adherent coils, and thus allowing pus to escape into the general peritoneal cavity. After removing the gauze around the mass, I plugged the abscess with a strand of iodoform gauze, and brought the end out through the incision in the abdominal wall. I also packed around this central strand of gauze with other strands, so as to shut off the peritoneal cavity, but they did not penetrate into the abscess sac. These were removed in forty-eight hours. On the fifth day after the operation a slough of the appendix an inch long was discharged from the abscess cavity, and the patient went out quite well a month later. She never had any signs of general peritonitis.

CASE II.—Wm. T., aged 8. In this case, the mass of adherent coils around the collection of pus was adherent at one place to the peritoneum of the anterior abdominal wall; but I had to open the peritoneal cavity just above, in order to see what condition I had to deal with, and in separating the adherent parietal peritoneum off the mass a little pus exuded. This was quickly sponged up, and after the opening had been enlarged with sinus forceps, I passed my finger in, the pus as it escaped being quickly absorbed by masses of gauze placed around. I did not feel the appendix, but the position of the abscess—at McBurney's point—left little doubt as to its origin. The abscess-sac was drained, and the general peritoneal cavity shut off as in the last case, with the same successful result.

CASE III.—C., boy, aged 16. In this case, on opening the peritoneal cavity, I found the mass on the outer aspect of the middle of the ascending colon, continuous with the lower end of the kidney. I plugged all round it with a quantity of iodoform gauze, and then separated adhesions, and evacuated some offensive pus and a typical appendix concretion. Before removing the temporary plugging, I inserted a strand of gauze into the abscess sac, and brought the end out through the incision in the abdominal wall. The temporary plug was then replaced by two strands of gauze, one placed on each side of the strand lying in the abscess sac, and the ends brought out through the abdominal incision. The temperature fell to normal after the operation, and there were no signs of general peritonitis; and in a month's time the boy's general condition was good, and only a sinus remained; but later on fresh abscesses (extra-peritoneal) formed and were opened, sinuses persisted, and the boy died nearly a year after the first operation. The parents refused to take the risk of an operation for removal of the diseased appendix.

The question has been much discussed during the last few years (especially by American surgeons) whether, in these cases of localised suppuration around an appendix, we should break down those adhesions on which the safety of the peritoneal cavity depends and remove the diseased part. The feeling of most surgeons, and certainly my own, is that the risk of setting up general peritonitis is too great. If the appendix is found lying loosely in the abscess sac, we should, I think, undoubtedly remove it; but we are not justified, I consider, in breaking down the adhesions between adherent coils of bowel which shut off the infected area, in order to remove it. Perhaps if we did remove the appendix in all these cases we might less often have troublesome sinuses after evacuation of an appendix abscess, but we might, I think, sacrifice the life of the patient; and these persistent sinuses are not very frequent, and only very rarely do they lead to any serious result. In the case which I now record, I advised that the appendix should be removed, when it became evident that it would cause chronic trouble, even though in the presence of septic sinuses the operation involved some risk.

CASE IV.—W. H. O., aged 10. In this case the collection of pus was situated in almost the same situation as in the last—outside the middle of the ascending colon, between the colon and the parietes; but it extended from this upwards, and was more difficult to reach. I was able to plug below it with a sponge packed in at the outer side of the cæcum, but could not push gauze or a sponge in above it, under the liver. The ascending colon formed a barrier to the entrance of pus into the general peritoneal cavity on the inner side. I turned the boy well over on his right side, and then, by separating adhesions, evacuated offensive pus. Nothing was seen of the appendix; but I had little doubt the abscess arose in connection with it, though not in the usual position for an appendix abscess. After thoroughly sponging out the abscess sac. I sponged out the fossa under the liver above the abscess sac, but found no pus there. The abscess sac was drained by means of Morris's wick drain, already described. Although the pus was evacuated, the boy's general condition got worse, and he died two days after the operation. At the necropsy, it was found that the abscess cavity had not only formed a considerable swelling within the peritoneal cavity by adhesions between the outer aspect of the ascending colon and the parietes, but had also eroded the peritoneum and the anterior aspect of the right kidney. The perforated tip of the appendix lay in the abscess sac. The abscess was, of course, primarily intra-peritoneal, and yet it had eroded the peritoneum over the kidney, and had not found an exit into the general peritoneal cavity, so great is the protecting action of adhesions within the peritoneal cavity in these cases. The necropsy showed that the evacuation of the pus had been accomplished without any infection of the general peritoneal cavity, for there were no signs of any general peritonitis.

I have operated on four cases of appendix abscess situated outside the middle of the ascending colon. Two are here recorded. In the other two the general peritoneal cavity had been shut off by adhesions at the time of operating, and therefore they do not come into this group. In one of these I found an appendix concretion in the abscess; in the other only the similarity in position, and the absence of any other obvious cause, led me to diagnose perforation of the appendix as the almost certain origin. No doubt in all the appendix lay directed upwards under the ascending colon (as was demonstrated in one of the cases), and the tip perforated in that position.

CASE V.—Boy, aged 16. A collection of pus was shut in by adherent coils of bowel, and omentum around a perforated appendix.

There were no adhesions to the abdominal wall. When the peritoneal cavity was opened, pus was found leaking out through a perforation in the omentum. The peritoneal cavity was washed out, but death from peritonitis occurred ten hours later. The necropsy showed that the peritonitis must have started before operation, as it was advanced in parts of the abdomen away from the focus of suppuration. An earlier operation would probably have saved the boy's life.

CASE VI.—A. B., aged 20. This was a case of large pelvic abscess, of doubtful origin; but I have included it amongst the appendicitis cases, as most probably it was due to a sloughed appendix, hanging over towards the pelvis. I have record of one fatal case of peritonitis from perforation of the appendix, in which the cavity of the true pelvis was full of pus, and there was no pus around the appendix; and yet a perforation of the appendix in the iliac fossa was clearly the cause of the peritonitis, for an appendix concretion was found lying there. In other cases we find the appendix hanging over the pelvic brim, with the perforated tip in the pelvic cavity. I believe the case to have been one of this kind, in which probably not only was the appendix perforated, but much of it had sloughed off. The patient presented a definite swelling just below McBurney's point, and a large pelvic swelling bulging into the rectum. I opened the abdomen over the abdominal mass, and found that it consisted of a mass of adherent bowel and omentum, which was only adherent at one or two spots to the anterior abdominal wall. I packed around the mass with iodoform gauze, and then broke down adhesions with my fingers, and tied and divided portions of adherent omentum, until the lower extremity of the cæcum was well exposed, but I could not find the appendix. While doing this, a little pus exuded from amongst the adherent coils. I then broke down the adhesion of the bowels on the deeper aspect of the mass, and thus worked into Douglas's pouch, and then a very free discharge of horribly offensive pus took place, and I found Douglas's pouch had been converted into a large abscess cavity, pushing forward the uterus. Before opening this up, the gauze packing was removed, as it was evidently impossible to protect the general peritoneal cavity from infection by its retention. I found the right Fallopian tube and ovary greatly swollen, and suspecting that the abscess might have arisen in a ruptured pyosalpinx, I removed them; but subsequent examination showed that although the tube contained lymph, its inflammatory condition was probably due to its having formed part of the wall of the abscess sac. No trace of the appendix could be discovered, but I thought there was an ulcerated area where it might have sloughed off. I very thoroughly flushed the whole peritoneal cavity with boiled saline solution, and placed a glass drainage tube in the pelvis, with a strand of iodoform gauze within it for a capillary drainage. The general condition improved very much after the operation, and the abscess sac continued to drain well; but another intra-abdominal abscess formed, a fortnight after the operation, on the opposite side of the abdomen above the level of the umbilicus, and when the pus was evacuated the knot of a sulpho-chromic catgut ligature came away in it, showing that it arose in connection with the primary seat of suppuration. After the opening of the secondary abscess, she made a satisfactory recovery. Although the general peritoneal cavity was infected by the offensive pus at the time of the first operation, yet by thorough flushing the onset of general peritonitis was prevented.

CASE VII.—Another case belonging to this group has already been published,[1] as one of recovery after draining a pyæmic abscess of the liver. A collection of pus was shut up around the diseased appendix, but there were no adhesions to the anterior abdominal wall. I removed the appendix, flushed out and drained the peritoneal cavity, and the boy did not develop any signs of peritonitis, and after evacuation of the pyæmic abscess in the liver, recovered.

Case VIII.—Evacuation of pus from the general peritoneal cavity, and drainage of ruptured pelvic abscess: recovery without peritonitis.

S. E., aged 36. On opening the peritoneal cavity just above the pubes, several ounces of very offensive pus escaped, and. I found a collection of pus shut up in the true pelvis by adhesion over the brim, and at one spot this had given way and the pus leaked out. The rupture through the adhesion was enlarged by my finger and the pus freely evacuated, the general peritoneal cavity well flushed with boracic lotion, and the abscess drained with a glass drainage tube, within and around which I placed strands of iodoform gauze. The cause of the abscess was probably suppuration in a Fallopian tube, as she had an offensive vaginal discharge. The rupture probably occurred two hours before operation, when she was seized with very severe pain in the abdomen. The glass drainage tube and the gauze-plugging around were removed in twenty-four hours after the operation and a rubber tube substituted. As the discharge remained offensive, I had the cavity frequently irrigated, and then it became sweet. The sinus persisted for several months.

Case IX.—Abscess in the mesentery: evacuation through peritoneal cavity without infection of peritoneum: death nine days after operation, from pneumonia.

J. P., aged 50. In this case there was a large swelling just below the umbilicus, with high temperature. The patient had been a heavy drinker. That there was an intra-peritoneal abscess seemed certain, but the cause was very obscure. On opening the abdomen I found a hard mass, the size of an orange, lying over the lumbar spine. It was covered by adherent coils of small intestine; but the great omentum passed over it without adhering to it. I very thoroughly packed all round the mass with iodoform gauze, and then broke down an adhesion between the adherent coils on the upper part, and thick offensive pus came out and was rapidly sponged up. My finger passed into a cavity amongst the adherent coils just like an abscess cavity from perforation of the appendix. After sponging up all the pus as it exuded, I plugged the cavity with gauze, and then withdrew the surrounding mass of gauze and passed small sponges on holders in various directions into the peritoneal cavity, but found no pus there. The strand of gauze which had been inserted into the abscess sac was then replaced by a large glass drainage tube, and around this, outside the cavity, was placed a mass of gauze to shut off the general peritoneal cavity while the abscess drained. It was removed under chloroform in forty-eight

---

[1] *Bristol M.-Chir. J.*, 1897, xv. 323.

hours. The progress of the patient, so far as his abdominal condition, was concerned, was most satisfactory; but he got lobar pneumonia, and died nine days after operation. At the necropsy the abscess cavity was found almost obliterated, and there was no trace of general peritonitis. It evidently had arisen in the mesentery, and probably from a limited necrosis, as a necrotic area was found in that structure. The appendix was normal.

Case X.—Collection of pus beneath adherent cysts in the pelvis: evacuation through peritoneal cavity without general infection of peritoneum.

E. S., aged 25. On opening the peritoneal cavity, I found a mass of adherent omentum and bowel around a small cyst of the left ovary, and a mass of small cysts firmly adherent in Douglas's pouch. On separating some omental adhesions, some serous fluid escaped, and then on passing my finger deeply into Douglas's pouch between the adherent cysts, some thick pus welled up and was caught on sponges. I freely flushed out the whole peritoneal cavity with sterilised saline solution. I did not remove any cysts, as to get the adherent mass away would have been a serious operation with suppuration in the pelvis. I left a large glass drainage tube in the peritoneal cavity, reaching down into Douglas's pouch. This was replaced by a rubber one forty-eight hours after. A fortnight after the operation another collection of pus formed higher up in the abdomen, but after incision and drainage the cavity closed. A sinus, however, persisted from the first operation, at the time she left the hospital, about four months after operation, but the discharge from it was very slight, and I believe it healed soon after her return home.

Case XI.—Intra-abdominal abscess in connection with a malignant growth in the bowel: drainage through the peritoneal cavity.

M. J., aged 50. The patient had a fairly large abdominal swelling to the right of the umbilicus, associated with marked pyrexia. On opening the abdomen over the swelling I came on a red hard mass, with the omentum adherent over it, and with adhesions here and there to the parietal peritoneum. On gently separating some omentum lying on it pus welled up, and this I caught on a sponge, and kept the sponge pressed against the opening until I got iodoform gauze plugged round. I then broke down the adhesions, and liberated some thick, very offensive pus. After the evacuation of the pus a portion of the swelling remained very hard. Before removing the gauze I passed a large glass drainage-tube into the abscess cavity. I then replaced the gauze by a fresh strand, the end of which was brought out of the opening in the abdominal wall with the end of the glass drainage-tube. It was removed in forty-eight hours, by which time the general peritoneal cavity had become securely shut off. Some fæcal discharge was observed on the second day. After temporary improvement, her strength failed, and she died a month after the operation. At the necropsy the abscess was found to be due to perforation of a malignant growth in the hepatic flexure of the colon. The growth was extensive, but had not blocked the lumen of the gut. The general cavity of the peritoneum had not been infected.

Case XII.—Evacuation of pus and fæces from the general peritoneal cavity: free irrigation: recovery.

Girl, aged 8. This case is a remarkable one, and was brought before the Bristol Medico-Chirurgical Society by Dr. Michell Clarke and myself some years ago. There were signs of an intra-abdominal abscess in the left iliac fossa. In fact, the case very much resembled an appendicitis abscess, except that the abscess was on the left side. On dividing the abdominal wall on the outer aspect of the swelling, *i.e.* just inside the anterior superior spine, I came down on what seemed to be greatly thickened peritoneum, and on gradually working through this with the point of a director some pus escaped. I dilated the track gently with my finger, and found a smooth-walled cavity the size of a hen's egg, out of which was an opening at the other end, through which my fingers passed into the peritoneal cavity, where free intestine could be felt. The wall of the abscess cavity seemed to be composed of adherent intestine. The general peritoneal cavity was washed out with a large quantity of hot boracic solution through the abscess sac. As soon as the irrigation was commenced, what appeared at first to be shreds of tissue from the interior of the abscess came away with the fluid, but they were quickly recognised as bile-stained, and were undoubtedly the contents of the first portion of the small intestine. The irrigation was continued until all this material had come away, and then a large-sized drainage tube was placed in the abscess cavity as far as the internal opening into the peritoneal cavity. The fæcal discharge of the same character persisted for some weeks, but there were no signs of peritonitis, and the child was discharged from the hospital six weeks after the operation.

The doubt as to the origin of the abscess was never cleared up. It must, I think, have given way into the peritoneal cavity just before the operation, perhaps during struggling as she went under the anæsthetic, and possibly a small area in one of the adherent coils of bowel, softened by inflammation, gave way at the same time, and hence the fæcal matter found in the general peritoneal cavity.

To these cases must be added two more. One of these I have already published.[1] A large abscess formed under the meso-colon from perforation by a fish-bone, which was found in the abscess sac. I was able to stitch the surface of the meso-colon to the parietal peritoneum before evacuating the pus and thus shut off the general peritoneal cavity from infection. The other case was one of enormous suppurating hydatid of the liver. There were no adhesions between the liver and the parietal peritoneum, but by stitching the liver surface to it around a small area, I was able to evacuate pus and an enormous number of daughter-cysts without infecting the general peritoneal cavity. The case will be published later on, with other cases of hepatic surgery.

[1] *Brit. M. J.*, 1894, i. 241.

SOME UNUSUAL OPERATIONS ON LUNATICS AND THEIR RESULTS.[1]

BY

J. PAUL BUSH, M.R.C.S. Eng.,
Surgeon to the Bristol Royal Infirmary.

———

I HAVE ventured to publish these five operation cases occurring in persons of unsound mind, as the cases are interesting not only to those working at surgery but also to those whose practice lies more especially in the treatment and diagnosis of mental cases; the recording of these cases may also raise the question, " What effects (if any) are produced on the mental condition after major operations on the insane? " These cases have all occurred within the past year, and I am glad to say, from a surgical standpoint, I am quite satisfied with the results. As time slips by one is rather apt to remember cases that have done well, while those that have done badly sometimes escape our memory. I therefore mention that the operations described below were consecutive ones, and in all of them improvement in the mental condition commenced shortly after operation, and this improvement continued till apparently the brain was restored to a healthy state, which, so far, has continued to be permanent in every case. In none of these operation cases was the bodily ailment even supposed to be a starting point for the deranged mental faculties, as in all the patients the unsound condition of the mind was manifest for months or years before the condition of the body, requiring the interference of the surgeon, was present.

E. K., a young lady whose mind had become unhinged,—it was thought through a love affair,—and who had been under restraint for three years, had two bad ingrowing toe-nails removed; she completely recovered her mental condition within three months.

G. D., a man aged 70, with cystitis and dysuria, was found to have a stone in his bladder. I operated by the supra-pubic method, and

———

[1] Read at the meeting of the Bristol Medico-Chirurgical Society, on April 12th, 1899.

extracted a calculus two inches long and one inch thick; in the centre of the stone was found a vulcanite pipe-stem. I had the bladder drained for ten days, on account of the cystitis; the abdominal wound was completely healed by the 17th day, the mental condition began to improve at once, and he was cured in body and mind within six months.

A. W., aged 44. This woman had been in an asylum for 2½ years with melancholia and severe suicidal impulses. On admission her physical condition was normal, a year after she had retention of urine and intermittent attacks of menorrhagia which continued for six months; when I saw her she was very anæmic, there was a large solid tumour reaching from the pubes to the level of the umbilicus, the os uteri was easily dilated, and I was able to reach and cut through a broad short pedicle attached to the side of the uterus. My trouble now began: the corkscrews used in the extraction of fibroids held well, but I was quite unable, on account of its size, to take away the tumour, which was now free in the uterus: as hemorrhage was taking place, I was afraid I might have, after all, to do an abdominal section and lay open the uterus, but by the timely arrival of a pair of midwifery forceps, and the exercise of some muscular energy, I was enabled at last to deliver the tumour, which, emptied of its blood, was somewhat larger in size than that of the fœtal head at the full time. The uterus was packed with iodoform gauze to stop hemorrhage; she made an uninterrupted recovery and was discharged mentally cured in some six months.

M. D., a woman aged 46. When first she came under notice there was nothing abnormal in her bodily condition; mentally she was acutely maniacal. When I saw her there was some history of a slight attack of jaundice seven weeks before, followed two weeks later by a sudden severe pain at the epigastrium, with temporary collapse, and afterwards a rise of temperature with diarrhœa: for ten days she seemed better, when the temperature suddenly rose to 104°, rigors came on, and a swelling was made out in the epigastrium, which was dull on percussion with an area of resonance above. I made a free incision, and after letting out about a pint of pus, I found the intestines matted together, the abscess sac being situated between the stomach and liver; I endeavoured to find what was evidently the cause of the abscess, namely, a perforated gastric ulcer; but the stomach was so coated by thick layers of lymph, that I contented myself with getting away as much of the septic *débris* as possible, sponged out the cavity, and packed it with iodoform gauze, leaving the ends outside the wound to act as drainage. The patient was much collapsed, and I must say I expected to hear she had died of septic peritonitis within the twenty-four hours. After some three weeks, during which time there were several attacks of sickness, the vomit containing pus and a watery fluid of a beautiful blue colour, she eventually made a complete recovery, and was mentally cured and discharged some seven months later.

This case was without doubt one of gastric perforation that had formed a residual abscess; whether the perforation was of traumatic origin, or whether it was originally an ulcer that had perforated, it is, I think, impossible to say. At my operation I looked for, but could not find, any trace of a foreign body which might have been the cause of the perforation.

M. R., aged 32. A woman suffering from melancholia with severe suicidal and homicidal impulses, had been under treatment for two years. A year before operation there was much abdominal pain, and a history of eating needles, but no physical signs were found at that time. Six weeks before operation patient complained of much pain over the stomach, there was vomiting at times, she was losing weight rapidly, but no tumour could be made out in the abdomen. Four days before operation the pain in the abdomen became general and more severe, and a hard tumour the size of a small orange was made out in the position of the pylorus; the emaciation was by this time marked; the woman now said she had eaten some hat pins, but statements by lunatics cannot always be relied upon. I saw her on November 30th, and from the symptoms and physical signs I thought I might find a malignant growth of the pylorus. I made a free incision into the abdominal cavity, and came down on a large mass of what looked like cancer involving the pyloric one-third of the stomach; on examining this with my finger, I found half a sewing needle. Having now something definite to guide me, I incised the mass, which was three inches thick and covered the whole of the anterior surface of the pyloric end of the stomach; it was hard and cut like scirrhus, the section, however, showing numerous points of hemorrhage with surrounding rings of various shades of yellow to red,—these were no doubt due to punctures by the hat pins. In one of these zones I could feel a sharp point. I deepened the incision and opened up the stomach, felt the head and extracted the first of the ornaments of the female head-gear. The rule which we follow after having removed a stone from the bladder occurred to me, and I decided to make sure there were no more foreign bodies in the stomach, and to explore the whole of this cavity I had to enlarge my opening, and after some delay I extracted the third and then the fourth offending member, the last being firmly fixed in the coats of the stomach. The heads of the pins prevented nature from expelling the unwelcome guests, but she had tried very hard to shut off the general peritoneal cavity by the deposition of so much fibrous tissue. I closed the stomach by three rows of Lembert sutures, and did not drain or wash out the peritoneal cavity. The operation was a long one, and the patient was much collapsed for forty-eight hours: she however recovered rapidly, the mental condition at once improving; she was up and eating light solid food in three weeks, and was discharged from the asylum three months after operation mentally and bodily cured.

It will be observed that the form of mental trouble in most of the cases was one in which we should not expect to find a rapid improvement, even if improvement at all took place under ordinary circumstances.

I am much obliged to Dr. Law Wade and to Dr. Sproat for the histories of some of the cases, and I feel sure that a good deal of the credit and the pleasing results of the cases under their care is due to the way the after-treatment was carried out.

After the reading of Mr. Bush's cases, Dr. J. H. SPROAT said that all the cases made good mental recoveries immediately after the operations. The cases of uterine fibroid and the gastrotomy more especially call for remark, as the prognosis of their mental disease was distinctly unfavourable on account of its duration and the constancy of their delusions. Analogous mental recoveries are seen when the insane suffer from severe attacks of acute bodily disease, such as pneumonia or erysipelas; impending dissolution frequently restores the mental condition, and cases of almost hopeless insanity die sane. Such results as accrued from the above cases should determine operation in doubtful cases, and no surgical condition should be allowed to exist in the insane simply because the person is a lunatic. The idea of suicide by swallowing hat-pins was originated in the above patient by reading the gruesome details of an operation for a swallowed hat-pin in one of our up-to-date dailies.—Dr. H. C. BRISTOWE said he had had some years of lunacy experience, but knew very little about surgical operations on the insane. The only case that came actually under his care was a tracheotomy for malignant disease of œsophagus and larynx; whether there was any improvement he could not say, as the patient did not live long enough. Mr. Bush's cases are, however, of great interest; but it was doubtful whether the mental recovery of those patients was due to the removal of the exciting cause, but rather to the mental effect that the operation had on the individual—the substitution of a healthy for an unhealthy introspection. It is a well established fact that in lunacy improvement takes place in the mental condition during an acute febrile disorder, but it is doubtful whether these cases can be included in the same category.—Dr. J. O. SYMES said that the sample of pus submitted by Mr. Bush, in addition to containing the bacillus of blue pus, contained also torulæ and various motile bacteria which were suggestive of its origin from the intestinal tract.

A SIMPLE FORM OF INFLUENCE MACHINE FOR X-RAY WORK.

BY

WILLIAM COTTON, M.A., M.D. Ed.

To get X-rays out of a suitable vacuum tube, it needs to be excited by an electric discharge at a tension of hundreds of thousands of volts. Such a discharge is furnished by the induction coil and by the static induction or "influence" machine, associated in its most elegant and effective form with the name of Mr. Wimshurst. In spite of the obvious advantages of the latter type of machine over the former, very little systematic X-ray work with the influence machine has appeared; and the greater number of the text-books of radiography pass the matter over with a general statement that the

Holtz or the Wimshurst machine from the steadiness and continuity of its discharge is specially fitted for work with the screen. It is possible, however, with a very simple form of influence machine to get good X-ray negatives. Such an apparatus is represented in Fig. 1.

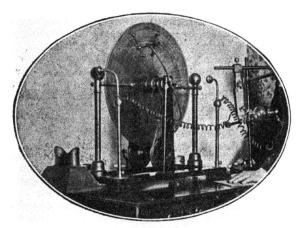

FIG. 1.

The essential part consists of two parallel circular discs of ordinary window glass, 22 inches in diameter, about $\frac{1}{8}$ of an inch thick, and $\frac{1}{4}$ of an inch apart, varnished with shellac. Being mounted centrally on independent wooden bosses, they can be rotated in opposite directions on a horizontal metallic spindle or axle, which pierces them and is supported at each end by a wooden upright springing vertically from a stout rectangular mahogany base. The lower parts of the two uprights support another horizontal axle, parallel to the main one, turned by a handle, with two wooden wheels on it, which by a crossed and an open strap act respectively on the bosses of the glass discs and thus supply the necessary motive power. The glass employed is of the gauge of 22 ounces per square foot. It must be of the highest dielectric quality; green glass and plate glass are found unsuitable, and of white glass of similar commercial standard some specimens are found on trial much fitter than others. Ebonite discs do very well, but exposure to vicissitudes of temperature causes them to bend and buckle, and in time the atmosphere affects them chemically on the surface and so deteriorates their insulating property.

At each end of the main axle where it projects through the supporting upright is metallically connected a movable brass rod, known as the neutralising rod. This rod is bent round at each end towards the surface of the adjacent glass disc, and has jointed to it at each end a straight piece about four inches long, radially disposed as regards the glass disc, parallel to its surface and just within the outer margin thereof. Each straight piece has attached to it at equal distances so as lightly to trail upon the surface of the glass three fine wire brushes. Thus we have two neutralising rods, a near one and a far one, each with two straight pieces, and each straight piece has three brushes, *i.e.*, there are twelve neutralising brushes in all. In Fig. 1 the greater part of the neutralising rod on the near side of the discs is seen, with its upper straight piece; the upper straight piece and brushes of the farther neutralising rod are dimly seen through the two glass discs.

Besides the wooden uprights, there are situated upon the rectangular base of the apparatus and towards its extremities three other pairs of structures. At the inside or far side of the base are two insulating cups or holders for a pair of Leyden jars, should it be thought advisable to join them up in the circuit. In front of each holder and opposite the right and left lateral rims of the glass discs are two stout vertical rods of ebonite or other insulating material, supporting a polished brass sphere about three inches in diameter—the prime conductors. From the metallic neck of each prime conductor there runs in horizontally for about four inches and exactly in the line of the horizontal diameter of the glass discs a pair of brass collecting rods—one rod in front of the near disc, the other behind the farther one. Each collecting rod has on it at equal distances eight trailing brushes similar to those on the neutralising rods. Thus we have two prime conductors—a right one and a left one—each with two collecting rods, and each collecting rod has eight brushes, *i.e.*, there are thirty-two collecting brushes in all. In front of the insulating supports of the prime conductors is a pair of more slender insulating rods to support the metallic stems of two approximately hemispherical knobs, somewhat smaller than the spherical heads of the prime conductors, which may be called the secondary conductors. The metallic stem is bent to a right angle. The supporting insulating rods can be rotated round the vertical axis and fixed at any point by a small set screw, so that the gap—the spark gap—between the prime and secondary conductor of each side is an adjustable one. It is on the management of these spark gaps, in series with the vacuum tube, that success or failure in the emission of X-rays from the tube mainly depends in the case of the influence machine.

The remainder of the apparatus as ordinarily joined up consists of two well-insulated thick copper wires or "leads," coiled *secundum artem*, running over from the brass stem of each secondary conductor to the external wire terminal of the indispensable Jackson focus tube on the same side. The stem of the tube is held by a specially designed well-insulated stand, with well-insulated ebonite rods to support the wire leads and to take the strain of them from off the external wire terminals of the tube. It is useful in some cases to have some arrangement for a second spark gap in series on each side of the tube; and it is always of importance to have the leads connected with the respective external wire terminals of the tube under cover of small hollow tunnelled brass spheres to minimise leakage of electricity from sharp points by brush discharge outside the tube. The internal resistance of the focus tube best suited for this machine is so great, that the distance apart of the external wire terminals of the electrodes into the tube should be greater than the spark length of the machine in air with tube away, with the same view of preventing brush discharge. To avoid the risk of puncture of the tube by sparking, the tube should have its external wire terminals at least eight or ten inches apart.

With the machine described a pair of Leyden jars may be used in two ways. *First:* The secondary conductors being disconnected from the tube and connected one to another by a thick copper wire between the brass stems, the spark gap between prime and secondary conductor on each side is left open, and the inside of each Leyden jar is put in direct communication with the adjacent conductor. Each jar is on its insulating cup, and has its outside coating connected by a thick copper lead to an external terminal of the tube. When the accumulated unlike internal charges of the Leyden jars recombine across the spark gaps and the wire uniting the secondary conductors, we have the reverse charges in the outer coatings recombining across the tube. As a result we have one or two explosive discharges per second, with deafening noise and an almost blinding yellow fluorescence of the tube; the screen lights up most brilliantly, but only for a moment. Owing probably to the higher quantity (amperage) of the electrical discharge, this method is dangerous to operator and patient, and very detrimental to the tube: it is only to be used with great caution in radiographing the thickest parts of the body. *Second:* When the apparatus is joined up in the ordinary way, a well-insulated Leyden jar (with the knob from its interior in contact with the adjacent prime conductor), at each side, having its outer coating removed, promises to be of great use. When this arrangement is made, the discharge across the spark gaps is white instead of violet, and is continuous. In this case the jars act as condensers or reservoirs of electricity.

The machine described, like other influence machines which have no metallic sectors, plates, buttons, or knobs upon the discs, is not (except under the most unusual climatic conditions) self-exciting—in other words, the discs are revolved with no electrical effect unless an initial charge of + or − electricity is communicated to one or other of the prime conductors. Once excited, it will not require re-excitement for a whole evening though revolved very slowly, or even allowed to be at rest for a little while. The most convenient method is to have a miniature influence machine, called the "Exciter," of the type which is the best known of Mr. Wimshurst's numerous modifications of the influence machine (shown in Fig. 2, in position to give a − charge of

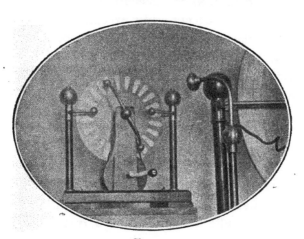

F̲ɪɢ. 2.

electricity to the left-hand conductor of its big relation). The sectors render it self-exciting—it has two glass discs seven inches in diameter, each with twenty-four tinfoil sectors on outside face, one brush on each neutralising rod to touch the passing sectors, and brushes on the collecting rods. There is a 1½-inch spark. For exciting purposes, only one prime conductor is needed on it; the other is superfluous.

16

It will at once be seen that structurally the two machines are almost identical. The influence machine described at length is a sectorless Wimshurst—it is a Wimshurst without sectors, with trailing brushes at the collecting and neutralising rods instead of points that are not in contact and brushes that merely touch the metallic sectors. In practice the sectorless Wimshurst is to be preferred to a sectored one of the same size for five reasons :—

(1) It is easier to construct and keep in order—it is simpler.

(2) It never reverses polarity during running—the other does so occasionally.

(3) It has a greater output of electrical energy—the tube lights up better with the same amount of mechanical energy expended on the handle.

(4) In a sectored Wimshurst, where there is a great resistance in the tube, the inner ends of the sectors leak towards the boss, as shown by a visible brush discharge.

(5) After prolonged use the friction of the brushes on the sectors as they pass leads to the formation of rings of metallic deposit, which break down the insulation.

On the other hand, except under exceptional circumstances, the sectorless Wimshurst is not, and the sectored Wimshurst is, self-exciting.

The sectorless Wimshurst having been carefully dusted, has a charge communicated by spark or contact from the exciter, and the discs are revolved. One soon learns which is the proper prime conductor to charge, according as the cathode or anode is left or right in circuit. Most operators find it convenient to turn the handle from left to right over the top of the circle. The energy to be expended is quite within the ability of an intelligent small boy. It is not a very high form of skilled labour to turn a handle steadily, and as a rule there is no lack of willing amateur assistance available, so that the medical man's attention can be entirely devoted to keeping the injured part and the patient steady. The most effective output of electricity is got when the winch is rotated eighty times a minute, giving 200 revolutions in the same time to each glass disc in opposite directions. The spark gaps are opened gradually from contact till the tube fluoresces brilliantly, which it never fails to do; unless there is actually damp deposited on the outside of the tube, the spirit lamp is entirely unnecessary. The focus tube to be preferred is one adapted for a nominally 10-inch spark induction coil: the sectorless Wimshurst gives with Leyden jars a maximum spark of 10½ inches; without, in favourable conditions of atmospheric dryness, a continuous brush discharge of 9½ inches in length between terminals when the tube is removed. All the brass work of the conductors should be of the highest finish, to avoid the formation of any pointed parts and consequent brush discharge owing to local increase of electric density; and for the same reason care must be taken that if any silk fastenings are made at the external terminals of the tube the knotted ends be cut short. Otherwise we shall get a large part of the discharge streaming away visibly. Bedclothes in the neighbourhood of the circuit should be put out of the way, for if they are heaped up towards the tube, the moisture in them streams up and locally breaks down the atmospheric insulation. The apparatus, joined up in the ordinary way, is free from noisiness—there is only a low-pitched hissing sound. The odour associated with the presence of ozone is very perceptible. It is found that the best results are obtained when the upper end of the nearer neutralising rod is situated 30° to the left of the vertical, and that of the farther one the same distance to the right (the " five minutes to five " position).

The self-excitement of the sectored Wimshurst on rotation is commonly explained by saying that when there are a number of metallic insulated plates scattered over a large non-conducting surface, one or other of them is pretty sure to be above or below the rest in electric potential. In other words, there is always an initial charge somewhere about. If the *rationale* of action of the ancestral electrophorus of Volta be kept in mind, it is comparatively easy in a general way to understand how by mutual induction (of each on all the rest) the metallic sectors of a sectored Wimshurst, one or other of which has a charge in it, can on rotation give rise to a continuous heaping up of + electricity at one prime conductor and of − electricity at the other, while the neutralising rods by the touch of their brushes on the passing sectors play the part of the touching finger on the "shield" of the electrophorus. The sectorless Wimshurst, once it has an initial charge given to one of its prime conductors, produces, in a manner that is very obscure, a similar heaping up of a + and a − electricity at opposite conductors. Mr. Wimshurst suggests that in the sectorless machine the trailing brushes (which ones?) act as sectors. Finally, the recombining electricities discharge across the vacuum tube put in the path of their reunion.

The results obtained by means of the sectorless Wimshurst described may be given under two heads.

I.—With the Screen.

I was able to see the shadow of a watch through the trunk of a thickset man; the heart with the pericardial bag was quite distinctly seen in outline suspended in the thorax of a boy of ten viewed from the back; in a young lady of twelve, the waves of contraction of the heart muscle on its left border were seen quite deliberately passing downwards in regular succession, viewed from the front of the chest; it was always possible with the Leyden jars joined up to get the fluorescent glow on the screen through the adult trunk. Every detail of the bones, even the fissure of a fracture if caught in its plane, could be seen in the hand, wrist, elbow, and ankle of the adult, and the shoulder and thorax of a young boy. In all these parts we get indications of soft tissues. The bones of the phalanges and metacarpus could be distinguished five' feet from the tube through a wooden door; and at the same distance the screen lit up through a brick partition.

It is an interesting point to note that the fluorescent screen glows with a light that has very little actinic power. Photographs with an ordinary camera of objects shadowed on the screen have been taken successfully, but I have never seen any, and have failed again and again to obtain a negative at different distances and with different kinds of plates, even after an exposure of ten minutes. On the other hand, it is easy to obtain a good photograph of a fluorescing focus tube with an exposure of a quarter of a minute; while everyone knows the electric spark under the same conditions photographs itself instantaneously.

FIG. 3.

OBLIQUE FRACTURE LOWER ⅓ OF TIBIA IN ADULT.

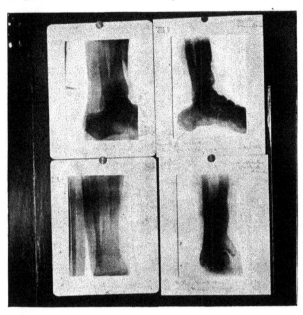

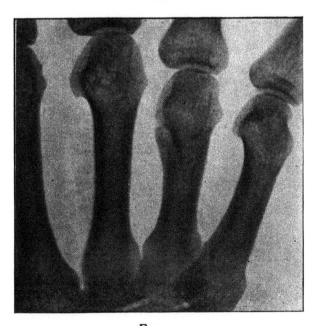

FIG. 4.

OBLIQUE FRACTURE OF METACARPAL BONE OF RING FINGER
(two months after injury).

To employ a screen to the best advantage the room must be darkened, and the eyes prepared by being kept in a dimly lighted room for ten or fifteen minutes. Daylight should always be religiously excluded.

II.—With the Photographic Plate.

The duration of exposure is somewhat long; about half the time would be sufficient where the detection of the presence only of a metallic foreign body is needed. We get pictures with detail and sharpness and quite a perspective effect, not mere shadowgraphs. To do justice to the negative, I always use gelatino-chloride paper, slightly undertone, and squeegee on polished glass. Shortness of exposure for its own sake is not much of an object when using the Wimshurst apparatus, as the patient keeps placid, and the operator is not obsessed by the haunting idea of impending collapse to one or more parts of a long train of complicated and costly apparatus. To give examples of the degree of detail, the sesamoid bones of the hand and foot (including that in the tendon of the peroneus longus as it crosses the sole of the foot) came out sharply, and we get details of all the bones of wrist, elbow, ankle, and knee, especially in the adult—the fibrous structure of the os calcis and astragalus is quite distinctly shown. Time of exposure: *Adult:* Fingers, 2 minutes; hand, 8—10 minutes; forearm, 10 minutes; elbow, 10 minutes; shaft of humerus, 10 minutes; shoulder (with clavicle, ribs, and scapula), 45 minutes; foot and ankle, 16—20 minutes; knee and leg, 20 minutes. *Aged 12:* Hip-joint, showing pelvic brim, 20 minutes. *Aged 6:* Femur, shaft, 18—20 minutes. *Fœtus, 6—7 months:* 15 minutes.

Among my own cases were fracture of upper part of ulna in a boy of 10; fracture of the shaft of the femur in a boy of 6 on the 24th day; oblique fracture of the lower end of tibia in an adult (see Fig. 3, where the two ankles above and below to the left were taken on the 29th day, the others on the 96th): fractures of the metacarpal bones of the thumb in adult and of the ring finger in adult on the 4th and 64th days (for this last see Fig. 4); in these and in others the fragments are seen in perspective and, as it were, one through another where they overlap. Those figured have been chosen to show the easily available range of the apparatus described. In two cases of suspected renal calculus, after two trials, in each case of about 35—45 minutes each, no stone appeared in the negative, only the indication of some ribs in the thinner (female) subject, and of the iliac crest in the other (a male). In both cases, at both trials, sufficient rays were got through to bring out the shadow of a coin lying on the envelope of the photographic plate. In the first case I was quite satisfied that if an oxalate of lime calculus—which is the most opaque of calculi to X-rays—had been present, it would have appeared on the negative. To be successful in these cases a more powerful apparatus is needed, say one with two pairs of discs 22 inches in diameter, or with two discs 36 inches in diameter; or possibly the same apparatus would do with a very soft tube.

In the cases enumerated, the average distance of the platinum plate from the photographic plate would be about 12 inches. At this distance a whole plate uses up only about $\frac{1}{15}$ of the available area of X-rays, and at 15 inches only about $\frac{1}{24}$, assuming the rays to radiate with equal intensity from the anti-cathodal centre of emission over just a little less than a hemisphere.[1] Some day we shall learn how to economise our X-rays a little better.

Dr. Monell[2] states that his apparatus (constructed originally for therapeutic purposes) consisted of an 8-plate 30-inch Holtz machine, not self-exciting, driven by a $\frac{1}{8}$-horse-power motor. He took a detailed radiogram (14 by 17 inches) of a fully clothed adult woman from a distance of twenty-five inches in five minutes. He undertakes to get negatives of the hip-joint, of renal calculus, or metallic bodies anywhere in the trunk of the adult in five minutes at twelve or fifteen inches distance. He publishes no radiogram, nor have I been able in any of the text-books, including those mentioned at the end of this paper, to find any radiogram avowedly obtained by means of an influence machine, except one[3] of a purse containing a key and

---

[1] " Further Observations on the Properties of X Rays," by W. C. Roentgen, translated in *Arch. Roentgen Ray*, 1898-99, iii. 80, 82.

[2] *Manual of Static Electricity in X-Ray and Therapeutic Uses*, 1897.

[3] *Roentgen Rays and the Phenomena of the Anode and Cathode*, E. P. Thompson, 1896, p. 99.

two coins obtained in sixty minutes, and another[1] of a bird showing excellent detail, and one[2] of a frog, of which the same may be said.

The ordinary process blocks of the periodicals are very unsatisfactory in reproducing the delicate gradation and detail of Wimshurst negatives. Lantern slides by reduction from the negative are also unsatisfactory. Lantern slides by contact are better; and lantern slides by reduction from a glazed silver print on gelatino-chloride paper are best of all. In this case, after taking precautions to avoid flares from the highly-glazed surface of the print, a quarter-plate process plate negative is taken in an ordinary camera; and the negative when developed for contrast is intensified slightly for the finer detail. Lantern slides are then taken from the process negative by contact, or prints may be got in miniature of the original ones. The method is further useful when we wish to show by lantern on the sheet a grouping together of different prints. After all, nothing comes up to the original highly finished gelatino-chloride positives. In every case the photographer must have the usual methods of negative development and intensification at his finger-ends to get the best results of his X-ray exposures.

The advantages of an influence machine in X-ray work may now be considered, taking as a standard of comparison an eight- or ten-inch spark induction coil, with special reference to the sectorless Wimshurst described.

(1) The primary inducing current of the coil and its appurtenances are abolished. There is no primary battery or accumulator, no interrupter, no primary coil, and consequently none of the uncertainties, annoyances, or risks of breakdown associated with the use of these pieces of mechanism. Further, the absence of Fizeau's condenser (a necessary part of the primary circuit to render the discharge of the secondary coil unipolar and to minimise the sparking at the platinum contacts of the interrupter) removes one source of "fault" development (and breakdown by sparking penetration of an insu-

---

[1] *The A.B.C. of the X-rays*, W. H. Meadowcroft.

[2] *Arch. Roentgen Ray*, 1898-99, iii. pl. LV.

lating partition) somewhere over its forty or fifty square feet of area—a fault that is difficult to locate, reach, or repair. A similar remark applies to the secondary coil of the induction coil proper, with its six or eight miles of fine insulated wire, which at any point, from overheating or mechanical injury or sparking perforation due to overdriving, may likewise develop a "fault." In place are substituted two glass discs in the open, easily removed and replaced if broken.

(2) Owing to the small amount of electricity, though at a high tension, passing continuously and regularly, the life of the tube as regards useful work is a prolonged one. There is none of the heating of the internal terminals of the tube under the heavy, interrupted, and it may be irregular discharges of the induction coil. The tube, not a very soft one to begin with, used for the last year with the sectorless Wimshurst has been under continuous discharge for a total of over 160 hours, and has only recently shown signs of "hardening." This hardening over its first condition is probably due to the use of the Leyden jars, for a few hours in the aggregate, by means of their outer coatings, in the manner described. When joined up in the ordinary way the tube never appears to heat and has never failed to respond promptly to the excitation of the discharge. The only difference to be noted is that the spark gaps have to be a little wider than they were a year ago. The tube has never turned sulky or needed to be coaxed with the spirit lamp or by any other of the empirical methods resorted to by the practical worker with the coil. It is probable that with the coil no tube after the first dozen hours of exposure to actual discharge but is perceptibly hardened, especially if the capacity of the apparatus is forced to its utmost. The sharpness of the Wimshurst negative is probably due in part to the quiet continuous discharge, the small emitting area not shifting, nor the original fine adjustment of the cathode and anticathode altered by irregular or extreme heatings under greatly varying discharges. To put the matter in a nutshell, it is hardly to be expected that any induction coil set, worked at a strain to perform some *tour de force*, however successful at the time, will repeat the performance, while a static induction machine

may be almost surely relied on to do again what it has once done.

(3) It is generally acknowledged that the continuous non-flickering, uniform discharge, varying only with the rate of rotation of the discs up to a maximum, of the influence machine renders it more suitable than the induction coil for work with the fluorescent screen. But, further, it is peculiarly fitted, especially if driven by a well-regulated electric or other motor, for delicate and prolonged experimentation, *e.g.* for photometric observation of the intensity of the fluorescence under different conditions ; for examining into the influence of X-rays on bacteria in the animal body or in cultures ; for testing the action of the rays on growing plants or germinating seeds. All such experiments when made with a coil labour under the fallacy that nothing certain is known quantitatively about the agent employed, except that it is on the whole after a short time irregularly diminishing in energy. The Wimshurst apparatus is the only one at present known in X-ray work that is adapted for the standardising of X-ray electrical, fluorescent and other physico-chemical effects.

(4) When joined up in the ordinary way without Leyden jars the static induction machine gives a discharge which is absolutely harmless to operator or patient, even if the live wires be purposely handled. A pricking sensation hardly amounting to pain and a fading of fluorescence in the tube is the sole result. There are none of the dangerous shocks to be apprehended from accidentally touching the circuit of the induction coil, on account of the small amperage associated with the continuous discharge of the former apparatus. No cases of eczema have been reported with the influence machine as yet ; it would be very interesting to test the matter by exposing to X-rays from a tube excited by an influence machine individuals who are known to be susceptible to X-rays and to have previously suffered from exposure to a tube excited by a coil. In demonstrating his fluorescent screen, the demonstrator has had to be exposed to the rays of the tube with his trunk in close neighbourhood thereto for four and a half hours without any inconvenience.

(5) In regard to portability, an important question as regards cases that have to be X-rayed in their own bedrooms, it may be mentioned that the sectorless Wimshurst weighs 28 lbs., the Leyden jars 3 lbs. each, the focus tube and stand 7 lbs., and the exciter 7 lbs.—in all 45 lbs.,—just a little over the weight of a six-celled charged lithanode accumulator; the jars are not indispensable, and in this case the apparatus weighs rather less. The whole apparatus can be packed in a box 39 × 19 × 14 inches, which can be used as a pedestal.

(6) The cost of an apparatus is about half or a third of a coil set giving the same length of spark; and there is no cost for maintenance or repairs, there being no accumulators to re-charge or parts to wear out.

The objection most urged against the influence machine is that it is liable to be much affected by damp and dust. Most certainly it is not more so than other electrical apparatus, and with ordinary care there is no great difficulty in keeping it in working order. Mr. Wimshurst says his machines work in the damp; he keeps them in glass cases permanently, to avoid dust and handling by the inexperienced. The sectorless Holtz is more susceptible to damp, and requires to be kept permanently in a case with a bowl of chloride of calcium, changed every six months, to keep the air dry. The sectorless Wimshurst described is kept in an ordinary room without any casing, and taken without packing in a cab to the patient's house; and if the night be damp, a little warming at a fire and dusting with a silk handkerchief is all that is required. On only one occasion I have seen it make a failure, and then it was on a very damp night in a long damp vault of a schoolroom, set up for use on a platform that had just been brought in from lying in the drizzle. Even under these circumstances we got a fair negative of metallic objects, and could see the bones of a man's fingers on the screen.

This paper has been written in collaboration with Mr. Thomas Clark, of Horfield, Bristol. He is almost entirely responsible for the electrical part of it. Some time ago he experimented successfully for X-rays with a sectored Wimshurst of his own construction, and was led to devise and construct the sectorless modification described above. His apparatus and some of the resulting radiograms were demonstrated lately by means of photographs and lantern slides before the Roentgen Society of London, and roused considerable interest among the electricians and medical men present. Having worked previously with coil and accumulator, I can speak from personal experience of the advantages and convenience of his system, especially in patients' own homes.

The Roentgen ray is the gift of Experimental Science to the Art of Medicine; it remains to be seen what uses the physician will make of this munificent present from the physicist. Simplicity of apparatus, provided we have efficiency and reliability for ordinary purposes, is the necessary condition for a general application of the new light to diagnosis by the practitioner. It is interesting to note that the evolution of the existing therapeutic influence machines for X-ray purposes has been in the direction of simplification, whereas the induction coil tends every day to become increasingly elaborate, complicated, and costly.

Mr. Wimshurst's latest expressed opinion is that "in a few years influence machines will be the only generators of electricity in use for X-ray purposes."

BIBLIOGRAPHY.

*References marked * I have been unable to verify myself.*

A. As regards the **history and theory** of the **influence machine**, a good deal of information is given in standard electrical textbooks. (The trade catalogues which electrical manufacturing firms give are interesting as regards the form of apparatus, and different forms of Wimshurst are described and figured in *Engineering*, vol. xxxiv., p. 323, May 21, 1886; vol. xxxv., p. 4, April 17, 1891; vol. xxxix., p. 60, May 5, 1893; vol. xxxix., p. 490, May 21, 1897; Oct. 6, 1882: and the *English Mechanic*, Nov. 14, 1884; Jan. 16, 1885; May 1, 1885; Oct. 10, 1885; Nov. 6, 1885.)

"Influence Electrical Machines," a lecture delivered by Mr. James Wimshurst to the Royal Institution, April 27, 1888.

"Influence Machines from 1788 to 1888," Prof. Silvanus Thompson: an address to the Society of Telegraph Engineers and Electricians, with discussion, *The Electrician*, June 8, 15, 22 and 29, 1888.

Electric Influence Machines, by J. Gray, 1890.

" Wimshurst Alternating Influence Machine," *English Mechanic*, Nov. 27, 1891.

" Alternating and Experimental Influence Machine," Mr. James Wimshurst, *Proceedings of the Physical Society of London*, Dec. 1871, and *Philosophical Magazine*, June, 1891.

" A New Form of Influence Machine," by James Wimshurst ; and

" An Influence Machine," by W. R. Pidgeon, *Proceedings of the Physical Society of London*, Dec., 1873.

B. As regards the **use** of the **influence machine** for **X-rays**.

Practical Radiography, by A. W. Isenthal and H. Snowden Ward, 1896, gives some practical details of early work with the Wimshurst machine.

* " Radiography," by W. Wilson, *Photography*, vol. viii., p. 708.

* " Experiments on Röntgen Rays," by T. C. Porter, *Nature*, 1896, liv. 149 ; 1896–97, lv. 30.

* " Production of X-Rays," by Prof. Oliver Lodge, *Nature*, 1896-97, lv. 100.

Manual of Static Electricity in X-ray and Therapeutic Uses, by S. H. Monell, 1897.

Radiography, by G. R. Bottone, chaps. vi. and vii., 1898.

" The Advantages of the Influence Machine for Lighting X Ray Tubes," by Mr. James Wimshurst ; paper read to the Roentgen Society, *Arch. Roentgen Ray*, 1898, ii. 83.

" The Influence Machine in X Ray Work," by Heber Robarts, M.D., abstracted in *Arch. Roentgen Ray*, 1898–99, iii. 104.

Progress of the Medical Sciences.

MEDICINE.

Common as **malaria** is in Bristol in returned sailors and soldiers, nothing is more remarkable than the disappearance of the home-grown disease from England in the last fifty years, and it is to be hoped that our neighbours in the marsh districts will exert themselves to discover whether those mosquito gnats have actually vanished from this country which have been shown to transmit it. Stephens found two species of anopheles here in 1825, and an investigation has been set on foot to determine whether they, like the malaria, have ceased to multiply on British soil.

Thin [1] points out that one great objection to the mosquito theory of malaria fell to the ground when it was shown that only certain species conveyed it, for both the fever districts and the healthy ones in Sicily swarm with mosquitos. Grassi [2] found that in Italy Culex pipiens swarmed in places where there was no human malaria; but where this disease existed the anopheles, or else the Culex penicillaris or Culex malariæ abound. Ross had already shown that C. pipiens was the form which produced malaria in sparrows, and had traced the development of the avian parasites in its body. The Italians did the same with the human plasmode in anopheles, and last autumn they produced malaria in a healthy man, who volunteered for the experiment, by shutting him up with these mosquitos which had been brought from an infected district. It has been shown that the young ones when hatched in a laboratory cannot convey the disease; but if they bite an affected person, and are kept some days in a warm temperature, they will then produce in a previously healthy person the exact type of malaria from which the first man was suffering. Thus experimental proof has been given of two points: the first, that the parasite can pass from the human body to a second host in certain mosquitos; and secondly, that mosquitos can produce the disease in men. Koch notices that in the central parts of Rome malaria does not appear, although the water comes from malarial districts; and Bignami and Grassi bring an argument against the theory of air-borne infection, showing that the plasmodes cannot bear the least desiccation. [3] Against the actual facts of the Italians, Lawrie's theoretical objections have little weight. So late as last December we find him asserting that the Laveran bodies are merely degenerate blood cells. [4] Thayer and Hewetson found them in every one of 616 cases of malaria except two or three convalescents. [5] Still, Ewing [6] acknowledges that occasionally they cannot be met with in a typical case of æstivo-autumnal fever; but even then a search in the spleen will sometimes reveal them, just as in similar cases of typhoid.

According to Ross, [7] the life history of the plasmode commences with its existence as an amœbula in a red cell which develops either asexually by spores for several generations in the same host; or, by gametocytes, such as the crescents, which, taken up by mosquitos, show male and female forms.

[1] Brit. M. J., 1899, ii. 349.
[2] Quoted in Editorial, Brit. M. J., 1898, ii. 1767.   [3] Ibid.
[4] Lancet, 1898, ii. 1468
[5] Johns Hopkins Hosp. Rep., 1895, v. 5.   [6] N. York M. J., 1899, lxix. 149.
[7] Nature, 1899 lx. 323.

Filaments from the male forms attack the female ones. The fertilised body is termed a zygote, which grows in the stomach-wall of the mosquito, and finally produces the flagellulæ or zygotoblasts. These pass into the salivary duct and stylet of the mosquito, and are introduced into a new host. If it can be shown that we can extirpate the malaria-bearing species of mosquito in a given locality, and that they are only a few out of many, the propagation of the parasites and of the disease may be stopped. It is claimed that their breeding places are comparatively few, and that the larvæ are killed by a few drops of paraffin thrown into the pool where they live. However, the subject is yet in its infancy, and one in which Bristol men may find an ample field for study.

*   *   *   *

Gastric ulcer is clinically accompanied in most cases by hyperchlorhydria, which, if not the cause, at any rate has great influence in prolonging the condition. Hence the value of **treatment directed against the excess of acid,** such as feeding entirely by the rectum and the use of the fixed alkalies, as magnesia and carbonate of bismuth, to neutralise the secretion without stimulating it as soda does. Milk, too, is valuable from its rapid combination with the free acid. Thus Frèmont[1] gives an ounce of warm milk with bismuth and magnesia every half-hour for twenty hours to be increased if the pain is not relieved. Olivetti[2] finds that the plan of giving massive doses of bismuth, 2½ to 5 drachms, every morning on an empty stomach, for which so much has been claimed, produces little change in the motility or secretions of the organ ; while Soupault declares that sodium chlorate in divided doses of two drachms daily, given when the stomach is empty, affords great relief in ulcer or hyperchlorhydria.

Tripier,[3] to cope with **hemorrhage,** employs rectal injections of hot water at a temperature of about 120° every few hours, and allows no food to be given by the mouth. A form of ulcer-ation, the minute erosion of gastric arteries, originally described by Murchison, is of interest from the absence of the usual dyspeptic symptoms beforehand. Dieulafoy and Lindsay Steven[4] have each pointed out that it may be the initial form of the ordinary round ulcer. The condition however has been rarely seen, and similar cases have been referred to vaso-motor disturb-ance. There is merely a small superficial abrasion with an opening into a vessel, easily overlooked. The hemorrhage may be extremely profuse; one of Steven's patients lost ninety-six ounces, and in another gastrotomy was unsuccessful from the difficulty of finding the bleeding point. The diagnosis would have to be made from ordinary ulcer, varix of the stomach or œsophagus, cancer, hyperæmia in heart disease, and duodenal ulcer.

*   *   *   *

[1] *Am. J. M. Sc.*, 1898, cxvi. 610.   [2] *Brit. M. J.*, 1898, ii. Epitome, p. 103.
[3] *Brit. M. J.*, 1899, i. Epitome, p. 12.   [4] *Glasgow M. J.*, 1899, li. 5.

Renal tuberculosis has been largely relegated to the care of the surgeon, partly as a local affection which should be removed as early as possible lest the bladder and general system should be affected, and partly from the little success which has attended medical treatment of tubercular diseases in the past. It is an interesting question, as our treatment of phthisis becomes more and more perfect, how far this view must be altered. In other words, can we expect such local affections, at least in their earliest stages, to disappear under the increased resisting power of the tissues brought about by fresh air, increased nourishment, climatic and other aids? How many instances of spontaneous cure and of recovery, more or less complete, under improved conditions of general health are on record? Enough to show that as great results may be hoped for with the improved methods as in phthisis.

The kidney is attacked either above from the blood-stream or below from the bladder, prostate, and testes, and practically never by direct invasion from a neighbouring tubercular focus such as a suprarenal one. In the **descending type** the first lesions are seen in the cortex or as minute tubercles under the mucous membrane of the pelvis,[1] and the disease may take the miliary or caseous form, or produce a pyelo-nephritis. The bacilli have been demonstrated in the glomeruli before any pathological changes were observable, and the possibility of their frequent passage in tuberculous patients through the kidney without injuring it is to be considered. Tilden Brown[2] seems to think this may sometimes be the case, but he does not give any instances where bacilli have been found in the urine and the kidneys after death proved to be normal. On the other hand, he points out that in descending tuberculosis the disease in the kidney may be far advanced before any symptoms appear.

The absence of symptoms in the descending form previous to an eruption into the calices is in marked contrast to the violent pain and dysuria which occur in early stages when the infection **ascends** from the bladder.

If, then, we have often no means of diagnosing an early attack, it may be asked whether we may expect the disease in any definite **percentage** of tuberculous patients. Chambers found it occurred in 18 per cent, Tilden Brown in 34, Collinet 5.5, and the Prague statistics give 5.6. But even if these figures were trustworthy they would be of little use, because the disease is so often the first or the only manifestation of tuberculosis, and we do not know the relative frequency of these primary and secondary cases. In doubtful instances some importance clearly attaches to a tubercular history or the presence of disease in the lungs, epididymis, bladder, peritoneum, or intestines; but it has been experimentally produced by

---

[1] Bryson, in *A System of Genito-Urinary Diseases* [etc.]. Edited by Prince A. Morrow, vol. i. part ii., 1893, p. 837.

[2] *N. York M. J.*, 1897, lxv. 377.

injection of bacilli into the aorta by Borrell, and the mode or
entrance into the system may be undiscoverable. We can only
say that renal tuberculosis has been found in from 1 to 2 per
cent. of all necropsies in 5,000 cases by Morris and Carmargo;
it is more common in men than in women, and rare in infancy.
In about half the cases both kidneys are affected, and at an
early stage the prostate will show one or two hard nodules
in almost every case, according to Bryson,[1] even when the
disease began in the kidney. The opinion is generally held
now that the descending form is the prevalent one, though
Rokitansky and many others took the opposite view. All
authorities however agree that the prostate rarely escapes,
and emphasise the importance of its examination. Hamill,[2]
who collected fifty-five cases in children under 14, finds that in
them the disease is almost always of the descending type,
genital tuberculosis as a starting point being certainly rare at
this age.

When **symptoms** do occur, they may include paroxysmal
or continued pain in any part of the urinary tract, hæmaturia
with acid urine, the presence of a tumour, the signs of bladder
irritation, and tubercle bacilli. Brown remarks, as important
in an early stage, the curious pallor of the face, a slight evening
rise of temperature, and an increase in the water excreted.
The last is probably compensatory to the destruction of part
of the kidney, as shown in Rose Bradford's experiments.
Casper[3] notes that there is sometimes an entire absence of
pyrexia throughout the disease, and quotes four such cases.
Generally in later stages, and with septic kidneys, marked
hectic with irregular chills occur, with emaciation and weakness. Tube casts are usually absent; albumin derived from the
blood and pus cells is found when actual erosions have taken
place into the urinary tract, but it is not in excess of that due
to the pus or hæmoglobin present. Occasionally it is found with
casts, but without blood, at an early stage from a secondary nephritis, but generally the remaining tubules do their work perfectly,
and Lacomb records a death from double renal tuberculosis where
no albumin had been present. Stress has been laid on the
increased frequency of micturition by night as well as by day
(Brown), but it is curious that nocturnal incontinence in
children never seems to be due to this disease. Of late years
the cystoscope has proved of the highest value in diagnosis,
showing lesions in the bladder and about the mouths of the
ureters, and enabling us to draw off the urine from one kidney
separately. This latter aim can be attained also by a simpler
instrument devised by Harris.[4] As to the hemorrhage, it
appears sometimes at an early stage from congestion,[5] and later
on from the erosions, and varies widely in amount. Unlike

[1] *Loc. cit.*   [2] *Internat. M. Mag.*, 1896, iv. 881.
[3] *Centralbl. f. innere Med.*, 1896, xvii. 471.
[4] *J. Am. M. Ass.*, 1898, xxx. 236.   [5] D. Newman, *Lancet*, 1898, ii. 14.

that caused by calculus, it is not increased by moving about. Sometimes by clots and sometimes from the *débris* of kidney tissue a ureter is blocked up, and thus we may find more or less complete retention alternating with profuse urination. This in turn may lead to hydronephrosis, but in other cases a tumour may be due to a collection of pus around the kidney, and often moderate enlargement of the organ takes place without suppuration.

If we turn to the question of the **bacilli,** there are two difficulties: first, their discovery at all, which may be impossible when there is much pus or blood present; and, secondly, their diagnosis from the smegma bacillus. Van Ketel[1] prefers to make a large number of specimens and stain twenty-four hours in an incubator with anilin water fuchsin, or if we can wait till the blood disappears the urine may be centrifugalised and stained rapidly with carbol fuchsin. If much pus is present, he shakes up with carbolic acid for five minutes, and allows it to settle, clearing the specimens by immersion in alcohol and ether. Von Jaksch recommends plate cultivations for separating the septic organisms present. For distinguishing the smegma bacillus, advantage is taken of the fact that it is decolourised by strong alcohol, while the tubercle bacillus is unaffected. Thus T. Brown, after Ziehl's fuchsin, employs a final bath of alcohol for more than five minutes; or we may counterstain with strong alcoholic methylene blue. Grünbaum finds the smegma bacillus in 50 per cent. of normal urines, and advises careful catheterisation to obtain urine free from it; but this seems hardly trustworthy, for the bacillus sometimes makes its home in the bladder.

With regard to **treatment,** pain is best relieved by codeia, according to Bryson,[2] who adds that cures are more often produced by antitubercular remedies than is generally believed. Among them he mentions sandal wood oil, cubebs, cod-liver oil, creasote, and especially change of climate. T. Brown has met with instances of surprising improvement even in advanced cases from rest, good food, change of climate, and large doses of creasote, and he claims that many early cases can be cured. Though, theoretically, it is desirable to get rid of a focus of disease in one kidney, yet the shock of operation may cause lesions elsewhere to spring into activity, and this point seems worthy to be taken into account. Savariaud[3] sums up the cases for operation as those where the patient is sinking from his sufferings or absorption of toxins, those where the kidney is practically destroyed by suppuration or where retention of urine or a peri-renal abscess exists, and finally some rare instances where hemorrhage or pain is so great that life is endangered. General miliary tuberculosis or advanced lung disease are a bar to operation, and all writers are agreed on the importance of avoiding catheterisation or washing out the bladder,

[1] Quoted by Webb, *Brit. M. J.*, 1898, i. 1202.   [2] *Loc. cit.*
[3] *Gaz. d. Hôp.*, 1898, lxxi. 821.

which is sure to aggravate the trouble even when antiseptic precautions are taken. The bladder irritation is often not due to infection, but merely to the passage of *débris* from the kidney. Israel[1] considers that the condition of the second kidney is of more importance than that of the bladder with respect to operation, and if not tuberculous it may show amyloid changes or chronic nephritis. In such cases the diagnosis is most difficult.

The **mortality under surgical treatment** has been urged against it. Thus Facklam's statistics recorded a death-rate after nephrotomy of 60 per cent., and of 28 per cent. after nephrectomy. To discuss this subject would, however, be out of place here, but I may mention that Bolton Bangs,[2] after analysing 135 recent cases, speaks strongly in favour of surgical intervention. He claims that the immediate results are brilliant in relieving pain and prolonging life, and that the remote results are better than those of medical treatment. His figures show a death-rate of 20 per cent, or 29.6 per cent. if we include the nine months after operation. However, the fact is that no statistics of other methods exist and few of the many recoveries are reported. It would seem probable that with better diagnosis and improved hygienic methods a vastly greater success might be obtained without surgical aid.

Both in medical cases and when the fitness of a patient to undergo an operation has to be decided upon, the question often arises whether the kidneys are acting normally and excrete effete matters in due quantity. The symptoms of kidney disease are not always trustworthy, and a test has been devised which may have a certain value. This is the **injection of methylene blue,** which in health colours the water in half an hour, and shows increasing effects for three or four hours.[3] In kidney disease, except in acute epithelial nephritis, a delay in the occurrence of the tint is constantly found. Failure of a functional character is also met with where no lesions after death are demonstrable, and conversely, if the lesion is small and much healthy tissue remains, permeability may be normal. To carry out the test 1 c.c. of a one in twenty solution of pure methylene blue (not methyl blue) is injected into the gluteal muscles, and the bladder is emptied at the same time and again in half an hour, and then every hour afterwards. A colourless derivative is sometimes passed before or together with the blue. If urine containing this chromogen is heated with acetic acid a green tint appears. Achard and Castaigne believe that if both the chromogen and the blue are absent in the first specimens permeability is very feeble, but if the blue alone is delayed there is only a functional failure. The test seems to be quite harmless, and may throw light on the

[1] *Deutsche med. Wchnschr.*, 1898, xxiv. 443 ; abstract in *Post-Graduate*, 1898, xiii. 1066.

[2] *Ann. Surg.*, 1898, xxvii. 14.

[3] *Bull. et Mém. Soc. méd. d. Hôp. de Par.*, 1897, 3ᵉ sér., xiv. 637 ; abstract in *Med. Rec.*, 1897, lii. 554.

condition of many patients whose symptoms are obscure.
Herter[1] thinks, however, that in advanced renal disease the
injection is not without danger, and finds that in most
individuals the colouration ceases in thirty-six hours. He adds
that the disappearance of the dye in that time shows probably
that the kidneys are normally clearing the blood of urea, salts,
and other matters, although the urine may show albumin and
casts. Numerous other papers have appeared on the subject.

* * * *

The vexed question, What are the effete matters retained in
uræmia? has had some light thrown on it by the experiments of
Monari,[2] who finds that when excretion is defective there is not
only an alteration in the density and corpuscles of the blood,
but that the bactericidal power is lessened, and an important
invasion of various microbes takes place. In 24 out of 30 cases he
was able to find the B. coli, staphylococci, and other organisms in
the blood, either alone or in combination. Thus uræmia is a
septicæmia produced by various infections when the blood cells
are weakened by the retention of any of the usual excreta, and
the toxins thus formed are the causes of the various uræmic
symptoms. Herter[3] points out that retention of potassium salts
cannot be a cause of the toxicity of the serum in this state, for
the serum contains very little of them. Nor is it due to urea or
extractives, for the toxicity is lost at a temperature which has
no effect on them. J. Rose Bradford, indeed, argues[4] that
laboratory results do not settle the question, for experimenters
can only by excision of the kidney produce "latent uræmia,"
such as is seen in suppression of urine either from obstruction
or from paralysis of the kidney, and in this form nearly all the
symptoms of true "acute uræmia" are absent. This absence
may, however, be due to the fact that life is not prolonged
sufficiently to produce the acute uræmia of Bright's disease.
The retention theory, he agrees, is disproved by many facts, but
he shows that there is a great disintegration of tissue in the
muscles from altered metabolism and a formation of broken-up
products in excess in the muscles. This, according to Monari,
is due to the bacterial invasion which he has discovered, and
it would seem that the toxins and not the urea and creatin are
the active poisons.

Two practical points follow. One is the great **danger of
massage** in gout and other quasi-uræmic states, because by it a
large quantity of toxins may be suddenly driven out of the
muscles into the circulation, producing what is known as
"massage kidney"; and the other is the **value of bleeding** in
uræmic asthma and allied conditions, if, as Herter says, the
heart is strong, the tension high, and the anæmia not too
profound. With it may be combined saline injections, at first

[1] *Phila. M. J.*, 1898, ii. 899.
[2] *Sperimentale*, 1897; abstract in *Brit. M. J.*, 1898, i. Epitome, p 52.
[3] *Med. Rec.*, 1897, lii. 280. [4] *Lancet*, 1898, i. 919.

in moderate amount, but afterwards increased if the kidneys are able to react to them. Booth and Huchard[1] gave as much as 2,000 grammes daily with brilliant success in a case of surgical kidney, and with permanent relief. Copious enemata were also employed; but only moderate hypodermic injections of saline were used at first, till it was seen that the kidneys were suffi-ciently active. With anasarca and scanty urine, there is a danger that the fluid may fail to pass away and only increase the existing evils.

*   *   *   *

Von Noorden,[2] in speaking of the **diet** desirable **in chronic kidney disease,** points out that the distinction of white and dark meats rests on no scientific basis, and the restriction of patients to the former interferes uselessly with their appetite and comfort, while the physiologists find that the highest creatin values are in the white meat of chicken and rabbits. A more important statement is that patients with contracted kidneys and dilated hearts are remarkably relieved by restricting the fluid they take. Cardio-renal asthma is, he finds, extraor-dinarily relieved by this method, and the dilatation of the heart is lessened. He adds that in no stage of this disease is the elimination of the important products of tissue change lessened by the restriction of the fluids taken to $1\frac{1}{2}$ litres daily. He bases this statement on long-continued experiments, though he confesses it is opposed to the generally received view that flushing the kidney with water aids the patient.

GEORGE PARKER.

SURGERY.

Catheterisation of the ureters is of extreme value in certain cases, but requires patience and practice in its performance. It probably has dangers of its own, although Casper thinks that with ordinary care the dangers are very few. He has catheterised the ureters over five hundred times without detecting any infection of the kidney thereby. He insists on the necessity of every precaution being taken, and only employing the method when it is really necessary for diagnosis and treatment.[3] David Newman is of opinion that the fullest possible information should be obtained by the cystoscope before resorting to catheterisation of the ureters as a last resort.[4] All are agreed that it should never be done if the bladder be septic.

Catheterisation of the ureters **in the female** has been rendered possible by Kelly's tubes. In a case of pyuria recently under my care, I was able to draw off turbid urine from one ureter which was found to contain tubercle bacilli. Urine from the **other**

[1] *Bull. gen. de Thérap.* [etc.], 1897, cxxxii. 75.
[2] *Internat. M. Mag.*, 1899, viii. 325.
[3] *Brit. M. J.*, 1898, ii. 1412.   [4] *Ibid.*, 1411.

kidney was healthy. This proved a certain and only guide, and the corresponding kidney was found to be tuberculous in an early stage. Briefly the method consists in placing the patient in the genu-pectoral position, or the dorsal position with the pelvis well raised, gauging the urethra, passing a speculum of corresponding calibre, deflecting it 30° to one or other side of the middle line, and searching for the ureteral papilla which betrays its position by an intermittent gush of urine. The orifice can be detected by a probe and the ureteral catheter passed in, often several inches and sometimes up to the pelvis of the kidney.

Catheterisation of the ureters **in the male** is beset with many difficulties. Dr. Willy Meyer has done much work in this· direction with instruments based on the principle of Nitze's cystoscope, although he prefers Casper's model[1] of ureter-cystoscope. The essentials are, that the urethral calibre must be adequate, the bladder must have a capacity of at least four ounces, and the fluid in the bladder must be and remain perfectly transparent. The patient is made to imbibe freely beforehand to increase the quantity of urine, then the following processes are gone through : (a) The bladder is washed out, cocainised and injected with six ounces of clear fluid. (b) The instrument is introduced, afterwards fully closing the lid. (c) The ureteral opening is approached, letting it appear at the very end of the cystoscopic picture. (d) The catheter is pushed forward parallel with the ureter for one or two inches. (e) The wire mandrel is withdrawn, and then the urine collected. Casper's cystoscope permits lateral deviation of the ureteral catheter ; but a great improvement seems to be effected in Albarran's instrument, in which the projected bent catheter can be flexed or extended, and so insinuated into the ureteral orifice with greater precision.[2] The application by Howard Kelly of his method to the male sex is strikingly novel, and very welcome in the fact that it does away with optical complications[3] which are always fatiguing. The speculum differs from the female type chiefly in its greater length ; viz., sixteen centimetres. The patient assumes the knee-chest position after the instrument has been introduced, the penis occupying an attitude of retroversion between the legs. The left forefinger or a speculum is inserted into the rectum to admit air. When the obturator is withdrawn the bladder also fills with air. The ureteral orifices are then inspected and dealt with as in the female. Kelly has devised a mirror on a handle for inspecting the bladder through the speculum, resembling a small laryngoscope mirror.

Analysis of the small quantities of urine obtainable **necessitates special methods.** Dr. Frederic E. Sondern estimates a sample of six cubic centimetres in the following way :—The

---

[1] *Med. Rec.*, 1897, li. 613.

[2] *Rev. de Gynéc. et de Chir. abd.*, 1897, i. 457 ; quoted by Valentine, *Med. Rec.*, 1898, liii. 573.

[3] *Ann. Surg.*, 1898, xxvii. 475.

specific gravity is estimated by a Westphal's specific gravity balance, and then the sediment obtained for microscopical and bacteriological examinations by centrifugalisation.   One cubic centimetre of the urine is used to test for albumin, and one for the Esbach's test.   If albumin be present, the remainder is boiled and filtered.   Of the filtrate, one cubic centimetre is used to test for urea, half a cubic centimetre for sugar, and the remainder serves for chlorides and other constituents.   Unfortunately the recorded results are discounted by fanciful observation such as " catarrh of the renal pelvis, probably a very moderate pyelitis and the cause of a very moderate renal hyperæmia ; moderate chronic cystitis ; excessive crystalline deposit, allowing suspicion of renal stone."[1]   This method may take as long as two hours to carry out and there appears to be some risk of false passage. One so called " perfectly successful catheterism of both ureters " involved a negative result on one side, and the catheter returned with the tip bent and the eye blocked by a clot.[2]

*   *   *   *

Air-inflation of hollow viscera has been employed in a passive way by Howard Kelly as an essential to his method of cystoscopy, and more recently by others for the active distension of hollow organs :

1. *The Bladder.*—This is passively distended by Kelly's method, both in the male and female, as soon as the obturator is withdrawn.   Cystoscopy by straight tubes was employed by Desormeaux in 1865, but the passive air-distension is the special feature of Kelly's method.   Active distension of the bladder by air instead of by water has been advocated by Dr. A. T. Bristow[3] and others.   Keen first employed the method in 1890.   It is claimed that air distension raises the peritoneum from the symphysis at least an inch more than water-distension does. One disadvantage in its employment formerly was the difficulty in estimating the amount of distension.   This has been overcome by an ingenious device by Dr. William Jepson.[4]   It consists in effect of two graduated bottles, one above the other, with necessary stopcocks.   The lower one contains air, and is connected from its upper part by a soft tube to the catheter. The upper bottle contains water, and is connected with the lower bottle by a tube with stopcock.   When it is required to distend the bladder with air, water is allowed to flow from the upper to the lower bottle, thus displacing an equal quantity of air into the bladder.   The bottles can be raised or lowered to meet hydrostatic requirements.   The chief points in this are, that the force is well regulated and perfectly controlled, and the air in the bladder is under a known pressure, but not rigidly confined.   This is obviously safer than using a pneumatic bicycle pump, since any extra tension in the bladder expends itself in the column of water above.

1 Meyer, *Loc. cit.*   2 *N. York M. J.*, 1897, lxv. 324.
3 *Ann. Surg.*, 1893, xvii. 667.   4 *Ibid.*, 1898, xxviii. 358.

2. *The Rectum.*—Kelly employs passive distensions of the rectum in his method of cystoscopy to depress the base of the bladder. It is particularly important for the male. Active distension was first used by Petersen in 1880 by means of his india-rubber bag, as an adjunct to suprapubic cystotomy. Kelly's tubes are now employed as proctoscopes with passive air-distension of the rectum, and Dr. James Tuttle speaks highly of them.[1] He claims even to have seen twenty to thirty-five inches up the lower gut by their means. By an ingenious method of using the fingers as retractors, combined with passive atmospheric dilatation of the rectum in the knee-chest position, Dr. T. C. Martin states that six or eight inches of the rectum can be easily inspected. The anæsthetised patient is balanced in position by an assistant, while the surgeon closes his fists, crosses his hands, and inserts both index fingers well into the rectum, retracting its walls as far apart as possible.[2]

3. *Gall-bladder.*—Weller Van Hook has recently advocated active air-distension in operations on the gall-bladder and ducts. He fits a nozzle into the gall-bladder, through which he inflates. The air acts as a probe and quickly finds its way into the ducts. It is of advantage in locating the seat of mischief, and subsequently in testing the accuracy of the suturing of the duct.[3]

*   *   *   *

Operative treatment of cirrhosis of the liver. An ingenious and somewhat successful attempt was made in 1896 by Dr. Drummond and Mr. Rutherford Morison, of Newcastle, to re-establish the portal circulation in cirrhosis by obtaining adhesions between the liver, spleen and omentum, and the parietes.[4] This was effected by vigorously rubbing the viscera and parietes with sponges. In one case the operation failed, in another it was very successful. It is premature to indicate the possibilities of this procedure, but of seven published cases two recovered, two were not improved, and three died from shock or sepsis. Weir has gone carefully into the matter, and cites a case, which, however, died on the 5th day from general peritonitis.[5] It appears that Eck, experimenting in 1877, made a series of anastomoses between the portal and systemic circulations in animals: but the results were disastrous, for seven out of the eight animals died within a week of the operation, Moreover, Hahn, repeating the experiments in 1892, found that in animals which survived for a time, the portal blood, passing directly into the systemic circulation, appeared to act as a direct poison, causing excitement, convulsions, coma, and death.

*   *   *   *

The toilet of the peritoneum, essential in its day, has largely given way before a knowledge of the capacity of the peritoneum

---

[1] *Med. Rec.*, 1898, liii. 527.   [2] *Columbus M. J.*, May 17, 1898.
[3] *Ann Surg.*, 1899, xxix. 137.
[4] *Brit. M. J.*, 1896, ii. 728.   [5] *Med. Rec.*, 1899, lv. 149.

for doing its own scavenger's work.   Three cases illustrating the remarkable **tolerance of the peritoneum** have been recently recorded.   One was that of a boy of 15, who was gored by a bull, about two inches above Poupart's ligament.   He arrived six hours afterwards with 1½ ft. of intestine protruding, smeared over with cow-dung, and covered with various leaves.   The parts were cleansed, the peritoneal rents sewn up, the intestines returned and less than three weeks afterwards the lad went home cured.[1]   A similar case is that of a woman aged 42 years, who was tossed by a cow early one evening and seen several hours afterwards.   Some twenty feet of intestine were protruding from the wound, and when they were returned she expressed herself as better, "now her bowels were in their places again."   The wound united by first intention, the temperature never reached 100° and she got up in less than a month.[2]   The third case concerned a dissolute married woman of 29.   A year previously she had had an abdominal operation preformed, and now the surgeon was sent for as she had "burst" in one of the slums. The surgeon regarded this with such incredulity that he did not visit her till the afternoon of the next day, when he found the woman lying on the floor in the corner of a common living room amongst a heap of straw and filthy rags.   She had indeed "burst," and in front of her was a heap of small intestines which had remained amongst the straw and dirt for twenty-four hours.   The bowels were washed with ordinary water drawn from a neighbouring tap, the guts were returned and a drainage-tube placed in the lower angle of the wound.   She made a rapid and uninterrupted recovery and remained free from recurrence of hernia for years.[3]

*   *   *   *

The great disadvantage of various bobbins and buttons for **intestinal anastomosis** is that they remain *in situ*, as foreign bodies, for some time after the operation.   Dr. Laplace has recently introduced ingenious forceps, by which the advantages of a bobbin or button are secured as regards facility of suture, and those of simple suture by their immediate removal at the end of the operation.[4]   The forceps combine to make two handled rings which are introduced into the intestine to be anastomosed, for fixation and support.   Each part is separable into two halves so as to be extricated just before completion of suturing.   A new feature thus introduced is the control of the operation given by means of the handles. The forceps are duplex, consisting of a semicircle on each half but when locked together they open as two rings, very much like a pair of tongue forceps.   Thus, after completion of suturing, the clamp on the forceps is removed, four sickle-shaped pieces have to be taken out and the site they occupied sutured.

[1] *Brit. M. J.*, 1898, ii. 897.   [2] *Lancet*, 1899, i. 290.
[3] *Ibid.*, 1898, ii. 74.   [4] *Ann. Surg.*, 1899, xxix. 297.

One ring of the forceps is inserted into the gut above, another into the gut below, and they are then approximated. The suturing is carried out with ease, and before the final stitch is tied the portions of the forceps are removed. The instrument is made in five sizes, the smallest being suitable for gall-bladder surgery. By its means end-to-end or lateral anastomosis, and also invagination, may be rapidly performed.

THOMAS CARWARDINE.

DERMATOLOGY.

At a debate of the Dermatological Society of London, November 9th, 1898, on **general exfoliative dermatitis or pityriasis rubra**, Dr. Walter G. Smith[1] said that in regard to nomenclature, etymology is a fallible guide in medical terminology, and he did not think it mattered much whether we choose to call it exfoliative dermatitis or pityriasis rubra, except that it would be well we should all agree, for convenience of reference, to adhere to the one designation, and the former term seems likely to prevail. Intense vivid redness he considers to be one of its most distinctive features; yet just as a zoologist finds no difficulty in acknowledging a white blackbird, so the dermatologist need not stumble at a white pityriasis rubra. Dr. Walter Smith is not aware that any important blood-changes have been made out in connection with dermatitis exfoliativa, although pseudo-leukæmia has been noted. Nor has the disease been proved to be due to a microbe, so we are left to mere conjecture. It has been suggested, especially by Mr. Hutchinson, that pityriasis rubra and other generalised forms of dermatitis are **etiologically related to the nervous system**, and may, in fact, be regarded as neuroses. In support of this view Mr. Hutchinson adduces the occurrence of joint-pains in many cases in the early stage, the occurrence of coma in one patient, and the fact that intolerable itching in the middle of the back ushered in the eruption in several cases. Hebra invokes the convenient hypothesis of vaso-motor disturbance. Dr. Crocker makes out a stronger case for association with rheumatism. He, by-the-by, prefers the term pityriasis rubra as being the original name, and thinks it better policy to stick to the old labels than to use new ones. He considered that pityriasis rubra represented a well-defined group of symptoms which might **develop primarily, or secondarily,** to some antecedent form of dermatitis, and that when the secondary cases were fully developed they were practically identical in their symptomology and course with the primary cases. The secondary cases might supervene not only upon almost any form of dermatitis, such as psoriasis, eczema, seborrhœic eczema, and lichen planus, in that order of frequency, but also, after the application of irritants to the skin, such as

[1] *Brit. J. Dermat.*, 1898, x. 437.

chrysarobin, arnica, and mercury. In the early days of the century, when mercurial inunction was used in a wholesale manner, this complication was not very rare. Clinically, many of the cases of the epidemic form described by Savill were indistinguishable from the non-contagious and classical form, and it showed that the presence of a special microbe was capable of producing the disease in some cases. Dr. Crocker had seen two cases in association with insanity, and he asked the members of the Society if they had had a corresponding experience. Dr. Walter Smith said that if dermatitis exfoliativa is recognised as a primary affection, and also as following upon such different affections as eczema, psoriasis, erythemata, lichen ruber, erysipelas, dermatitis herpetiformis, pemphigus, and perhaps, in children, syphilis, and if, further, it is allowed that this condition may be started by strong external irritants, and perhaps by internal remedies, *e.g.* chloralamide,[1] then in the absence of any uniform etiological factor, it is more rational to consider it as an accidental phenomenon, or as an evolution of some other affection, rather than an independent entity. Pityriasis rubra has been observed to supervene upon psoriasis, and when the pityriasis rubra got well the psoriasis resumed its normal course. As to frequency of primary and secondary cases of exfoliative dermatitis, Stephen Mackenzie's statistics give a nearly equal frequency (eleven primary and ten secondary). Moreover, although the first attack may be plainly secondary to some existing cause, yet it may be impossible to discover any adequate cause for subsequent recurrences. Dr. Smith considers that no certain boundary line can as yet be drawn between acute general eczema—possibly, also psoriasis—and exfoliative dermatitis. Dr. Galloway believes the secondary forms of the disease most commonly succeed psoriasis, and he considered that there was some danger in producing this grave secondary state by over-medication. He thought the histological alterations were distinctive, although they did not throw much light on the pathology of the disease, except to emphasise, what was pretty clear from clinical observation, that the poison which caused the disease was from within and not from without. Dr. J. J. Pringle's remarks pointed strongly towards the probability of the existence of **changes in the central nervous system,** possibly of toxæmic origin, as the determining factor in the production of general exfoliative dermatitis. These were: (1) the frequently neurotic character of the persons attacked; (2) the rapidity with which the condition develops and generalises itself; (3) the prominence of extreme itching, insomnia, and insanity among the leading symptoms; (4) the marked susceptibility to changes of temperature, and the instability of the peripheral circulation; (5) the remarkable changes occurring in the skin appendages—hair and nails. He considered that the prominent

[1] Pye-Smith, *Guy's Hosp. Rep.*, 1877, 3rd Ser., xxii. 151;
1881, 3rd Ser., xxv. 205.

rôle played by alcohol, at all events as a predisposing cause, had been generally underestimated, and that the existence of **albuminuria** always constituted a grave complication. As to treatment, arsenic was deleterious in the early stages of the disease, and he suspected that it was often responsible for its supervention upon cases of psoriasis. Dr. Leslie Roberts thought that the process of dermatitis exfoliativa was not purely ectodermal, but rather a neuro-ectodermal process in which the sensitive matter of the cerebro-spinal axis operated with or upon the epithelium and underlying vessels and nerves. He had come to this conclusion after careful consideration of certain clinical and histological facts; to wit, the almost startling suddenness with which the entire epidermis became altered in character, the predominance of nervous complications in the course of the disease, and the very characteristic inward growths of the epithelial cones. He considered that the morbid epithelial changes in dermatitis exfoliativa were certainly under some powerful nerve-influence; but he could not say, in the light of present evidence, how this influence occurs. Mr. Malcolm Morris thought the disease was peculiar for the reason that, in spite of the great redness and desquamation present, there was an entire absence of thickening; indeed there seemed to be rather an atrophy of the corium present, as shown by a slight thinning of the skin when picked up between the fingers. He considered that the presence of albumin in the urine was a factor justifying the utmost caution in regard to prognosis, and that in his experience such cases were often fatal.[1]

*   \-   *   \-

Pityriasis rosea, though a comparatively rare disease, occurs more frequently than is generally supposed, for cases are often overlooked or incorrectly diagnosed. A typical case runs a very clear and definite course. Without any previous symptoms, there appears on the trunk, somewhere in the region of the waist, as the "herald" of the disease, a reddish-yellow spot which expands into a patch, circular in form, very little elevated, with a rosy-red border and a yellow centre. The shade of yellow which forms the centre is sometimes described as fawn-coloured; frequently it very closely resembles the colour of chamois leather. Often enough this patch is entirely overlooked, and the first the patient knows of the disease is about a week later, when the whole trunk is covered with a profuse eruption of spots similar in nature to, though smaller in size than, the original one. All do not expand into circles; many remain as spots, and to this variety of the disease the name pityriasis rosea **maculata** is applied. When they do expand into circles, the adjective **circinata** is employed instead. Too much stress must not be placed on the identification of the "herald"

[1] *Brit. J. Dermat.,* 1898, x. 463.

patch; in the majority of cases it is not discoverable. The eruption is almost limited to the trunk. A few spots may be found about the shoulders, and a few on the thighs; but it is rare on the face and on the distal ends of the limbs, though it may be limited to them. In spite of the name, there is not often much scaliness. After a duration of from five to eight weeks the eruption gradually disappears. The cause of the disease is unknown. No organisms have been found which could be definitely associated with it. Dr. Norman Walker gives[1] a picture which is an admirable illustration of this disease.

The numerous reports from foreign sources which ascribe to the **X-ray therapeutic properties**, and give the results produced in cases of cancer and lupus vulgaris, and also claim for it a retarding action upon the growth of bacteriological cultures, have led Dr. Charles Leonard to study the electrical conditions present in order to determine whether the results obtained cannot be more reasonably explained by the action of physical and physiological forces the properties of which are perfectly known and understood. His conclusions are that the X-ray "burn" is not the result of the action of the X-ray, but the dermatitis produced is the result of the static currents or charges induced in the tissues by the high-potential induction field surrounding the X-ray tube. The therapeutic properties attributed to the X-ray do not belong to it, but are due to the static charges and currents induced in the tissues, which have long been known to be capable of producing similar results.

The dermatitis, which has been called an X-ray "burn," is the result of an interference with the nutrition of the part by the induced static charges. The patient may be absolutely protected from the harmful effects of this static charge by the interposition between the tube and the patient of a grounded sheet of conducting material that is readily penetrable by the X-ray; a thin sheet of aluminium or gold-leaf spread upon cardboard is an effectual shield.[2]

Dr. S. Pollitzer, of New York, says[3] that the peculiar yellow plaques and nodules in the skin known as **xanthoma** have been the subject of extensive studies on the part of pathologists and dermatologists, ever since they were first described by Addison and Gull in 1850. The greatest diversity of opinion exists as to their nature. The clinical grounds for separating xanthoma of the eyelids from multiple xanthoma are as follows: The nodules of xanthoma multiplex are firm, round, elevated papules; the patches of eyelid xanthoma are soft plaques on the level of the skin. Eyelid xanthoma persists through life; multiple xanthoma sooner or later undergoes involution. Eyelid xanthoma is quite common; multiple xanthoma is extremely rare. If the eyelids were in this preponderating degree the seat of predilection for a common xanthoma, we should expect to

---

[1] *An Introduction to Dermatology*, 1899.   [2] *N. York M. J.*, 1898, lxviii. 18.
[3] *Tr. Am. Dermat. Ass.*, 1897, 21.

find the eyelids affected in every case of multiple xanthoma; but, as a matter of fact, the two forms are rarely associated in the same individual. The author has been able to show that common eyelid xanthoma is not a new growth, but is due to a degeneration of pre-existing embryonally misplaced muscular tissue. The so-called xanthoma cell is a fragmented muscle fibre in a state of granulo-fatty degeneration, with proliferation of the muscle-nuclei. This explanation of the origin of eyelid xanthoma harmonises with a number of hitherto unexplained clinical and pathological facts, *e.g.* the absence of any clinical signs of tumour; its almost exclusive occurrence in the face, where peculiar muscular conditions prevail; its heredity; its usual development after middle age, when degenerative processes are apt to occur; the peculiar yellow pigment that is always present in muscles undergoing fatty degeneration, etc. The structure of multiple xanthoma is shown to be wholly different from that of eyelid xanthoma. It forms a sharply circumscribed tumour in the cutis. It is an irritative hyperplastic development of connective tissue, whose cells produce fibrous tissue on the one hand, or undergo fatty degeneration on the other. In diabetic xanthoma the process is a little more diffuse and the tendency towards fatty degeneration more marked. In both, irregular patches of granulo-fatty matter, interspersed with cellular detritus, occur in the middle of the nodules as the results of the fatty degeneration of the cells. In over 85 per cent. of the recorded cases of multiple xanthoma, far too large a number to be accounted a mere chance, there was either diabetes or some severe lesion of the liver with jaundice. The author thinks it likely that research may show that the fibrous nodes and fusiform enlargements of tendons in chronic rheumatism are to be placed in the same general class as the nodes of xanthoma. We should then have a large group of diseases, hepatic, diabetic, rheumatic, all characterised by toxæmic conditions, in all of which irritative connective-tissue lesions occur in the skin and elsewhere. At one end of this series we should have the persistent fibrous node of rheumatism; at the other, the transient nodules of diabetic xanthoma, while between them, intermediate in its tendency toward the formation of fibrous tissue and fatty degeneration, ultimately undergoing involution, would stand the nodule of common multiple xanthoma.

HENRY WALDO.

Reviews of Books.

Charles Darwin and the Theory of Natural Selection. By
EDWARD B. POULTON, F.R.S. Pp. 224. London: Cassell
and Company, Limited. 1896.

An American naturalist has well described this little book
as one of the minor classics of evolutional literature. Admirable
in its clearness and lucidity, admirable in the evolution of its
evolutionary theme, admirable in its portrayal not only of the
central figure but of his environment, it is above all admirable in
the skill with which it depicts the combined insight and patience,
breadth of view and minute attention to detail, strength of
intellect and lovable simpleness of character, perseverance and
strength of will in one who for long had every excuse to be a
confirmed invalid, which characterise Charles Darwin. Professor Poulton's book should appeal not only to biologists, but
to all who would gain strength and inspiration from the life-
work of a man of whom England may well be proud.

Darwin's relations to Mr. Alfred Russel Wallace afford a
lesson which smaller men might do well to lay to heart. Inspired
by the work of Malthus on Population, Darwin brooded over
the subject of competition and struggle for existence for twenty
years; he pondered over the store of facts he had amassed
during the voyage of *The Beagle*, ransacked the literature of
natural history, tested everything by observation and experiment, discussed the developing theory of natural selection with
a few chosen friends such as Lyell and Sir Joseph Hooker, and
still refrained from publishing. Mr. Wallace, inspired by the
germinal idea derived from the same source, thought out the
whole of his theory in a couple of hours, and completed his
essay in three days. It was sent to Darwin with the request
that if he thought well of it he should send it to Lyell for perusal.
Through the urgent persuasion of Lyell and Hooker, Darwin
was induced to publish, at the same time as Mr. Wallace's
essay, an abstract of his views, together with a letter to Asa
Gray in which they were summarised. "I was," he says, "at
first unwilling to consent, as I thought Mr. Wallace might consider my doing so unjustifiable, for I did not then know how
generous and noble was his disposition." May we not regard
with pride these two great men—for Mr. Wallace is great with
another greatness—for whom such an incident was not a nucleus
of jealousy and bitterness, for it laid the foundations of a life-
long friendship, strengthened by mutual confidence and esteem?

Alike to those who know their Darwinian literature and
have read Mr. Francis Darwin's worthy life of his father,
and to those who desire a short but sufficient sketch in clear

perspective, we recommend Professor Poulton's book, confident that they will not be disappointed and that they will endorse our high opinion of its merits.

A Manual of the Practice of Medicine. By FREDERICK TAYLOR, M.D. Fifth Edition. Pp. xvi., 1002. London: J. & A. Churchill. 1898.

This popular text-book has been carefully revised, some sections have been largely re-written, and notices of many diseases have been added. Amongst the newest chapters are those on glandular fever, divers' paralysis, erythromelalgia, angeio-neurotic œdema, hypertrophic pulmonary osteo-arthropathy, and tubercle of the skin. A separate section is devoted to diseases of the mediastinum; and filarial disease and hæmoglobinuria have been transferred to diseases of the lymphatic system and of the blood respectively. It is difficult to compress the facts of medicine within the limits of a volume such as this, but the issue of five editions in eight years shows that the attempt has been much appreciated.

Contributions to Clinical Medicine. By T. M'CALL ANDERSON, M.D. Edited by JAMES HINSHELWOOD, M.D. Pp. x., 415. Edinburgh: Young J. Pentland. 1898.

One who has been a hospital physician and clinical teacher for upwards of a quarter of a century must always have something worth relating. This volume will be specially welcome to Dr. M'Call Anderson's old students. Some of the papers are a little scrappy, and some rather old; but they are of worldwide interest, and they are all presented in good form, well printed on thick paper, easy to read, and well worthy of any time which may be spent upon them.

Die Störungen des Verdauungsapparates als Ursache und Folge anderer Erkrankungen. Von Dr. HANS HERZ. Pp. xviii., 543. Berlin: S. Karger. 1898.

The plan of this book is original, and we know of no work in English that covers exactly the same ground. The author's idea is to consider the disorders of the alimentary tract and its accessory glands as they occur in the course of general diseases and of diseases of other organs. In this way a broad general view may be arrived at of the modes in which the digestive apparatus is affected in diseases which have no causal connection with it. At the same time the reverse of the picture is taken into view, and the digestive organs considered as the seat of origin of disease. Thus throughout the volume two points of view are consistently regarded: firstly, the alimentary tract considered as the primary seat of each disease or group of diseases; and secondly, the secondary disturbances of this tract which occur in the same diseases when they own another source of origin. We may take the acute infectious diseases as an example. The share of the digestive tract in the etiology of these diseases is first discussed, with an appendix on the occurrence of fever in disorders of the alimentary canal, and then the secondary disturbances of this tract which occur in the course of these fevers are systematically described and grouped under the heads of symptoms referable to the mouth, pharynx, stomach, intestines, liver, spleen, pancreas, peritoneum, and mesenteric glands. Again, in syphilis and tuberculosis the clinical and pathological history is given of the cases in which these infections obtain entrance to the system through the alimentary canal, and then of the secondary disturbances of the latter when an entrance of the poison is gained through some other channel.

The author points out that although much has been and is still to be gained by differentiation and distinction in the consideration of diseases, less has been done—and there is probably almost as much information to be gathered—by putting together like things. His book is to be regarded as an effort in this direction, a contribution to homogeneity in medicine, an example of how light may be thrown on obscure processes of disease in one system of organs by comparing their disorders as they occur in different diseases. Nor is it to be supposed, and the work under notice is a striking example to the contrary, that such a consideration of the disorders of one system by itself must necessarily lead to a narrow specialism, to a limited grasp or one-sided view of the problems of medicine. Rather the effect should be to widen and enlarge one's ideas, for in this particular instance of the digestive system, as one reads on one realises with increasing force how intimately this system is bound up with the rest, and how impossible it is to treat its disorders scientifically without a full appreciation of the mutual interdependence of organs upon each other, and of the fact that no one system can be disturbed without affecting to a greater or less degree every other; that, in clinical language, the patient and not the disease is to be treated.

Enough has been said to show that this book is written in a scientific spirit, and approaches its subject from an aspect that is novel and capable of throwing new light upon what may be already familiar to the reader. But in addition there must be very much that is actually fresh to most readers, and more that is new in the sense that it is now first collected in a readily accessible form. Obviously the labour of writing a book dealing with diseases of the digestive apparatus on such a plan must be very great, and the author displays in the prosecution of it immense erudition and research. When we consider the extensive literature of the primary digestive disorders by themselves alone, and then that of the secondary disorders as met with in all other diseases, we can appreciate the magnitude of the task. So far as we have been able to ascertain, the author has carried out his plan remarkably well, and his work is a storehouse of recorded facts and observations on the pathology and symptoms of every affection of the alimentary tract. It thus forms a valuable work of reference which contains a quantity of information that otherwise would have to be laboriously sought out in scattered papers. Not that we mean to imply that the book is a mere compilation; far from it,—it is written with critical insight, and bears the stamp of experience and sound judgment. There is one point on which we disagree with the author; in his preface, he states that he considers an index unnecessary, as he has given a very full table of contents. We think, however, that to bring out the full value of his book as a work of reference, it requires a copious index as well.

Diseases of the Heart and Aorta. By GEORGE ALEXANDER GIBSON, M.D. Pp. xx., 932. Edinburgh: Young J. Pentland. 1898.

A mastery of all that it seems capable of knowing in connection with diseases of the heart is displayed in this admirable treatise. A reference to standard works for information on some particular point as often as not fails to give satisfactory aid. In this book, however, we consider that not only knowledge, but exceptional judgment has been displayed. The mass of facts the book contains has been most ably handled, and rarely have we been disappointed in search for fresh light on a subject, or felt disposed to criticise where there is a summary of varied opinions.

One will always find points of minor importance with which one may not fully agree, such as the statement that when myocarditis is associated with pericarditis, " only the superficial layers of the heart " are affected. On two occasions during the past year we have seen myocarditis associated with rheumatic pericarditis extending through the wall of the left ventricle to the endocardial surface, where in one instance the speckled appearance produced by the degenerative changes was very marked. We refer to this point, because the subject of the power of rheumatism to attack the heart-muscle has recently been brought into prominence. We do not consider myocarditis associated with pericarditis to be due to direct spread of the inflammation from the pericardium inwards.

The varied aspects of disease are so numerous, that it must be rare to find descriptions that fully satisfy all observers. Dr. Gibson's book, however, seems to us to be as infallible as it is possible for a work of the kind to be.

18

The Cold-Bath Treatment of Typhoid Fever. By F. E. HARE, M.D. Pp. xii., 196. London: Macmillan and Co., Limited. 1898.

It seems remarkable that the medical profession of this country should be charged with inertia, because the cold-bath treatment which has been in vogue for some thirty years should not be universally adopted. It is true, as Dr. Hare remarks, that the difficulties in the systematic adoption of the method have been greatly exaggerated; the plan of procedure which he describes (page 18) makes the whole thing easy for hospital wards, and there can be no reason why the bath should not be of far more general use if its absolute necessity is demonstrated. There are, however, other antipyretic methods, and it is only occasionally that the bath has to take precedence of these.

In a consecutive series of 1902 cases treated at the Brisbane Hospital in Queensland, Dr. Hare claims to have reduced the mortality from 14.8 per cent. in the years 1882 to 1886, to an average of 7.5 per cent. for the years 1887 to 1896, an improvement amounting practically to 50 per cent. This result harmonises with Osler's dictum : " The cold-bath treatment, rigidly enforced, appears to save from six to eight in each century of typhoid patients admitted to the care of the hospital physician." Any fallacies which tend to inhere in an enquiry of this sort are as far as possible minimised or eliminated, and it is argued by the author that the difference in mortality for the two periods is not due to any other accidental variations, but simply and entirely to the systematic use of cold bathing. We congratulate the author on his persistent and successful efforts.

Clinical Lectures on Mental Diseases. By T. S. CLOUSTON, M.D. Fifth Edition. Pp. xii., 727. London: J. & A. Churchill. 1898.

We know of no book which better deserves its popularity than this one. Designed as a clinical manual for students of mental diseases and general practitioners, the book forbears intimate discussion on many vexed questions, and hence does not invite, in greater part, the criticism which awaits the propounder of hypotheses. The author has advanced, almost of necessity, certain assumptions which may invite discussion amongst his fellow-alienists; but it would be straining the function of criticism to raise this here whilst there is so much matter of the highest value to receive comment; it should be said, that to no debatable opinions of his own does Dr. Clouston give undue or misleading prominence.

There is evidence in this work of acute observation, large and shrewd views of sane as of insane humanity, unsurpassed experience and versatility of treatment. In our opinion no modern physician has better conceived and practised, in its widest sense, the treatment of insanity; from the aspect of therapeusis alone the book is of great worth. Exceptional, too, are the powers of graphic description, of harmonious groupings of varied clinical pictures, and of sound generalisation, and as the result there is aroused a vivid interest in the cases described. Of especial utility will be found the sections relating to the examination and certification of persons of unsound mind, together with the various contingencies arising in connection with these procedures.

This edition has received important addition in the excellent plates and descriptive letter-press which demonstrate some most recent processes in microscopic technique. In short, anyone who digests this book will have acquired a valuable knowledge of the clinical aspects of insanity, and despite the endless variety of these will always find typical descriptions, ripe experience, and happy suggestions to guide him.

A Manual of Modern Surgery. By JOHN CHALMERS DaCOSTA, M.D. [Second Edition.] Pp. 911. London: Henry Kimpton. 1898.

In the new edition of this book no attempt has been made to alter the character or to change the purpose of the manual, about which we have already spoken favourably. Some new articles have been added and many of the former ones enlarged or otherwise altered to meet modern requirements. Among them may be mentioned the following: Sections have been added upon the surgery of the liver and gall-bladder, wounds inflicted by modern projectiles, and the use of the Röntgen rays. The following modern operations have been described: Resection of the Gasserian ganglion, methods of gastrostomy, use of the Murphy button, various modern operations upon the intestines, &c., &c. All of these have been well done, and, so far as was possible in the limited space, they have been fully described. The style of the author is simple and unpretentious, and he has succeeded in producing a handy volume which well meets the requirements of students reading for examination or practitioners wishing to refresh their knowledge.

On the Origin and Progress of Renal Surgery. By HENRY MORRIS, M.B. Pp. viii., 288. London Cassell and Company, Limited. 1898.

The Hunterian Lectures which Mr. Morris delivered in 1898 form the greater portion of this admirable volume, which is about equally divided between descriptive matter and tabulations of cases. It is impossible to praise too highly this masterly exposition of the recent advances in renal surgery, which is embellished by excellent figures. It is indicative of an immense amount of labour and research, as well as of personal experience. Although every section is of importance to the surgeon, that dealing with the surgery of the ureter is particularly so, since it emphasises the most important of recent advances. The Heinecke-Mikulicz suture for the relief of ureteral stricture, and the methods of ureteral anastomosis, are deserving of careful study.

Mr. Morris's theory, like his practice, is of a distinctly conservative type; and as he was one of the pioneers in boldly attacking the kidney, so he is the foremost in advocating conservative methods. Surgeons and patients will alike benefit from a study of the work.

Traumatic Separation of the Epiphyses. By JOHN POLAND. Pp. xxxi., 926. London: Smith, Elder, & Co. 1898.

This is a most exhaustive treatise, and is the result of investigations by the author, which have been carried on for many years, both in clinical and in anatomical work. We could not have imagined that so large a book could have been written on the subject. It is one to which all surgeons may from time to time turn for information, if they suspect the injury from which their patient suffers to be of this nature, and they will certainly not be disappointed by the information they will receive. Illustrations are very abundant, and most of them very good, and there can hardly have been a book yet published with so many illustrations of skiagrams. Some of these are very clear, but in a few we must say we fail to see a demonstration of the lesion. We would suggest to the author that a series of skiagrams of the normal epiphyses of all the bones of the extremities would be a very valuable addition to the next edition of the book, for in skiagraphic work the picture of a normal part is of very great assistance. Nineteen skiagrams of the normal epiphyses of the hand and wrist at various ages are given, and one or two of each of the long bones would be a great gain. The author first considers traumatic separation of the epiphyses in general, and then describes in a most thorough way the pathology, signs, and treatment of those lesions in the various bones. He has collected an enormous number of cases to illustrate the subject.

The book is issued in a state of magnificence that has rarely been equalled in medical work, and we feel sure that it will be the standard English work on the subject; our knowledge regarding it has been very greatly increased by the author.

Tropical Diseases. By PATRICK MANSON, M.D. Pp. xvi., 607. London: Cassell and Company, Limited. 1898.

This manual covers the whole field of the diseases of warm climates, and is of an eminently practical nature. Chapters are devoted to fevers, diseases of undetermined nature, abdominal diseases, infective granulomatous diseases, animal parasites, skin diseases, and local diseases of uncertain nature, such as goundou and ainhum. The subject of malaria is dealt with most fully and successfully. With regard to the part played by the mosquito in the etiology of malarial infection Dr. Manson, whilst not accepting the theory as proved, recognises its importance, and thinks that every effort should be made to establish or confute it. Hæmoglobinuric fever, concerning the etiology of which there has been much discussion, will, Dr. Manson thinks, be found to be dependent on a form of malarial parasite peculiar to itself. The book is profusely illustrated, and the coloured plates of the malaria parasites are very finely executed. We can recommend the work to all students and teachers of tropical medicine.

An Atlas of Bacteriology. By CHAS. SLATER, M.B., and EDMUND J. SPITTA. Pp. xiv., 120. London: The Scientific Press, Limited. 1898.

The value of this excellent book, which consists, in addition to its pages of letterpress, of a collection of one hundred and eleven full-page original photo-micrographs, is much enhanced by the brief introductory description of the method by which the pictures have been produced, a method which is in complete accord with the published experience of some of the most accomplished operators in this field of work. The saving of time, labour, and money resulting from the immediate possession of a knowledge of the best available means of obtaining satisfactory representations of the bacteria will render the acquisition of this volume a very profitable transaction on the part of anyone entering upon this fascinating study, although some acquaintance with the manipulation of microscope and camera will be required to put into practice the terse directions of the authors.

The perfection of the methods adopted is best attested by the beauty of the pictures, the truthfulness of which makes them very valuable companions to the text-book. A word of commendation is also due to the short descriptions of the organisms which accompany the illustrations, and which, without being overloaded with detail, furnish a fairly complete account of the leading features of the various species.

Ueber die Wirkung des neuen Tuberkulins TR auf Gewebe und Tuberkelbacillen. Von Dr. H. STROEBE. Pp. 114. Jena: Gustav Fischer. 1898.

Although the practical results of this last tuberculin have been hitherto almost *nil*, we welcome the record of Dr. Stroebe's careful investigations on its true properties and reactions. If any progress is to be made in applying this and similar remedies to the cure of human and animal tuberculosis, or in preventing its spread, the result can only be obtained by an exact study of its effects.

We find here details of researches on healthy and tubercular animals, and on the degree of immunity conferred by the new remedy; and if the results, both in the way of cure or in the production of immunity, are directly opposed to those of Koch, the sooner a dangerous treatment is abolished the better. The writer, we may remark, obtained in no case a complete cure of experimental tuberculosis in guinea-pigs by the use of the tuberculin, and he seems likewise to have failed to produce immunity by its means. He gives also a review of some of the chief investigations which have lately appeared, and of the controversy arising from them.

The Ferment Treatment of Cancer and Tuberculosis. By HORACE MANDERS, M.D. Pp. xix., 251. London: The Rebman Publishing Co., Limited. 1898.

Giving a clear exposition of a fresh development of therapeutics, this book brings forward certain new and important facts. It explains thoroughly the treatment of various diseases by "pure ferments," and the *rationale* of it; but it is disfigured by too much padding *de omnibus rebus et multis aliis*. If we had been spared thirty pages on cells and bacteria, twenty-eight on the pathology of tuberculosis, with the symptoms and modes of infection, and a vast amount of information easily obtainable from text-books, but having no connection with the subject, the interest of the book would have been greater, for in its main thesis it is sound.

The chief practical result so far of bacteriology has been serum-treatment. Dr. Manders shows that there is another, the ultimate importance of which may be far greater. Living yeasts act as phagocytes and destroy pathological bacilli. He shows that absolutely pure yeasts can be introduced into the human body, and can multiply there for a time without injury, causing leucocytosis, converting some of the sugar derivatives into alcohol (which he has measured so far as excreted by the lungs) and destroying certain pathological bacteria. Thus in phthisis the cells may be found in the expectoration enclosing degenerate bacilli. Of these important facts he gives convincing proofs; and, in addition, he believes that the cells, having done their work, are of nutrient value, supplying nuclein, succinic acid, and certain mineral substances.

Dr. Manders employs the pure yeast or backérine as a hypodermic injection, as a powder upon ulcers, and occasionally by the mouth, rectum, or as a spray for diphtheritic throats. The hypodermic dose is 1 c.c. at intervals of a week or longer.

There is a sharp reaction followed by improved appetite, and in phthisis a diminution of bacilli and night-sweats with general improvement. Yeast seems to inhibit altogether the growth of the typhoid bacillus *in vitro*, and it has been used with some benefit in typhoid fever. In future papers the writer promises abstracts of the cases of phthisis, typhoid, and septicæmia in which he has used it with advantage. We hope his materials will be put together in a better form. The method deserves careful examination and testing.

Operative Gynecology. By Howard A. Kelly, M.D. Vol. I., pp. xvii., 563. Vol. II., pp. xiii., 557. London: Henry Kimpton. 1898.

We have frequently in these columns expressed our admiration of the work of those associated with the Johns Hopkins Hospital, and Dr. Kelly's admirable book reflects the highest credit upon himself and the institution with which he is connected. The object of the writer has been to set forward his own experiences, and to record those methods of procedure which he has found to be trustworthy and best, and we hail with the greatest satisfaction the ability to read for ourselves the masterly exposition of one so famed in the gynæcological world as the author. The work is large, but a considerable amount of space is occupied by the twenty-four plates and five hundred and fifty original illustrations with which it is embellished. Of the letterpress as a whole we may say at once that it is clear and incisive, and free from verbiage, carrying its own conviction as the work of one whose experience and judgment are of the highest order. The illustrations too are masterpieces of execution, and render the book one of the most beautifully adorned works of its kind.

In the first volume, the three opening chapters deal mainly with the question of sepsis, antisepsis, and bacteriology. Every detail of the disinfection of the patient, surgeon, and appliances is carefully described, and a brief account is given of the chief organisms (and the methods of staining them) met with in gynæcological practice. For disinfection of the hands before operation the author prefers the use of permanganate of potash and oxalic acid. Then follow chapters on topographical anatomy, the method of making a gynæcological examination, the use of local and general anæsthesia, and the general principles involved in plastic operations.

Chapter IX. treats of diseases of the external genitals, and several plastic operations for the removal of large portions of these parts for tubercular disease, pruritus vulvæ, &c., are described. The plastic art of the surgeon is still further brought out in Chapter X., which deals with rupture of the recto-vaginal septum and relaxed vaginal outlet, and here we can find a lucid account of the true principles underlying a successful operation for these conditions

—an operation which has suffered much from the incorrect and unintelligible descriptions which are often met with. Operations on the vagina is the subject of Chapter XI., the most important being those necessary for traumatic affections as the result of injuries incurred in labour. Chapter XII. treats of affections of the urethra and bladder, and Chapter XIII. of affections of the ureters, and it is in the diagnosis of these conditions in the female that Dr. Kelly has worked so laboriously and successfully in perfecting his methods, which are universally recognised to be of the greatest value. These methods, which have long been known from his other writings, have been largely instrumental in making a reputation which is world-wide and well-deserved. In connection with large vesico-vaginal fistulæ, we are glad to see that the author regards the operation of kolpo-kleisis as a thing of the past. The final chapters (XIV.—XIX.) deal with operations upon the cervix of the uterus, including dilatation and curettage; prolapse of the uterus; vaginal hysterectomy; vaginal extirpation of submucous myomata and polypi; and certain conditions in which the uterus acts as a retention-cyst. The account of the examination of uterine scrapings after curettage bears witness to the care and exactness with which Dr. Kelly's work is performed. We regret that nothing is said of the results of vaginal hysterectomy for cancer, for the author's large experience and opinion would have been of great value in estimating the much-discussed value of this operation.

The second volume opens (Chapters XX.—XXII.) with an account of the general principles and complications common to abdominal operations; the care of wound and patient up to recovery; and complications arising after abdominal operations. These chapters deal in a most complete manner with the subjects of which they treat, and give much reason for reflection, and, if space permitted, for discussion also. Each surgeon doubtless falls into certain routine treatment in the after-management of abdominal sections, and consequently the practice of others may appear to be wanting in certain ways. Hence we feel disposed to point out the great value which we attach to the treatment of tympanites by turpentine enemata, and to the use of strapping over the dressings to support the abdominal muscles as it were in a splint, neither of which appears to find a place in the author's practice. Of still greater importance, however, is it for us to raise a protest against the restriction of all fluids by the mouth for the first twelve hours or more after operation. This would seem, in face of the intense thirst which often exists, to amount to an unnecessary piece of torture (the word is not too strong in many instances), for we have long been in the habit of allowing tablespoonful doses of hot water at frequent intervals, and can unhesitatingly say that we have never known it productive of harm. Chapter XXIII. deals with tubercular peritonitis, and we note with satisfaction that the author agrees in abandoning all drainage in these cases. In Chapter XXIV. the author describes his method of suspension of the uterus by attaching the posterior surface of the uterus to the abdominal wall, and though we cannot accept this as the best operation, we would admit that the author's experience has shown that it is less open to objection. than many others. Chapter XXV. treats of conservative opera-- tions on the tubes and ovaries. This is one of the signs of the times, and is an important contribution to the subject which all operating surgeons would do well to consider. Salpingo-oöphorectomy is considered in Chapter XXVI.; vaginal drain-age and enucleation for pyo-salpinx, &c., in Chapter XXVII., and abdominal hystero-salpingo-oöphorectomy in Chapter XXVIII. To those who are not familiar with the life-saving advantages of vaginal drainage in certain cases, this portion of the book may be commended. Ovariotomy is the subject of Chapter XXIX., and abdominal hysterectomy for carcinoma of the uterus is the subject of Chapter XXX. In the latter chapter the author gives excellent reasons for his preference for the abdominal rather than the vaginal route, and after giving certain rules for the prevention of cancer, he says: " If these rules were conscientiously observed, there can be no doubt but that thousands of lives would be saved yearly in this country alone,"—a statement which amounts to a grave (and not alto-gether undeserved) indictment against both the profession and the public which it is well that both should consider. Chapter XXXI. gives an account of myomectomy, and hystero-myomec-tomy, and the latter operation is confined to the retro-peritoneal method. Chapters XXXII.—XXXIV. are taken up with opera-tions during pregnancy, Cæsarean section, and extra-uterine pregnancy, and Chapters XXXV. and XXXVI. deal with the radical cure of hernia and intestinal complications. These last cover a wide area, and are comparatively briefly treated, and rightly so, for they only indirectly concern the gynæcologist. The final chapters (XXXVII. and XXXVIII.) describe the more remote results of abdominal operations and the conduct of autopsies.

We have spoken of the contents of the book in some detail, to show what an extensive ground is included thereby. Such a work must long remain as a standard book of reference, and will always be a lasting memorial of the labours of the author both in deed and word. The one weak spot is in the index, which might be considerably enlarged, and so further enhance the value of a work of which we have little to say except in appreciation.

Ovariotomy and Abdominal Surgery. By HARRISON CRIPPS. Pp. 624. London: J. & A. Churchill. 1898.

The main part of this book runs to 422 pages, the rest being taken up with an appendix of selected cases which are out of place and in no way enhance the value of the work. We hope that in any future edition this space will be taken up by a greater elaboration of the details described in the earlier part of the volume; for the fault of the book as a whole lies in the insufficiency of description devoted to the various subjects. The author tells us that his chief object is to record such methods as he has found valuable in his own experience; but the addition of a chapter of "Anatomy of the Abdomen" (which is beautifully illustrated by coloured plates), mainly from the pen of Mr. H. J. Waring, and others on the "Surgery of the Kidney' and the "Radical Cure of Hernia," by Mr. Bruce Clarke and Mr. C. B. Lockwood respectively, indicate that there was also a desire to make the book complete and of general use. In this, however, we do not think the author has fully succeeded, owing to the want of detail. The only chapters which have received sufficiently full treatment are those on "Ovariotomy" and "Inguinal Colotomy." Our objection is rather with what has been left unsaid than with what has been actually written, and the incompleteness of the work renders it of comparatively little value to those seeking information on abdominal surgery. This could be altered, without increasing the size of the book, in the way already suggested.

A Clinical Treatise on Diseases of the Breast. By A. MARMADUKE SHEILD, M.B. Pp. xvi., 510. London: Macmillan and Co., Limited. 1898.

It would be a mistake to think all pathology had been omitted from Mr. Sheild's book because he calls it a "clinical treatise," but the work is eminently one for the guidance of the surgeon in the many difficulties he has to encounter both in the diagnosis and the treatment of diseases of the breast. Mr. Sheild has written an admirable and a very readable book—the style is good, and the information clearly given. Coloured plates abound, and we have hardly ever seen morbid conditions so clearly represented. We must, however, make an exception of Plate XIV., which we think does not represent the scirrhus-growth as nearly white enough.

The results of operations for cancer of the breast are given with a clearness and fulness which make this part of the work of much value. This we might expect, for it is not long since Mr. Sheild brought the matter before the Royal Medical and Chirurgical Society, and elicited the opinions and experiences of both the senior and junior surgeons in London, some of whom adopted very different lines of practice. We cannot help saying that we consider there is one fault in the book, which, however, is not confined to Mr. Sheild's writings or sayings. It is the idea implied now and again in this work that a London surgeon has special opportunities for arriving at a right conclusion on some disputed facts. This all depends on the amount of clinical or pathological material available by the individual surgeon. Many surgeons attached to large provincial hospitals have much greater experience of diseases than surgeons on the staff of some of the London hospitals.

All that is best in recent periodical literature on the subject on which Mr. Sheild writes is referred to by him. Duct cancer, a subject about which so much has been written of late, and of which various descriptions are still given, is clearly described, and its distinction (which is so great) from ordinary cancer is well given. Beatson's method of treating cancer by oöphorectomy receives some notice, and also the treatment of malignant disease of the breast by Coley's fluid. Reference is of course made to Mr. Gould's very interesting case, in which an undoubted recurrent cancer of the breast and glands entirely disappeared. Mr. Sheild is sceptical as to the spontaneous disappearance of fibro-adenomata of the breast. He thinks such swellings have probably been sclerosing mastitis or cysts with indurated breast-tissue around. He says fibro-adenomata roll about in the breast. This is a very common statement; but we should like to know how the movement takes place. There is no space for them to roll about in. The finger receives the sensation as if they were rolling about in the breast, but that is because the part of the breast in which, or on which, they lie can be so readily moved on the other portions of the organ. A full and instructive account is given of Paget's disease of the nipple, or " dermatitis maligna " as Mr. Sheild calls it, in which the relation of the disease to psorosperms is discussed.

We can strongly recommend the book, not only to the busy practitioner who needs to refer to some modern work for guidance in dealing with diseases of the breast, but also to the operating surgeon, for the problems which he has to face are clearly and ably discussed.

System of Diseases of the Eye. Edited by WILLIAM F. NORRIS, M.D., and CHARLES A. OLIVER, M.D. Vol. III.—*Local Diseases, Glaucoma, Wounds and Injuries, Operations.* Pp. xii., 962. Philadelphia: J. B. Lippincott Company. [1898.]

A considerable departure has been made from the original forecast of the contents of this volume. The articles on diseases of the cornea, diseases of the lens, and errors of refraction have been deferred to the fourth volume. On the other hand, Dr. G. C. Harlan, in addition to his chapter on " Diseases of the Eyelids," contributes forty-four pages on " Operations performed upon the Eyelids," a useful section, which was not specified in the original programme, and which adequately describes all the best-known expedients. For want of space a critical reference to the various articles is impossible, but some 160 pages at the end of

the volume on "operations usually performed in eye-surgery,"
deserve special mention.   The author, Dr. Herman Knapp, is
so well known as a master of this subject that his dogmatic
statements are more than justified, though all may not agree with
them.   For example, to cleanse the eye before operation he uses
bichloride of mercury, 1 to 5000, with which he mops the everted
palpebral conjunctiva, while in cataract operation he advocates
operating on the patient in his bed.   His style is terse; but the
meaning is precise, and the article covers an immense amount
of ground.   Recognising the risks of a needling operation, but
at the same time its almost inevitable necessity, he performs his
extractions specially with that end in view, and takes particular
care to avoid any unnecessary mangling of the iris, or injury to
the lens capsule.   The disastrous suppuration which is occasionally seen to follow discission of secondary cataract he attributes
not to direct inoculation from the needle, or immediate infection
of the wound, but to the awakening of pyogenic germs which
had been previously introduced, and were lying dormant.

The volume on the whole is remarkably free from errors.
We notice, however, on page 261, in speaking of pupillometers,
a correct description is given of the Keratometer, invented by
Mr. Priestley Smith some fifteen years ago, which the writer says
may be used as a pupillometer.   But by accident it is called a
Tonometer, and as a result a picture of the tonometer, invented by
Priestley Smith in 1866, is dragged in " to render the working of
the tonometer clear to readers."   It is incredible that the authors
of the article should be responsible for the whole of this blunder.
The chapter on glaucoma by Priestley Smith, in which the
tonometer is again depicted and correctly described, is admirable
in every way, and the wood-cut illustrations are all that could
be wished.

In reference to the illustrations of the volume generally, it
must be said that they are on the whole disappointing.   Some
are very good.   Some are pretentious, but convey no particular
information ;   whilst   others,   particularly   those   illustrating
ophthalmoscopic appearances, are quite unworthy of being
included in so important a work.   The article on diseases of the
retina is marred by such plates as XII. and XXVII.   The section on diseases of the choroid has no illustrations of the fundus
oculi, and so does not suffer in this respect, but it is only fair
to say that the illustration of the fundus facing page 768 leaves
nothing to be desired.   _____

A Treatise on Aphasia and other Speech Defects.   By H.
CHARLTON BASTIAN, M.D., F.R.S.   Pp. viii., 366.   London:
H. K. Lewis.   1898.

Dr. Bastian is so high an authority on aphasia that this
book, which gives a complete and authoritative exposition of
his views on the subject, will be read with great interest.   The

remembrance of the admirable Lumleian lectures of 1897, dealing with "some problems in connection with aphasia and other speech defects," will arouse favourable anticipations with regard to the present volume, which are not disappointed in it. Dr. Bastian is well-known for the lucid manner in which he presents to his readers some of the most intricate problems with which medical men have to deal. He has wisely in this book illustrated his observations with reports of typical cases, well chosen, and for the most part completed by a necropsy. The careful study of such reports gives great help in the actual working out of the problems involved in cases of aphasia, and brings out more clearly the basis of fact on which the theories of speech-defect are founded. The book is also free from the tendency found in some writers on aphasia to construct elaborate classifications, which have very little to support them in the way of proved pathological or psychological data. We are grateful to the author for the simple nomenclature which he adopts, and which is easily understood.

Besides expressing his own views as to the nature and origin of aphasic defects, Dr. Bastian gives throughout the book a very fair presentment of the views of other writers, especially on the points in which they differ from him. It would be impossible within the limits of this notice to enter into any discussion of the many vexed questions which beset the subject. Dr. Bastian attaches special importance and brings forward a number of cogent arguments for the activity of the word-centres in the right as well as in the left hemisphere, and for the compensatory action of the former in disease affecting the latter; this possibility, first advanced as a probable explanation of the preservation of slight or disordered speech after destruction of the left auditory word-centre, was originally due to him. But for this and the many other difficult and interesting points connected with the disorders of speech we must refer the reader to the book itself, in which he will find that they receive a full and adequate discussion.

The work can be confidently recommended as a trustworthy guide by the hand of a master. The excellent introductory chapters deserve special mention; and the final chapters on etiology, diagnosis, prognosis, and treatment of speech-defects are particularly good, and will be found of much value in practice. Where necessary the text is illustrated by clear diagrams, and a carefully thought-out scheme for the examination of patients is given.

Diet and Food, Considered in Relation to Strength and Power of Endurance, Training and Athletics. By ALEXANDER HAIG, M.D. Pp. vi., 86. London: J. & A. Churchill. 1898.—Dr. Haig's views on uric acid are now well-known, but the world has not yet sufficiently realised that "in diet lies the key to nine-tenths of the social and political problems that vex our nation and time." The universal experience of mankind for many centuries counts for nothing : "Diet, as at present used, is often the product of a vast amount of ignorance; it is the cause of a hideous waste of time and money; it produces mental and moral obliquities, destroys health and shortens life, and generally quite fails to fulfil its proper purpose." How to remedy all this, to show how diet may be easily made to fulfil its proper purpose, is the author's object in this little book, the work of an enthusiast in the subject and a radical reformer of diet both in health and disease.

Wie ist die Fürsorge für Gemüthskranke von Aerzten und Laien zu fördern? Von Prof. Dr. C. Fürstner. Pp. 64. Berlin: S. Karger. 1899.—This is a pamphlet dealing with some aspects of the care of the insane in Germany. The author advocates the formation of special departments in general hospitals for treatment of mental diseases (such as, for instance, exists at St. Thomas's Hospital), and then points out some legal difficulties which have arisen, in Germany, in the transference of patients from such clinics to asylums. He also discusses from what class nurses should be drawn, and recommends, as far as possible, the substitution of female for male nurses.

Minutes of the General Medical Council for the Year 1898. Vol. XXXV. London: Spottiswoode & Co. 1899.—No one, until he has looked through the various reports and recommendations of the numerous committees and branch councils, has any idea of the vast amount of work done by the General Medical Council. The public generally, and the medical profession in particular, ought to be most thankful that they are represented by such an able body of men, who at times may be a trifle too unprogressive and make some blunders, but who are altogether doing a very useful work.

Aids to Examinations. Part II. By T. Reuell Atkinson, M.D. Pp. 170. London: Baillière, Tindall & Cox. [N.D.].— If this book is really an "aid to examinations," so much the worse for the examinations. It is a curious medley of medicine, surgery, midwifery, pathology, anatomy, and physiology. No attempt has been made to arrange it in any order, so that the reader jumps from a question in medicine to another in anatomy. We recommend students to acquire their knowledge in a manner different from this, and not trust to such miscalled "aids."

Epidemic Cerebro-Spinal Meningitis and its Relation to Other Forms of Meningitis: A Report of the State Board of Health of Massachusetts. By Dr. W. T. Councilman, Dr. F. B. Mallory, and Dr. J. H. Wright. Pp. x., 5—178. Boston: Wright & Potter Printing Co. 1898.—This is a valuable contribution to the study of this disease, and gives the most complete account of the pathology. It deals with 111 cases of the recent epidemic in the New England States, and these were fully investigated. It is the more interesting as the true nature of the recurring epidemics of cerebro-spinal meningitis appears to have been first recognised in Massachusetts. Short accounts of the clinical history of each case are given, with, in many instances, charts of the pulse and temperature. The general result of this enquiry is to confirm the diplococcus of Weichselbaum as the cause of the disease; it was found in 31 out of 35 fatal cases in cultures taken from the exudations after death. Stress is laid on the importance of spinal puncture in diagnosis. This procedure gave a positive result in 38 out of 55 cases, and it is pointed out that from this source fresh light may be anticipated on the sporadic cases of the disease. The organism is not very viable outside the body; inoculation into animals was only once successful in producing meningitis, in the case of a goat. In the meningeal exudation large cells were found, often containing many leucocytes, and were derived from the cells of the con-nective tissue, and from those lining the lymph spaces. Amongst other changes in the brain, chiefly secondary to the meningeal inflammation, we notice the pronounced changes in the neuroglia, consisting of swelling and proliferation in the glia cells. All the changes in the brain-substance were very marked around the ventricles. The authors found that lesions of nerves were very common—of the cranial nerves, especially the second, fifth, and eighth;—and lesions of the spinal nerve-roots, varying in intensity, were found in every case in which they were examined. With regard to the important question of the distinction from pneumococcus meningitis, the authors say that without being warranted in making extensive generalisations, the absence or slight development of symptoms pointing to extensive infection of the meninges, of the cord and spinal roots, and extension of infection along the cranial nerves point to the pneumococcus infection. A series of good coloured plates of the most important bacteriological and pathological appearances is given, and the work affords the best account of the disease, derived from original observations, known to us, and has been admirably done in every respect.

The Schott Treatment for Chronic Heart Diseases. By RICHARD GREENE. Second Edition. Pp. 16. London: The Scientific Press, Limited. 1898.—This brief account of the treatment of heart disease at Nauheim is of value to those who do not wish to buy a more expensive book. The number of patients visiting Nauheim continues to increase, so apparently the interest in the treatment is not materially abating.

How to Avoid Tubercle. By A. T. TUCKER WISE, M.D. Pp. 15. London: Baillière, Tindall and Cox. 1898.—The size of this booklet shows what the power of condensation is able to effect. Dr. Wise emphasises the fact that many household pets, such as canaries and parrots, may be a source of tubercle dissemination, and considers that in regard to health a household is safer without any pets—except, perhaps, the cat and dog.

A Synopsis of Surgery. By R. F. TOBIN. Pp. xx., 3—277. London: J. & A. Churchill. 1898.—This book, the author states, is a collection of leaflets of synopses of lectures delivered by him at St. Vincent's Hospital, Dublin. It is not illustrated, save for a few temperature charts; and the subject matter, which is interleaved with blank paper, is little more than a tabulation of facts "to lessen for the students the trouble of taking notes." For this purpose it will, no doubt, be useful, as the facts may be generally accepted and they are concisely stated. Externally the book resembles an *édition de luxe* of a devotional work.

An Investigation on the Influence upon the Vital Resistance of Animals to the Micro-organisms of Disease brought about by Prolonged Sojourn in an Impure Atmosphere. By D. H. BERGEY, M.D. Pp. 10. Washington: The Smithsonian Institution. 1898. —The experiments here recorded were undertaken with a view to determining whether impure atmosphere produces detrimental effects upon the animal organism as shown in greater susceptibility to certain diseases. Owing to technical difficulties, results were obtained in only one series of experiments. In these it was shown that guinea-pigs living in an atmosphere containing a larger amount of carbonic acid than normal succumbed more quickly to tuberculosis when inoculated than did control animals.

A Text-Book upon the Pathogenic Bacteria. By JOSEPH McFARLAND, M.D. Second Edition. Pp. 497. London: Henry Kimpton. 1898.—The second edition of this work does not present many new features, the most important being additional chapters on whooping cough, mumps, yellow fever, hog-cholera, and swine-plague. The general scope of the volume remains very much as in the first edition, a favourable notice of which has already appeared in this *Journal*.

A Synopsis of the British Pharmacopœia, 1898. Compiled by H. WIPPELL GADD. [Third Edition.] Pp. 183. London: Baillière, Tindall & Cox. 1898.—In this edition some fresh information is added, and the doses as expressed in metric equivalents are now given only approximately and not precisely exact; this arrangement, however, is much more practically useful. We can now repeat even more warmly the praise which we bestowed upon the first edition.

Chloroform: Its Absolutely Safe Administration. By ROBERT BELL, M.D. Pp. 40. Glasgow: Robert Love Holmes. 1898. —Whilst we entirely agree with Dr. Bell as to the desirability of using some form of graduated inhaler for the administration of chloroform, we doubt very much whether his pamphlet will in any way conduce to a general acceptance of his views. In a work avowedly written for and in the interests of the public, it is to be regretted that there should occur such a statement as the following: "Each death which occurs [in the administration of chloroform], to put it mildly, should in justice be described as one of culpable homicide." The statement, too, that in medical journalism there is an organised opposition to the facts of the chloroform controversy being known is without foundation. From a scientific standpoint this monograph is worthless, and it is calculated to do much harm by alarming and misleading the public.

Diseases of the Skin. By MALCOLM MORRIS. New [Second] Edition. Pp. xv., 589. London: Cassell and Company, Limited. 1898.—That there is a demand for this useful book is shown by this considerably enlarged edition. It seems almost superfluous to say that, upon the whole, the work is an excellent one for the busy practitioner as well as for the student. It is concise and clearly written. To some minor points only should we take exception. We have seen cases of "verruca necrogenica" amongst men who have had nothing to do "with handling dead tissue," and we are of opinion that one attack of erythema nodosum is, comparatively, rarely followed by a second one. Herpes zoster, in our opinion, is not such a right-sided affair as the author states ("the right side being far more often affected than the left," p. 158). We have investigated returns of our cases extending over nearly ten years, and out of 206 cases of zona the right side was affected in 100, the left in 93, and in 13 cases the incidence was unrecorded. We have seen a statement that zona occurs nineteen times on the right side to one on the left side of the body. On the other hand, amongst the older writers, Reil observes that he has always found it on the left half of the body. In looking over our statistics we do find sometimes a remarkable run, first upon one side and then upon the other; and we can well conceive that one observer, in the chapter of coincidences, might meet with a long one-sided succession. We have gone into this question before, and we believe the incidence would be, in a large number of cases, as much in favour of one side as the other. The index, printed in unnecessarily small type, is good, but has faults. "Rodent ulcer" should be p. 558, not 556; and on p. 138 we do not find a word about lichen planus. We congratulate the publishers on the improved external appearance of this edition.

Essentials of the Diseases of the Ear. By E. B. GLEASON, M.D. Second Edition. Pp. 206. London: Henry Kimpton. 1898.—We are not surprised that this little book has so rapidly reached a second edition. It contains in a small compass a large amount of useful information; and it is written in such a bright and easy manner that it forms a most readable work, notwithstanding the fact that it is arranged in the usually objec-

19

tionable form of question and answer. The present edition contains a good account of the principal modern surgical procedures in intra-cranial complications of ear diseases; these are well illustrated and are plainly described. We know of no other small work on ear diseases to compare with this either in freshness of style or completeness of information.

Transactions of the Clinical Society of London. Vol. XXXI. London: Longmans, Green, and Co. 1898.—This volume contains a most interesting and varied collection of clinical reports on medical and surgical cases. Dr. Calot himself contributes a paper on his treatment of Pott's disease, and there are others—all more or less favourable to Calot's method—on the same subject. The report of the Committee on the antitoxin of diphtheria is also added, and the results of their investigation tend to show that by the use of antitoxin the general mortality is reduced by one-third.

Transactions of the Royal Academy of Medicine in Ireland. Vol. XVI. Dublin: Fannin and Co., Ltd. 1898.—A noteworthy paper in this volume is that on "Pneumonia: a Multiple Infection," by Dr. John W. Moore, who submits "that there is clinical evidence to show that a true pneumonitis may occur in . . . erysipelas, influenza, tuberculosis and enteric fever. Further, it is reasonable to suppose that in each case the pneumonitis is directly due to a localisation of the specific poison of the disease in the lung, whether that poison be a micro-organism itself or a toxin derived therefrom." Dr. W. R. Dawson, writing on membranous colitis, remarks: "The lesion is of the nature rather of a slight annoyance rather than a serious malady, and hence does not appear to demand any more energetic interference" than enemata, especially glycerine injections of about a couple of drachms, which appear to have been found most satisfactory. The "Clinical Report of the Rotunda Hospital" is, as usual, full of interest.

Transactions of the Grant College Medical Society. Bombay: The "Tattva-Vivechaka" Press. 1898.—These *Transactions* are for the most part a summary of a series of papers on the therapeutics of Indian drugs, of many of which we have never heard. The various meetings at which these papers were read must have been somewhat tame, but Dr. Dhargalker appears to be a host in himself, and scarcely any other topics were needed. Twenty or so new drugs at a meeting must give our Indian *confrères* abundant food for therapeutic investigation. The booklet is very unattractive in appearance.

Transactions of the Iowa State Medical Society. Vol. XVI. Burlington: The Keehn-Hafner Mfg. Co. 1898.—The Society whose transactions are here recorded has reached the 47th year of its existence. Many of the papers are on topics of general interest, and are worthy of a very wide circulation. The book would be all the better if more attention were given to the proof-reading. We noticed "Kraska," "chololithiasis," "serum-theraphy."

Transactions of the Medical Society of the State of New York. Published by the Society. 1898.—The present issue contains the usual amount of valuable material which is to be found in these volumes, and is in every way equal to its predecessors. We would notice particularly the excellence of the articles on the use of the X-rays in medicine and surgery.

Transactions of the Ohio State Medical Society. Cleveland: J. B. Savage Press. 1898.—The Society contains 903 members and is evidently doing good work. The discussions on the various papers read at its fifty-third annual meeting are fully reported and are full of interest.

Transactions of the South Carolina Medical Association. Charleston : Walker, Evans & Cogswell Co. 1897.—This is the report of this Association's forty-seventh annual session. It shows that the South Carolinians are aspiring to be at all times up-to-date, and are working with the motto which their president wished them to keep continually before their eyes, " High endeavour and concerted action."

Transactions of the American Surgical Association. Vol. XVI. Philadelphia: William J. Dornan. 1898.—The most notable articles in this volume are on " The Etiology and Classification of Cystitis," by N. Senn ; " The Question of Operative Interference in recent Simple Fractures of the Patella," by C. A. Powers; " The Use of Animal Toxins in the Treatment of Inoperable Malignant Tumors," by G. R. Fowler ; and " A Clinical and Histological Study of Certain Adenocarcinomata of the Breast," by W. S. Halsted. Dr. Senn gives a most exhaustive account of his investigations into the subject of the various forms of cystitis, chiefly bacteriological, but partly also clinical, by which he proves that the essential or exciting cause of cystitis is invariably the presence of microbes in the tissues of the bladder. He describes the various forms of microbes met with, and discusses their mode of entrance into the bladder. The article well deserves a careful study. Dr. Powers has made a collective investigation among the Fellows of the American Surgical Association, the Members of the New York Surgical Society, and of the Philadelphia Academy of Surgery as to the advisability of operating on recent simple fractures of the patella, the form of operation preferred, and the number of cases operated on, with results. He gives a summary of the replies, and we are astonished at the conservative feeling manifested by the majority of these surgeons on the subject. Four would actually use Malgaigne's hooks in suitable cases where the fragments cannot easily be approximated. Seventeen are opposed to operation in any case. Nine would operate in all cases in which no distinct contraindication exists and in which the surroundings are satisfactory. Forty-one would operate on selected cases. Very high praise is given to the so-called "Dutch" method of treatment by massage. This is not half so well known in this country as it should be, and we refer our readers to this article for an admirable description of it. The article by Dr. Halsted contains his latest views and statistics on the methods and results of the supraclavicular operation and other operations for the removal of cancer of the breast, and we are appalled at the radical nature of the operation now advised by Dr. Halsted. The operation as now performed by him occupies from two to four hours and requires highly trained and skilful assistants. So much skin is removed that grafts have to be cut from the patient's thigh as large as or larger than one's hand to cover the raw surface. The neck is operated on in every case. Both pectoral muscles are removed. The axillary, subclavian and internal jugular veins are stripped clean. The supra-clavicular fossa is cleaned out. All fat is removed from the subscapular region and also from the supra- and infra-clavicular regions, while the nerves and vessels of the axillary cavity are stripped as clean as possible. After this extensive operation Dr. Halsted has met with an astonishing degree of success. One hundred and thirty-three cases have been operated upon; there have been only thirteen local and twenty-two regionary recurrences, while of seventy-six cases operated on more than three years ago, thirty-one are living without recurrence. This is far better than any results that have hitherto been shown, and it looks as if the day of the old operation had gone for ever.

The Transactions of the Edinburgh Obstetrical Society. Vol. XXII. Edinburgh: Oliver and Boyd. 1897.—Apart from the usual subjects of clinical interest which the *Transactions* always contain, there are in the present volume many papers on the speculative and scientific side of the subject, such as the question of the existence of a positive pressure in the growing pregnant uterus and the causation of twins. These are well worth reading, and will be found to contain many valuable suggestions.

Transactions of the Ophthalmological Society of the United Kingdom. Vol. XVIII. London: J. & A. Churchill. 1898.— In his Bowman Lecture, Mr. Priestley Smith, amongst many original observations, suggests that ordinary convergent strabismus, bearing as it does but little relation to the degree of the hypermetropia, is due to the "overaction of a motor centre which has escaped from conscious control." He lays stress on the necessity for "educative" treatment in addition to spectacles and operative measures. The elaborate report of the sub-committee on excision of the eyeball and the various operations which have been substituted for it occupies more than seventy pages. On the whole, the verdict is in favour of simple excision, with the addition in suitable cases of the insertion of a glass globe into Tenon's capsule. Mr. Gunn's very able paper on the ophthalmoscopic evidence of arterial disease is the outcome of an immense amount of careful observation. The diagnostic value of the conditions he depicts and describes, especially. perhaps in cases where there is *no* albuminuria, is only just beginning to be recognised. In his paper on epithelial xerosis of the conjunctiva, Mr. Sydney Stephenson concludes that the disease is not usually due to the so-called xerosis bacilli, which are invariably present and are microscopically indistinguishable from diphtheria bacilli, but is caused by the irritation of spring and summer sunlight acting on the conjunctiva of anæmic and ill-nourished children. Upwards of a dozen cases are related of the successful detection of foreign bodies in the globe or orbit by the aid of the X-rays, and some good reproductions are given of Mr. Mackenzie Davidson's skiagrams.

The Transactions of the Society of Anæsthetists. Vol. I. London : The Medical Publishing Company, Limited. 1898.— The transactions of this infant Society deal chiefly with debatable points. Attention may be directed to Mr. Walter Tyrrell's. suggestion to add ether vapour from a second bottle to the chloroform vapour from a Junker's apparatus; and to the address of Dr. Waller on the dosage of anæsthetics, embodying his conclusions from experiments on nerve. He lays stress on the great fact that the lethal dose of chloroform is only twice the anæsthetic dose. The book is sent out in an unattractive dress, and has neither table of contents nor index.

Annual and Analytical Cyclopædia of Practical Medicine. Vol. III.—*Dislocations to Infantile Myxœdema.* Philadelphia: The F. A. Davis Company. 1899.—Dr. Sajous, the editor of this stupendous work, states that the kind reception afforded the first two volumes has been the source of much gratification. The plan of the work has met the wants of the general practitioner, while preserving for authors and teachers the leading advantages of the older annual. On reading through several of the articles, *e.g.*, epilepsy, exophthalmic goitre, infantile myxœdema, hypnotism, and hysteria, we have found them to be very accurate and complete monographs on the respective subjects.

E. Merck's Annual Report [of New Medicinal Preparations] on the year 1898. Pp. 185. Darmstadt: Eduard Roether. 1899. —The composition and action of many modern drugs are here described, together with an original communication on the action of some morphia derivatives. The well-known name of Merck requires no commendation; but many of these preparations, though interesting from the chemical standpoint, are too much in advance of the Pharmacopœia to be of great utility to other than the experimental therapeutist. Our patients commonly will not be satisfied to spend time and money on drugs whose reputation has not yet borne the test of time.

Therapentic Notes. London: Parke, Davis & Co.—Dated July, this is the first number of a serial which is a simple advertisement, bright, crisp, and up-to-date, of some of the preparations of this enterprising firm.

The British Physician. London: The Sanitary Publishing Co., Ltd.—This new monthly journal aims at a more or less distinctive character, and "while admitting contributions on any and every branch of medical science and practice, will be more closely concerned with therapeutics and pharmacology." It will avoid matters of purely surgical interest. We trust that the editor will be able to carry out his views and will have the support of a large staff of scientific contributors, both metropolitan and provincial.

The Caledonian Medical Journal. Glasgow: Alex. Macdougall. —This new exchange contains the proceedings of the Caledonian Medical Society—which is peripatetic, holding its annual meetings in various towns. The editors are Dr. Macnaughton of Stonehaven, and Dr. Andrew Little of Burnley, who inform us that the reputation of the *Journal* is steadily increasing, and that no pains will be spared to make it bright, interesting, and readable. If the members of this Society are not immortalised by their professional doings, they will be borne in mind by an amused posterity, for a picture of them at dinner is given as a frontispiece to this number.

The Edinburgh Medical Journal. New Series. Vol. V. Edinburgh: Young J. Pentland. 1899.—We have in this publication a nicely printed volume of 648 pages, containing a large number of original articles, many reviews of recent books, and a monthly account of the recent advances in the various departments of medical science. Those who do not see the monthly numbers of the *Edinburgh Medical Journal* would do well to peruse the six-monthly volume, which contains the views of the best authorities on many modern topics.

A Year's Work in Medical Defence, 1898. London: 4 Trafalgar Square.—From the annual report of the Medical Defence Union we learn that the condition of the fund is satisfactory, and that the Union continues to gain members. Of its utility, if proof were needed, the present report is evidence. We cannot help regretting that the Council have decided not to proceed further in the prosecution of quacks, although we believe such a duty is one that naturally devolves upon the General Medical Council, but that body seems to prefer to obtain convictions for qualified men. We may call attention to the change of address, so that medical men wishing to join should now write to the address given above.

Archives of the Roentgen Ray. Vol. II. London: The Rebman Publishing Company, Limited. 1898.—Vol. ii. of this interesting chronicle of skiagraphical progress, though it has no very remarkable development of its subject either in theory or practice to record, contains nevertheless particulars of a good deal of important work which has been done with the object of enlarging the possibilities and ensuring the success of X-ray diagnosis. Two questions of special practical moment are conspicuously to the fore. The first is the exact localisation of foreign bodies when surrounded by a great thickness of tissue, and this receives a good deal of attention, several methods of procedure, both with the photographic plate and with the fluorescent screen, being described. The other question is the structure and efficiency of that most essential of all the items of skiagraphical equipment—the X-ray tube. This is also dealt with at considerable length, and considering how fickle and untrustworthy, for the most part, the average tube proves when put to the test of serious use, such investigations into the conditions of maximum efficiency as are here recorded are of the highest value. In addition to the letterpress, the volume contains numerous well-executed reproductions of skiagrams. Many of these are interesting, though none present features of special novelty, except perhaps Dr. W. J. Morton's skiagram of the whole of an adult, taken by a single exposure of thirty minutes.

Burdett's Official Nursing Directory, 1899. London: The Scientific Press, Limited.—The second year of the *Nursing Directory* differs little from the previous one, which we noticed a year ago. Testing it by reference to the various institutions we know locally and elsewhere, we find it correct, and the information as complete as required. Perhaps we shall some day have the legal status of a nurse defined, and then the *Directory* will really be of "official" value. We still think it desirable that there should be local lists.

Year-Book of the Scientific and Learned Societies of Great Britain and Ireland. Sixteenth Annual Issue. London: Charles Griffin and Company, Limited. 1899.—It seems strange that the compilers of this book will not increase its value by providing a more comprehensive index, which should include references to the papers read before the societies. Some of the slight errors in its pages might be removed if a proof was sent to the numerous secretaries of the societies recorded.

Knowledge. June, 1899. London: T. Thompson.—We are glad to see this old-established journal showing such sustained vigour. The number of interesting original scientific articles is remarkable, and the illustrations are good. As a result of a careful study of the Hereford earthquake of 1896, Dr. Charles Davison puts forward an ingenious theory of the origin of the double focus in earthquakes. A map shows the large area affected by this disturbance, which acted over probably 100,000 square miles. There are charming papers on certain crustacea which grow to fit the habitations they adopt, and on the organisms to which flint is originally due; while the column of ornithological notes will attract many lovers of rural sights and sounds. A paper by Professor A. Thomson gives us in graphic form the proportions of the limbs and trunk of the human subject in different races. The long arms and long legs of the negro, the shortness of the upper in contrast with the lower limb of the white man, and the long legs and short body of the Australian are strikingly displayed. The ultimate reduction of the great existing mass of anthropological data to some useful form seems to depend on the adoption of some such method as this.

Physicians' Book for Private Formulæ: with Posological Table. Bristol: John Wright & Co. [1898.]—Those who have short memories may find this little book useful for recording formulæ, the details of which they have difficulty in carrying in their heads. The blank pages for this purpose, together with the doses of the last *British Pharmacopœia* preparations and much other useful information, make up a tiny but elegant volume which can really be a waistcoat-pocket companion whose society may often be of value to the doctor.

Programme of the Inauguration. Wellcome Club and Institute, June, 1899.—The enterprise of the firm of Messrs. Burroughs, Wellcome, & Co. is not limited to providing facilities for the prescribing doctor, but has an ever watchful care for the well-being of those whom it employs. The last practical shape which this has taken is a Club and Institute at Dartford, which, to judge by the illustrations given in the booklet, must be a truly delightful place.

Motes on Preparations for the Sick.

The annual museum of the British Medical Association usually gives an excellent opportunity of learning what new things there are in food and physic; the recent display at Portsmouth was no exception to the rule. We propose to notice a few of the things which attracted our attention.

The **Somatose** group (BAYER & Coi), including Ferro-Somatose and Lacto-Somatose, which we have noticed on previous occasions (September, 1895, and March, 1899), appear to be establishing themselves as very useful manufactured foods in the convenient form of powders. Fairchild's **Peptogenic Milk Powder**, about which we said something last September, is also well known as a means for the production of normal mother's milk for infants. One of the most interesting series of food products has as its basis a powder prepared from milk, containing the milk proteids. It is called **Protene** (THE PROTENE

COMPANY), and may be regarded as a dried milk from which the fat and sugar have been eliminated. It is obviously not a complete milk food, but is practically a pure proteid, which will keep for any length of time, can be added to or combined with a great variety of other foods, and cannot fail to be most valuable to the diabetic and the corpulent. A great variety of biscuits made with the protene flour as a basis provides suitable food for many different purposes and various tastes.

The use of a powder like protene, with the addition of cream and sugar, goes far towards the abolition of the morning and evening importation of so many tons of water inside the milk cans, which are such an annoyance diurnally at most of our railway stations. Why should not the milk be at once concentrated, and be kept in the house ready for use at any time by the mere addition of water? The ordinary condensed milks have not been as great a success as they deserve; possibly a milk powder would be more likely to attract the public fancy. Is not this the best solution of the difficulty as regards the prevention of tuberculosis by the sterilisation of milk? The abolition of the uncooked milk, and the sole use of the manufactured product, would reform the milk trade and be greatly to the advantage of the consumer. A milk powder, which may form the basis of a great variety of milk drinks, gives great scope for an indefinite production of products suitable to the needs of the invalid of the future.

The products of the AYLESBURY DAIRY COMPANY, HENRI NESTLÉ, and the ANGLO-SWISS MILK COMPANY are now well known to be perfectly trustworthy.

Several varieties of **Foods for Special Invalids** were exhibited by Messrs. CALLARD & Co., who provide not only for the diabetic but for the obese, the gouty and the rheumatic. They have also a special food to counteract constipation, a palatable, moist brown bread, a marmalade made with glycerine, and an infants' food described as non-farinaceous.

Mellin's Food products were much in evidence, including our old familiar friends the Mellin's Food Biscuits and the Cod Liver Oil Emulsion.

The **Beef Peptonoid** powder of Messrs. CARNRICK & Co., and the **Liquid Peptonoids** prepared from it, are beginning (though somewhat slowly) to be appreciated. The powder is efficiently sterilised during manufacture, and in the liquid preparation this aseptic condition is maintained by the addition of sufficient alcohol to preserve it. The combination with Coca is a palatable predigested fluid having much nutritive value.

The **Bovril** preparations are maintaining their reputation. One of the best of these is the raw **Meat Juice** expressed in the cold, and which is of the highest nutritive value.

Of the numerous preparations exhibited by Messrs. ALLEN AND HANBURYS the most interesting and novel were two combinations of Creasote: one, the phosphate, called **Phosote**, and the other, the tannophosphate, called **Taphosote**. They are best administered in capsules, each containing half a gramme. Six grammes have been given daily, and with a good result.

Hommel's Hæmatogen (NICOLAY & Co.) is a solution of Hæmoglobin, and should be an ideal blood-maker in cases where anæmia is a prominent feature, and more especially in cases where the inorganic preparations of iron are not proving satisfactory. In rickets, scrofula, and wasting diseases of childhood this fluid has given good results.

The **Hunyadi János Mineral Water** (ANDREAS SAXLEHNER) is too well known to require description. Its especial value at the present time is due to its presumed utility as an intestinal antiseptic in catarrhal gastro-enteritis of influenza type. It is recommended that it should be given freely, a pint on an empty stomach at the onset, and a glassful (1) on several consecutive mornings. The patient, purged of the influenza poison, is expected to escape all subsequent tendency to inflammatory complications, together with the adynamia and muscular debility.

The Library of the Bristol Medico-Chirurgical Society.

The following donations have been received since the publication of the list in June :

August 31st, 1899.

L. M. Griffiths (1)	56 volumes.
F. E. Hare, M.D.	1 volume.
Official Board of Advertising for the Isle of Man (2)	1 ,,
Medical Faculty, McGill University (3)	1 ,,
Norske Medicinske Selskabs Bibliotek (4)	35 volumes.
Editor of *The Railway Surgeon* (5)	1 volume.
Royal Medical and Chirurgical Society (6)	5 volumes.
R. Shingleton Smith, M.D. (7)	1 volume.
Editor of *Virginia Medical Semi-Monthly* (8)	1 ,,
Cyril H. Walker, M.B. (9)	1 ,,

Unbound periodicals and a framed picture have been received from Mr. L. M. Griffiths. Unframed pictures have been presented by Dr. J. O. Symes and Mr. Cyril H. Walker.

THIRTY-THIRD LIST OF BOOKS.

The titles of books mentioned in previous lists are not repeated.

The figures in brackets refer to the figures after the names of the donors, and show by whom the volumes were presented. The books to which no such figures are attached have either been bought from the Library Fund or received through the *Journal*.

Allbutt, T. C. [Ed.]	*A System of Medicine.* Vol. VII.	1899
Anderson, J. W.	*The Power of Nature in Disease*	1899
Anstie, F. E. ...	*Notes on Epidemics* ... ... (1)	[1866]
Armitage, T. R....	*Hydropathy as applied to Acute Disease*... ... ... (1)	1852
Baden, G. L. ...	*Lægevidenskabens Historie* ... ... (4)	1823
Bauke, A. C. ...	*Medical Officer* ... ... (1)	1860
Beil, B.	*A System of Surgery* (1) Vols. I., New Ed., 1790, II., 3rd Ed., 1787, III., 4th Ed., 1789, IV., 3rd Ed.	1789
Blundell, J. ...	*Vorlesungen über Geburtshilfe* (Deutsch bearbeitet von L. Calmann). 2. Hauptabth. ... ... (4)	1838
Boeck, W.	*Recherches sur la Syphilis* ... ... (4)	1862
Bonorden, H. F....	*Die Syphilis* ... . (4)	1834
Briggs, F. H. and H. F.	*Advanced Scientific Dentistry* ... ... (1)	[N.D.]
Brindel, [—] ...	*Des Lésions de la Table interne du Crane dans les Suppurations de l'Oreille moyenne*	1899
Brodie, [G. J.] Guthrie und [B. C.]	*Vorlesungen über die vorzüglichsten Krankheiten der Harnausführungsorgane und des Mastdarms* (Deutsch bearbeitet des F. J. Behrend) ... ... (4)	1836
Browne, L.	*The Throat and Nose, and their Diseases* .. 5th Ed.	1899
Bruel, W.	*Praxis Medicinæ, or, The Physicians Practise* (1) 2nd Ed.	1639
Burns, J.	*Handbuch der Geburtshülfe* (Herausgegeben von H. F. Kilian) ... ... (4)	1834
Buxton : its History, Waters, Climate, Scenery, etc....	[N.D.]
Carlsbad, Guide to ... ... (1)	[1886]
Carus, C. G. ...	*Lehrbuch der Gynäkologie.* 2 vols. ... ... (4)	1820
Clutterbuck, J. Wardrop und H.	*Blutentziehungen in Krankheiten* (Deutsch bearbeitet des F. J. Behrend) ... (4)	1840
Coblentz, V. ..	*The Newer Remedies* ... ... 3rd Ed.	1899
Creuznach-Spa and its Environs	1899
Dick, R.	*Diet and Regimen* ... ... (1) 2nd Ed.	1839
Dover, T.	*The Ancient Physician's Legacy to his Country* (1) 8th Ed.	1771
Druitt, R.	*Haandbog i Chirurgien* (Oversat af A. Arndtsen) (4)	1856
[Dutt, W. A.] ...	*Lowestoft as a Winter Resort*...	1899
Elder and J. S. Fowler, G.	*The Diseases of Children*	1899
Ellis, H.	*Mescal : A New Artificial Paradise*	1898
Encyklopädie der gesammten Medicin. (Herausgegeben von C. C. Schmidt) (4) 6 bd. 1841-42, Supplementbd. I., 1843, II.—IV. 2. Aufl.	1849
Erichsen, J. E. ...	*Praktisches Handbuch der Chirurgie* (Übersetzt von O. Thamhayn). 2 vols. ... ... (4)	1864
Fitzgerald, J. ...	*Pyorrhœa Alveolaris*	[1899]

Foster, M. ... ... *Recent Progress in Physiology* ... .- ... ... 1898.

Fowler, G. Elder and J. S. *The Diseases of Children* 1899

Fry, D. P. ... ... *Law of Vaccination* .. .. (1) 5th Ed. 1872

Gant, F. J. ... ... *Guide to the Examinations by the Conjoint Examining Board in England.* 7th Ed. (Ed. by W. Evans) 1899.

Goodhart, J. F. ... *The Diseases of Children* ... ... 6th Ed. 1899

Gräfe, E. A. ... *Neues pratisches Formulare und Recepttaschenbuch* (4) 1834

Grafstrom, A. V. *Medical Gymnastics* 1899

Gregory, J. ... ... *Conspectus Medicinæ Theoreticæ.* (Translated) (1) [2nd Ed.] 1833.

Guthrie und [B. C.] Brodie, [G. J.] *Vorlesungen über die vorzüglichsten Krankheiten der Harnausführungsorgane und des Mastdarms* (Deutsch bearbeitet des F. J. Behrend) ... ... (4) 1836.

Harrison, R. ... *Stone, Prostate and other Urinary Disorders* ... ... 1899.

Herschell, G. ... *Constipation* ... ...- 2nd Ed. 1899

Hewer, Mrs. L. ... *Our Baby* ... ... 6th Ed. 1899

Hooper, R. ... :.. *Medical Dictionary* ... ... (1) [wants title]

Hudson-Cox and J. Stokes, F. *The Pocket Pharmacopœia* 1899

Isle of Man, The—Official Guide .. .. (2) 1899.

Johnson, G. ... *On Epidemic Diarrhœa and Cholera* ... ... (1) 1866

Kingscote, E. ... *Asthma* 1899

Külz, E. ... ... *Klinische Enfahrungen über Diabetes mellitus* ... ... 1899.

Landerer, A. ... *Treatment of Tuberculosis with Cinnamic Acid.* (Translated) ... ... [N.D.]

Latham, P. M. ... *Diagnostik durch das Gehör bei Krankheiten der Brust* (Deutsch bearbeitet des F. J. Behrend) ... (4) 1837

Lexicon of Medicine and the Allied Sciences (New Syd. Soc.). Vol. V. ... 1899.

Liebig, J. ... ... *Chemistry in its Application to Agriculture and Physiology.* 2nd Ed. (Ed. by L. Playfair) ... (1) 1842

Lisfranc, [J.] ... *Krankheiten des Uterus* (Deutsch bearbeitet des F. J. Behrend) ... ... (4) 1839.

Lockwood, C. B. ... *Aseptic Surgery* ... ... 2nd Ed. 1899.

Lumley, W. G. ... *The Medical Officer's Manual* ... ... (1) 3rd Ed. 1871

M., G. E. F. ... *Medical Missions* ... ... [N.D.]

McCaw, J. ... ... *Aids to the Diagnosis and Treatment of Diseases of Children (Medical)* .. .. 2nd Ed. 1899.

Mac Donald, A. ... *Experimental Study of Children* 1899

Macilwain, G. ... *On the Unity of the Body* ... ... (1) 1836

Mackintosh, D. J. *Skiagraphic Atlas of Fractures and Dislocations* ... ... 1899.

Magendie, F. ... *Vorlesungen über organische Physik* (Deutsch bearbeitet des F. J. Behrend) ... ... (4) 1836.

... *Vorlesungen über organische Physik* (Uebersetzt von G. Krupp) Band III. ... ... (4) 183

... *Vorlesungen über das Blut* (Aus dem Französischen von G. Krupp) ... ... (4) 1839.

Moer, T. H. Pearmain and C. G. *Aids to the Analysis of Food and Drugs* 2nd Ed. [1899]

Morellus, P. ... *The Expert Doctor's Dispensatory.* (Translated) (1) 1657

Morison, A. ... *The Nervous System and Visceral Disease* 1899

Moullin, C. M. ... Enlargement of the Prostate ... ... 2nd Ed. 1899
Nederlandsch Gasthuis voor Ooglijders, Utrecht, De Voltooiing van het ... (9) 1899
Niemeyer, F. v. ... Lehrbuch der speciellen Pathologie und Therapie.
2 vols. ... ... (4) 7th Ed. 1868
Nurses, The Pocket Case Book for ... ... [N.D.]
Parham, F. W. ... Thoracic Resection for Tumors growing from the Bony
Wall of the Chest 1899
Pearmain and C. G. Moor, T. H. Aids to the Analysis of Food and Drugs
2nd Ed. [1899]
Petit, [C.-A.] ... Sur la Cure à Royat 1899
Plenck, J. J. ... Novum Systema Tumorum ... ... (1) 1767
Quinn, J. H. ... Manual of Library Cataloguing 1899
Rieder, H. ... ... Atlas of Urinary Sediments. (Tr. by F. C. Moore.
Ed. by A. S. Delépine) 1899
Shaw, J. ... ... Golden Rules of Psychiatry ... ... [1899]
Siebold, E. C. J. von. Lehrbuch der Geburtshülfe ... ... (4) 2nd Ed. 1854
Smith, H. ... .. Hæmorrhoids and Prolapsus of the Rectum (1) 3rd Ed. 1862
,, ... The Surgery of the Rectum ... ... (1) 1865
Squire, P. ... ... Companion to the British Pharmacopœia. 17th Ed.
(Revised by P. W. Squire) 1899
Stokes, F. Hudson-Cox and J. The Pocket Pharmacopœia 1899
Taylor, J. W. ... Extra-Uterine Pregnancy 1899
Thompson, Sir H. Urinorganernes Sygdomme (Pa Dansk ved J. Blicher)
(4) 1871
,, Modern Cremation ... ... 3rd Ed. 1899
Thomson, StC. ... The Cerebro-Spinal Fluid 1899
Treves, F. ... ... Intestinal Obstruction ... ... [2nd Ed.] 1899
Typhoid Fever in the Metropolis of Sydney, N.S.W., The Sanitary Value of
the Operations of the Board in Reducing and
Avoiding the Mortality from ... ... [1898]
Vegetable Physiology and Botany ... ... (1) 1842
Venables, R. ... Elements of Urinary Analysis and Diagnosis ... (1) [1850]
Walker, N.... ... An Introduction to Dermatology 1899
Walshe, W. H. ... Lungernes Sygdomme (Oversat af J. Blicher) ... (4) 1861
Wardrop und H. Clutterbuck, J. Blutentziehungen in Krankheiten
(Deutsch bearbeitet des F. J. Behrend) ... (4) 1840
West, C. ... ... Fremstilling af Børnesygdommenes (Bearbeitet af F.
V. Mansa) ... ... (4) 1855
,, ... Fremstilling af Qvindens Sygdomme (Bearbeitet af F.
V. Mansa) ... ... (4) 1860
Wilson, E. M. ... Notes on Malaria in Connection with Meteorological
Conditions at Sierra Leone. 3rd Year 1899
Xeroform ... ... [N.D.]
Ziekenverpleging en de zorg voor de openbare gezondheid in de laatste 50 jaren, De 1899

TRANSACTIONS, REPORTS, JOURNALS, &c.

American Association of Obstetricians and Gynecologists, Transactions of the ... ... Vols. IX.—XI. 1897-99
American Gynæcological and Obstetrical Journal, The .. Vol. XIV. 1899

American Journal of Obstetrics, The ... ...   Vol. XXXIX.   1899
American Journal of the Medical Sciences, The   .. ... Vol. CXVII.   1899
American Laryngological Association, Transactions of the   1899
American Public Health Association, Reports and Papers of the
                                                             Vol. XXIV.   1898
Archives cliniques de Bordeaux   ... ...   Tome VII.   1898
Archives of Clinical Skiagraphy ... ... [Vol. I.]   1896
Archives of Pediatrics, The ... ...   Vol. XV.   1898
Archives of the Roentgen Ray   ... ... Vol. II.   1898
Boston Medical and Surgical Journal, The   Vols. CXXXIX., CXL.   1898–99
Bookseller, The ... ...   (1) 1884–98
Bristol Port Sanitary District—Annual Report for 1898   1899
British Gynæcological Journal, The   ... ...   Vol. XIV.   1898
British Medical Journal, The ... ...   Vol. I. for   1899
Bulletin de l'Institut international de Bibliographie   1897
China Medical Missionary Journal, The   ... . Vols. XI., XII. 1897–98
Cincinnati Lancet-Clinic, The   ... ...Vol. LXXXI.   1899
Dermatological Society of Great Britain and Ireland, Transactions of
       the ... . Vol. IV.   1898
Dublin Journal of Medical Science, The   ... ...   Vol. CVII.   1899
Edinburgh Medical Journal, The ... ...N.S., Vol. V.   1899
Gazette de Gynécologie ... ...   Tome XIII.   1898
Giornale internazionale delle Scienze mediche   1898
Glasgow Medical Journal, The   ... ... Vol. LI.   1899
Gloucester Court Guide and County Blue Book, The   1899
Grant College Medical Society, Transactions of the...   1899
Hospital, The   ... ...   Vol. XXV.   1899
Hospitals—
       Glasgow Hospital Reports ... ... Vol. I.   1898
       King's College Hospital Reports   ... ... Vol. V.   1899
Indian Medical Gazette, The ... ...   Vol. XXXIII.   1898
International Directory of Laryngologists and Otologists   1899
International Medical Congress, 1881.—Catalogue of Temporary
       Museum ... ...   (1) 1881
Johns Hopkins Hospital Bulletin, The   ... ... Vol. IX.   1898
Journal de Neurologie   ... ...   Tomes II., III.   1897–98
Journal of Experimental Medicine, The   ... ...Vol. III.   1898
Journal of Nervous and Mental Disease, The ... ...   Vol. XXV.   1898
Journal of the American Medical Association, Vol. XXXII., 1899;
       General Index to Vols. I.—XXIV.   1896
Journal of the Sanitary Institute ... ...   Vol. XIX.   1898
Lancet, The... ... ...   Vol. I. for   1899
Library Association Year Book, The   1899
Library World, The ... ...   Vol. I.   1899
London, Report on the Sanitary Condition of the City of, for 1898 (7)   1899
McGill University, Faculty of Medicine, Calendar of the   ... ... (3)   1899
Medical and Surgical " Review of Reviews," The ... ...   Vol. I.   1898
Medical News, The ... ...Vols. LXXIII., LXXIV.   1898–99
Medical Press and Circular, The ... ... [Vol. CXVIII.]   1899
Medical Record ... ...   Vol. LV.   1899

Monthly Cyclopædia of Practical Medicine, The ... ... Vol. I. 1898
Münchener medicinische Wochenschrift 1898
New York Medical Journal, The ... ... Vol. LXIX. 1899
Obstetrical Transactions ... ...Vol. XL. 1899
Philadelphia Medical Journal, The ... ...Vol. III. 1899
Practitioner, The ... ... Vol. LXII. 1899
Railway Surgeon, The ... ... (5) Vol. V. 1898–99
Retrospect of Medicine, Braithwaite's... ... ... Vol. CXIX. 1899
Royal Medical and Chirurgical Society of London, Proceedings of the
    Vols. I.—IX., 1857–82 ; N.S., Vol. I., 1885 ; (6) 3rd Ser.,
        III., IV., 1891–92, VI., VII., 1894–95, IX. 1898
St. Petersburger medicinische Wochenschrift 1898
Sanitary Record, The ... ... Vol. XXIII. 1899
Scottish Medical and Surgical Journal, The .. ..Vol. IV. 1899
Virginia Medical Semi-Monthly ... ... (8) Vol. III. 1899
Year-Book of Scientific and Learned Societies 1899

Local Medical Notes.

BARNSTAPLE.

PUBLIC HEALTH.—Dr. Mark Jackson has been re-appointed Medical Officer of Health. Dr. R. Gooding has been appointed Medical Officer of Health for the Barnstaple Port Sanitary District, *vice* Mr. E. Rouse, deceased.

VACCINATION RETURNS.—At a meeting of the Board of Guardians held on July 21st, the Chairman remarked that vaccination was on the increase in their union ; in one district £9 were paid for vaccination fees during the past quarter, whereas in 1898 only £15 were paid for the whole year.

BARRY.

NEW NURSING HOME.—With the rapid growth of Barry, the work of the nursing staff has steadily increased, and the New Victoria Jubilee Nurses' Home, which has just been completed, was very badly needed. It is a handsome and commodious structure, and has been erected entirely by means of voluntary subscriptions.

BATH.

PUBLIC HEALTH.—Dr. W. H. Symons has been appointed Medical Officer of Health for the City and County of Bath. At a meeting of the Town Council it was decided to increase the salary of the medical officer from £200 to £435 per annum.

PREVENTION OF CONSUMPTION.—At a meeting of the Sanitary Committee on June 26th the Medical Officer of Health (Dr. Symons) presented a report, in which he stated that there were last year 59 deaths from phthisis, and from other tuberculous diseases 28. In 1868 the deaths from phthisis in Bath numbered 132, and from other tuberculous diseases 70. This saving from death and from illness was probably due to sanitary and social improvement. Their death-rate from phthisis is now less than that for England and Wales ; but they ought not to be satisfied as long as any persons died of phthisis. It had been decided to form a branch of the National Association for the Prevention of Consumption for the Counties of Gloucestershire, Somerset, and Wilts. Other large towns were falling in with the movement, and Dr. Symons hoped Bath would not be behindhand. So far, he thought, they were doing more than was being done in many places. They disinfected after deaths from phthisis wherever they could get permission to do so, and they always visited the houses and left circulars as to the means to be adopted to avoid the disease. They had not yet got regulations under the Dairies, Cowsheds, and Milkshops Order, but these were now under consideration. As to the practical results likely to follow the new movement, it appeared to him that they might teach persons suffering from phthisis how to carry out successful treatment at home by giving them a few weeks' treatment in a public institution where every detail was under medical supervision. Recent results showed that phthisis could be cured as well in England as elsewhere.

ROYAL UNITED HOSPITAL.—Mr. Frederick C. Forster has been appointed House Surgeon.

EASTERN DISPENSARY.—Mr. D. Leslie Beath has been appointed Honorary Medical Officer.

OBITUARY.—The death is reported of Mr. John Terry. The deceased qualified as M.R.C.S. in 1844, and L.S.A. in 1845. Mr. Terry was a very old member of the Bath and Bristol Branch of the British Medical Association, and for many years served on the Council. He was a constant attendant at the meetings, and took an active part in discussions relating to mental diseases, in which, as proprietor of Bailbrook Asylum, he was most interested.

BRENTRY.

HOME FOR INEBRIATES.—At the meeting of the Bristol Town Council held on June 14th, it was decided to make a conditional grant of £2,000 to the Royal Victoria Home for Inebriates at Brentry. The Cardiff Watch Committee, at their meeting on June 14th, decided to accept the offer of the authorities of the Inebriates' Home at Brentry, and to send patients there at a cost of £10 a year each, with 3s. 6d. per day for maintenance, such provision to be for not less than five inmates and for five years.

BRISTOL.

HAM GREEN FEVER HOSPITAL.—On the invitation of the Health Committee, a large number of medical men visited the new Corporation Fever Hospital at Ham Green, on July 14th. As a pamphlet containing full information on the structure of the pavilions aud other buildings was presented to each present, there is no need to go into details ; it will suffice to say that the wards are a model of what a hospital should be, the bed-space being more than ample, the sanitary arrangements and conveniences perfect, and every possible care taken to render the place suitable for the reception of sick people. Of the surroundings nothing could have appeared on that day more charming, the beautiful lawns, magnificent cedars and other trees, and the charming views made the visitors almost wish they were convalescents, and compelled to stop there for some weeks at the city's expense. The latest report is that some patients are already there, but, as the Medical Officer of Health said, the less the place is used the better he will be pleased, as it will indicate an absence of infectious diseases in the city. We cannot conclude without congratulating Mr. Yabbicom, Dr. Davies, and the Hospital Sub-committee on the satisfactory completion of their. labours, for they have supplied Bristol with a Fever Hospital second to none in the kingdom.

INFIRMARY NURSES' HOME.—The Carnival at the Zoological Gardens held to raise enough money to furnish the Nurses' Home at the Royal Infirmary was one of the most, if not the most, successful entertainment of that sort ever held in Bristol, and what is more gratifying, everybody was pleased, and more than sufficient money was received, though we have no doubt some worthy object will be found at that Institution for the surplus. Firstly, the weather was all that it should be, the gardens were at their best, and the willing band of ladies who took stalls or helped in the refreshment places, the medical students and many gentlemen who helped at the shooting galleries and Aunt Sally booths threw all their energies into "the cause," and extracted the not unwilling pence from the spectators. The bicycle gymkhana was very entertaining and some wonderful riding was shown by a company of ladies and gentlemen from Weston. Lastly, but by no means leastly, the maypole dance by small children was very pretty, and elicited hearty applause at each performance.

CARDIFF.

PUBLIC HEALTH.—A deputation from the Cardiff Medical Society has informed the Health Committee of the Cardiff Corporation that the members of the Society were prepared to notify to the Medical Officers of Health cases of tuberculosis coming under their notice, with a view to infected rooms and articles being disinfected by the Authority. No fee will be paid by the Corporation for the information.

The Public Health Laboratory, which was established last year by the Glamorgan County Council, will in future be under the joint charge of the Medical Officers of Health of Cardiff and of the county, under the name of the "Cardiff and County Public Health Laboratory." A bacteriological laboratory has been erected and fitted up by the County Council at a cost of about £500, and the current expenses of the institution will be shared during the next two years by the two Authorities. A bacteriologist is to be appointed at a salary of £300 per annum, and he is to have a qualified assistant. It is expected that arrangements will be made with the authorities of University College whereby the bacteriologist appointed may become a Professor of the College and give lectures on hygienic subjects.

INFIRMARY.—Dr. W. M. Stevens has been appointed Pathologist.

CHEPSTOW.

PUBLIC HEALTH.—Mr. G. Lawrence has been appointed Medical Officer of Health, vice Mr. E. P. King resigned.

CHELTENHAM.

HOSPITAL FOR SICK CHILDREN.—Mr. C. E. Lansdown has been appointed Surgeon.

CHIPPING SODBURY.

PUBLIC HEALTH.—Mr. A. D. Parr-Dudley has been appointed Medical Officer for the Fifth Sanitary District.

VACCINATION LITERATURE.—At a meeting of the Chipping Sodbury Board of Guardians a letter was read from Dr. F. T. Bond, Honorary Secretary of the Jenner Society, enclosing specimen tracts and leaflets on the subject of vaccination. One of the members thought they

20

should also have some of the large posters issued by the Society placed in two villages where information was much needed upon the matter. It was decided to purchase some large posters and copies of several of the tracts and leaflets.

DEVONPORT.

ROYAL ALBERT HOSPITAL.—At a meeting of the Subscribers of this Institution it was decided to erect a new Nurses' Home at a cost of £2,200, and to provide isolation wards, consulting rooms for the medical staff, etc., at an estimated expenditure of about £1,500.

INFIRMARY.—The Infirmary Committee of the Devonport Board of Guardians, in an exhaustive report on the nursing staff and the management and general condition of the infirmary, suggest that the Local Government Board should be urged to issue an order directing that matrons of workhouses should have no jurisdiction in infirmaries, but that the superintendent nurse should exercise paramount authority.

MEMORIAL TO THE LATE MR. L. P. METHAM.—At the annual meeting of the Royal Female Orphan Asylum it was decided to perpetuate the memory of the late Mr. L. P. Metham, M.R.C.S.Eng., L.S.A., who had been Honorary Secretary to the institution from its foundation, by raising a fund, to be called the "Metham Endowment Fund," for the maintenance of five beds to be filled by children nominated from time to time by his two daughters.

HONORARY FREEMANSHIP TO A MEDICAL MAN.—On July 25th the honorary freemanship of the borough of Devonport was presented to Alderman Joseph May, F.R.C.S.Eng., L.S.A., J.P. The certificate presented to Mr. May contained sketches of the municipal and other public buildings, made allusion to the "eminent services rendered to the borough" by him, and recorded his municipal appointments as follows : Commissioner, 1840-94 ; councillor, 1861-63; alderman, 1868-99; mayor, 1870-71, 1871-72, 1872-73, 1875-76. The casket was of silver-gilt, richly embellished and suitably inscribed.

EXETER.

DEVON AND EXETER HOSPITAL.—T.R.H. the Duke and Duchess of York visited the Devon and Exeter Hospital on July 4th. Afterwards a garden party was held in the grounds, and 120 little girls presented the Duchess with purses of £5 each, on behalf of the hospital.

GLOUCESTER.

PUBLIC HEALTH.—In his annual report, Dr. Bond, the Medical Officer of Health to the Gloucestershire Combined Sanitary District, states that the birth-rate was 26.4 per 1,000 of the estimated population. The general birth-rate has varied during the last ten years beween 29.6 and 25.9, but with a distinct tendency to decline, as might be expected in a district which is so largely agricultural in its character. The total number of deaths registered during the year was 1,264, being a diminution of 137, or 9.7, on the mortality of the previous year, and giving an average death-rate of 12.9 for the whole district, the best for the last quarter of a century.

HELSTON.

VACCINATION.—At the meeting of the Board of Guardians held on July 22nd, it was reported that the vaccination expenses for the last quarter amounted to £107, being £72 in excess of the preceding quarter. The Clerk stated that at present the cost of vaccination would average about £180 yearly, while under the old system it never exceeded £50 per annum. The Guardians decided to petition the Local Government Board to reduce the minimum fees to be paid to Public Vaccinators.

ILFRACOMBE.

PUBLIC HEALTH.—Dr. E. Slade-King has submitted to the Devon County Council his annual abstract of the reports made by the Medical Officers of Health at the close of the year 1898, relative to the several rural and urban districts of North Devon, together with his comments. He says: " The standard reached by the majority of the reports is excellent, and is the outcome of earnest, practical work, conducted on the lines of skilful sanitary training. The vital statistics for North Devon are: Birth-rate, 24; death-rate, 14.5; zymotic death-rate, .9; infant death-rate per 1,000 births, 112.5; notification of infectious disease per 1,000 population, 3.2. The vital statistics for England and Wales are: Birth-rate, 29.4; death-rate, 17.6; zymotic death-rate, 2.22; infant mortality per 1,000 births, 161."

KEYNSHAM.

SEWERAGE SCHEME.—The Keynsham Rural District Council has received a letter from the Bristol Sanitary Authority to the effect that the Sanitary Committee of the Council of Bristol was preparing a scheme to divert the sewage of Bristol from the river Avon, and to discharge it into the Bristol Channel at Avonmouth. The proposed outfall sewer of the Corporation could easily be made available for the use of the inhabitants of all the areas draining into the rivers Avon and Frome, up to and including Bath; and it appeared to the Corporation that drainage by means of such a sewer would be more efficient and less costly than by systems of sewage treatment adopted independently by the several Local Authorities. The Keynsham Rural District Council was invited to discuss terms with the Bristol Corporation for the use of the proposed sewer. The Keynsham Council decided that this invitation should be accepted.

TUBERCULOSIS.—The Keynsham Board of Guardians, at a recent meeting, supported a resolution from the St. Saviour's Union, Surrey, urging the Local Government Board to make an exhaustive inquiry into the causes and treatment of tuberculosis.

MILLBROOK.

MEMORIAL TO THE LATE DR. A. B. CHEVES.—Some friends have placed a beautiful stained-glass window in the side chapel of the parish church as a memorial to the late Dr. Alexander Bruce Cheves.

NEWPORT.

WATER-WORKS.—The expenditure on the Wentwood Water-works up to the present has been £160,000, and it is estimated that the works will not be completed for another two and a half years. The original estimate was £120,000, and the contract was let for £93,000, but the Newport Corporation subsequently undertook the work themselves.

NEWQUAY.

PUBLIC HEALTH.—The report of the Medical Officer of Health indicates that sanitary matters are well attended to at this popular

seaside resort. The death-rate for 1898 was 14.7. A small epidemic
of scarlet fever was promptly and efficiently dealt with, and the
isolation hospital proved of great value in limiting the outbreak. In
the Meteorological Report we notice the equable character of the
temperature; and the fact that the lowest recorded temperature was
32.9° shows the mildness of the climate.

NEWTON ABBOT.

VACCINATION.—At the meeting of the Board of Guardians held on
July 12th, the Vaccination Committee reported that the new Act had
cost the Guardians during the past half-year £168 more than the old
Act in the corresponding half of last year. The public vaccinators
received £192 for 591 cases, as against £45 for 437 cases in the corresponding period of the preceding twelve months; the average cost of
each case being 6s. 6d. against 2s. 1d. of last year. The Chairman of
the Committee stated that the medical officers were dissatisfied with
their fees, and he thought that the Committee would be compelled to
recommend the Guardians to increase the fees from 6s. to 7s. 6d.
per case.

PENARTH.

DIPHTHERIA.—The District Council have decided to convert the
upper portion of the Council offices into a temporary hospital for the
isolation of cases of diphtheria.

PENZANCE.

PUBLIC HEALTH.—Mr. R. D. Boase has been appointed Medical
Officer by the Port Sanitary Authority.

REDRUTH.

WEST CORNWALL WOMEN'S HOSPITAL.—The children's ward recently
added was formally opened by Mr. Passmore Edwards on May 17th.
The ward is to commemorate the Queen's Diamond Jubilee.

SALISBURY.

INFIRMARY.—Dr. Edmund T. Fyson has been appointed Physician.

STRATTON.

PUBLIC HEALTH.—Mr. S. H. Rentzsch has been appointed Medical
Officer of Health for the South District of Stratton Union.

SWANSEA.

GENERAL HOSPITAL.—The annual meeting was held on July 13th.
The report for 1898 showed 1,307 in-patients had been admitted during
t he year. The average length of stay of each was thirty days, and the
daily number of occupied beds was eighty-four. 4,636 out-patients
had been treated. The financial statement showed that the ordinary
ncome amounted to £4,761, being an increase of £272 as compared
with 1897. The ordinary expenditure was £4,906, a decrease of £118
with the previous year. It was decided to spend £1,000 in extending
the heating arrangements of the hospital. On May 18th the Mayor
of Swansea (Mr. R. Martin) opened the Victoria Nurses' Home, erected
in connection with the Swansea General Hospital, at a cost of £1,800,
in commemoration of the Queen's Diamond Jubilee.

THORNBURY.

VACCINATION FEES.—At a meeting of the Thornbury Board of Guardians, held on May 26th, a communication was read from two of the medical officers, asking that the vaccination fees might be on a higher scale than those fixed by the Local Government Board. The majority of the Guardians were of opinion that they had acted fairly to the medical officers by fixing the fess above the minimum laid down by the Act, and as these officers had appealed to the Local Government Board, it was decided that the fees should, therefore, remain the same as suggested by the Local Government Board.

TIVERTON.

PUBLIC HEALTH.—Mr. J. R. R. Pollock has been appointed Medical Officer of Health.

SEWERAGE SCHEME.—A Local Government Board inquiry was recently held at Tiverton into the Town Council's application for sanction to borrow £6,750 for purposes of sewerage and sewage disposal. Mr. J. Siddalls described the scheme of sewerage. The district (West Axe) to be sewered contained a population of about 2,800. As the district was low-lying, it had been found necessary to divide it into two portions.

INFIRMARY.—The recent bazaar held in aid of the Tiverton Infirmary Building Fund, after paying all expenses, realised nearly £600.

TORQUAY.

SEWERAGE SCHEME. — Recently Major General Carey, Chief Engineering Inspector of the Local Government Board, presided at a Conference between Torquay Town Council and St. Marychurch District Council relative to the discharge of additional sewage by St. Marychurch into the Torquay sewers. Mr. F. S. Hex, Town Clerk, acted on behalf of Torquay Town Council, and Mr. Grant Wollen for St. Marychurch. Both Councils were strongly represented. St. Marychurch Council had prepared a new drainage scheme that will carry additional sewage into the Torquay main, and the Torquay Council protested.

TOTNES.

COTTAGE HOSPITAL.—Drs. J. L. Cuppaidge, G. J. Gibson, Mr. J. L. C. Hains, and Dr. K. R. Smith have been re-appointed Medical Officers.

TROWBRIDGE.

PREVENTION OF TUBERCULOSIS.—A small but influential meeting, under the auspices of the West Wiltshire Branch of the National Association for the Prevention of Consumption and other Forms of Tuberculosis was held on July 29th. Captain Chaloner, M.P., presided, and was supported by the Bishop of Salisbury, Dr. E. Markham Skerritt, Dr. F. R. Walters, and others. Dr. Markham Skerritt, alluding to a special report on tuberculosis presented to the Health Committee of the Bristol Town Council by Dr. Davies, said that during the last ten years the seven principal zymotic diseases caused 4,673 deaths in Bristol, while 3,520 were credited to pulmonary consumption alone, and the deaths from tuberculosis as a whole amounted to 4,876 in the same period, or more than those for the zymotic diseases put together. One death in every nine was due to some form of tuberculosis, and one in every twelve to consumption of the lungs. The Bishop of Salisbury also spoke, suggesting the Wiltshire Downs as an admirable site for a sanatorium. On the motion of Mr. C. Awdry, seconded by Sir John Wallington, it was agreed to amalgamate Gloucestershire, Somerset-shire, and Wiltshire, for the purpose of making a joint effort against tuberculosis.

TRURO.

PUBLIC HEALTH.—Mr. C. P. Mathew has been appointed Medical Officer for the Tregony Sanitary District.

TUBERCULOSIS.—At the last meeting of the Cornwall County Council it was resolved :—" That the objects of the Devon and Cornwall Branch of the National Association for the Prevention of Consumption are deserving such support as the County Council can give, and, pending the further consideration of the matter, we recommend the Council to bear the cost of publishing throughout the county information with regard to these diseases and their prevention."

WARMLEY.

PUBLIC HEALTH.—Mr. F. W. S. Stone has been appointed Medical Officer for the Bitton Sanitary Distict.

VACCINATION RETURNS.—At a meeting of the Board of Guardians held on July 18th, it was reported that the number of successful vaccinations for the half-year ending June 30th, 1898, was 106, and for the first six months of 1899 it was nearly double that amount—viz., 208.

WELLS.

PUBLIC HEALTH.—Dr. C. G. MacVicker has been appointed Medical Officer and Public Vaccinator for the Fourth Sanitary District, vice Dr. F. J. Malden resigned.

Congrès International de Médecine Professionelle et de Déontologie Médicale.

In connection with the Exposition Universelle in Paris, it is proposed to hold an International Medical Congress from the 23rd to the 28th of July, 1900. The members alone will have the right to take part in the discussions, and a fee of 15 francs will be required. The Editor of this *Journal* will be glad to receive the names of any persons in this district who may wish to be enrolled.

The College of Physicians of Philadelphia.

The William F. Jenks Memorial Prize of Five Hundred Dollars will be awarded to the author of the best essay on "The Various Manifestations of Lithæmia in Infancy and Childhood, with the Etiology and Treatment." The essay must be sent before January 1st, 1901, addressed to Richard C. Norris, M.D., Chairman of the Committee. Dr. James V. Ingham, the Secretary of the Trustees, will send full information concerning the conditions.

SCRAPS

Clinical Records (28).—This conversation is said to have taken place in the out-patient department of an East-end hospital:—House-Surgeon : " Come, now, tell the officer who did it. Was it your husband ? " Patient : " No, he wouldn't a done it—he 's more like a friend than a husband ! "

Modern Therapeutics.—*The Post-Graduate* says that those who fear that since the times of Addison and Macaulay, the age of fine writing is past, may comfort their anxious souls, by reading the following extract from a medical paper in a recent number of one of our great journals :

" He who has watched for the past decade that jostling horde of barbaric drugs which, emerging from the sulphurous mists of the chemist's laboratory, have swept across the medical horizon in unbroken column, only to disappear in the silent caverns of oblivion, will hardly care to attack the statement that permanency is not the most obtrusive characteristic of prevailing methods of treatment."

Provincial Medical Schools.—Writing on the advantages of provincial medical schools, the *Medical Press and Circular* says : " Among the smaller provincial schools, Bristol, one of the oldest, has always been distinguished for the quality of its teaching. Of late years the status of the school has been materially advanced by its affiliation with the University, and the erection of handsome new buildings. Quite recently another great step has been taken to increase the facilities of students in obtaining clinical material. The Royal Infirmary, dating from ancient times, has lately joined forces with the more modern Bristol Hospital, so far as the training of students is concerned. A large surgical practice is always to be witnessed at both institutions, owing to the position of the town as a large manufacturing centre and seaport."

Examination Papers. —The following are taken from some reported answers :—

The stomach is the most diluted portion of the elementary canal.

Hygiene is all that you can tell about that which is asked.

The doctrine of evolution began with the beginning of life, and grew higher and higher, until it regenerated into monkey. This process was slow—so slow that neither the monkey nor the man knew anything about it.

A germ is a name applied to a particular particle, tiny subbacterial organism, which, when demonstrated, causes disease.

A germ is a tiny insect sometimes found in diseases or organs—that is why diseases are contagious. It is so small that it can be seen only with a telescope. Then it appears like the head of a pin, but it goes floating around into the atmosphere.

The germ theory of diseases is continually floating around in the air, and is very dangerous, especially when the atmosphere is unwholesome.

The Experience of an Army Surgeon.—*The Doctor's Factotum* says that the following verses, dedicated to the editor of the *Medical Standard*, were read by Dr. Jay at the Phi Rho Sigma Interchapter " Smoker," at the Grand Pacific Hotel banquet-hall. Dr. Jay assures the editor that the verses contain more truth than poetry :

" Some of these dysenteric germs
   Into my food had stolen,
And soon were where they love to roam—
   Within a human colon.
They thought my cæcum should be red,
   And this they did inflame ;
They discovered my appendix,
   And they colonised the same.

" They travelled through the sugar
   Down in the crypts of Lieberkühn
Explored the Peyer's patches,
   And more ambitious soon,

They dug in the mucosa,
   Where they licked the phagocytes,
As the cowboys licked the Spaniards
   Upon El Caney heights.

" Then over to my sigmoid
   Some millions emigrated
And everywhere my colon
   They with ulcers decorated.
They dug those ulcers deeper
   Than the muco-fibrous juncture,
And every time I had the cramp
   I thought it was a puncture."

Obstetrics Home and Foreign (6).—"In the Injunctions at the Visitation of Edmunde (Bonner) Bishop of London from September 3d, 1554, to October 8th, 1555, 4to., we read: 'A mydwyfe (of the diocese and jurisdiction of London) shal not use or exercise any witchecrafte, charmes, sorcerye, invocations or praiers, other than suche as be allowable and may stand with the lawes and ordinances of the Catholike Churche.'

"In the Articles to be enquired in the Visitacyon in the fyrst yeare of Queen Elizabeth, 1559, the following occurs: ' Item, whether you knowe anye that doe use charmes, sorcery, enchauntmentes, invocations, circles, witchecraftes, southsayinge, or any lyke craftes or imaginacions invented by the Devyl, and *specially in the tyme of women's travayle*.' It appears from Strype's Annals of the Reformation, i. 537, under 1567, that then midwives took an oath, inter alia, not to ' suffer any other bodies child to be set, brought, or laid before any woman delivered of child, in the place of her natural child, so far forth as I can know and understand. Also I will not use any kind of sorcery or incantation in the time of the travail of any woman.'"—Brand's *Popular Antiquities*, ed. Bohn, 1849, vol ii., p. 69.

"The *Yi* of India, the *Dye* of Syria, the herb-knowing hag of Mexico, and the midwife of the Bible are very much the same in their habits, their qualifications, and their knowledge. It is the same habitual old woman who figures in all countries and at all times, and with whose peculiar qualifications we are quite familiar. In cases where the midwife is at a loss, the aid of the medicine man is sought. The Baschkirs rely upon their 'devil-seer,' who discovers the presence of the evil spirit and drives him away if rewarded by the present of a sum of money or a fat sheep. Among others a priest is called who hastily mumbles a few verses of the Koran, spits into the patient's face, and leaves the rest to nature."—Engelmann's *Labor Among Primitive Peoples*, 1882, p. 131.

Medical Philology (XXXI.).—The *Promptorium* gives " Dyndelyñ, *Tinnio*," and the *Catholicon Anglicum* "to Dindylle. *Condolere*" or " *Errobare*."

In his note, Mr. Way points out that these are somewhat different senses, the *Catholicon* equivalent signifying " suffering acutely." He adds: " Brockett gives to dinnel, or dindle, to be affected with a pricking pain, such as arises from a blow, or is felt by exposure to the fire after frost. In the Craven dialect to dinnle has a similar signification. Langham, in the Garden of Health, 1579, recommends the juice of feverfew as a remedy for the 'eares ache, and dindling.' Dutch, tintelen, to tingle."

Mr. Herrtage in his *Catholicon* note says: " In Jamieson we find ' To dinle, dynle. (1) To tremble. (2) To make a great noise. (3) To thrill; to tingle.' ' Dinle, *s*. (1) Vibration. (2) A slight and temporary sensation of pain, similar to that caused by a stroke on the elbow.' Cotgrave gives '*Tintillant*. Tinging; ringing; tingling, *Tintoner*. To ting or towle often; to glow, tingle, dingle.' ' Hir unfortunat husband had no sooner notice given him upon his returne of these sorrowfull newes than his fingers began to nibble . . . his ears to *dindle*, his head to dozell, insomuch as his heart being scared with gelousie . . . he became as mad as a March hare.'—Stanihurst, Descrip. of Ireland in Holinshed's Chronicles (1576), vol. vi. p. 32, § 2.

> ' The birnand towris doun rollis with ane rusche,
> Quhil all the heuynnys *dynlit* with the dusche.'
>   Gawin Douglas, *Eneados*, Bk. ix. p. 296, l. 35."

The *New English Dictionary* says that the derivation of the word is obscure, and that it is probably onomatopoeic. It will be seen from the references to Jamieson that it is well known as a Scottish word. Some of the quotations given above show that in some instances it had a special medical significance.

In June, 1894, I quoted from a note in Mr.·Way's edition of the *Promptorium* a prescription containing feverfew, which Langham recommends as a remedy for the dindling. Feverfew has been for ages the popular name of *Pyrethrum Parthenium*, which was also called *Matricaria* because, as Turner says, "The new writers hold . . . that feverfew is better for weomen." (*Herbal*, ii. 796, quoted by the *New English Dictionary*.)

The Bristol
Medico-Chirurgical Journal.

DECEMBER, 1899.

MEDICAL BRISTOL IN THE EIGHTEENTH CENTURY.

The Presidential Address, delivered on October 11th, 1899, at the Opening of the Twenty-sixth Session of the Bristol Medico-Chirurgical Society.

BY

W. H. HARSANT, F.R.C.S. Eng.,

Surgeon to the Bristol Royal Infirmary.

ALTHOUGH I have been a member of this Society for twenty-three years, and during that time have been actively engaged in the practice of surgery, I am conscious that such a period is not long enough to justify me in inflicting upon you anything in the nature of reminiscences, or of comparisons between the state of our knowledge at the commencement of my career and our more enlightened condition at the present time.

I cannot, like some of my predecessors in this chair, go back to the pre-anæsthetic period and draw attention to the wonderful advancement made in surgery since that time, and although I might tell much of the pre-antiseptic days and recall many of the glorious improvements which have been effected by the introduction of the antiseptic and aseptic treatment of wounds, it seems to me that such a subject is somewhat

21

hackneyed; it has been done so many times before by abler
hands than mine, that I prefer to address you to-night in a
lighter vein, and if possible to interest you for a short time in
some of the doings and sayings of our predecessors who fretted
their time upon the stage in Bristol before any of us now
present had arrived upon the scene.

I have lately had the opportunity of looking through some
old manuscript volumes of "Biographical Memoirs," written
by Richard Smith, a surgeon who lived in Bristol at the
beginning of the present century, and I thought that inasmuch
as these volumes, fifteen in number, were never published, and
are inaccessible to many of the members of this Society, some
account of their contents might be of interest. I therefore
purpose to dive into their pages and to extract some of the
interesting gossip which they contain about the medical profession in Bristol during the latter half of the eighteenth
century. And first I would say a few words about the
writer of the volumes. He says little about himself. Although
he took infinite pains to gather particulars of his contemporaries
and predecessors, we are left to other sources to find out what
we know concerning the author.

He was the son of a former Richard Smith, surgeon to the
Infirmary from 1774 to 1791. He himself was surgeon to that
institution from 1796 to 1843, a period of no less than forty-
seven years, so that father and son continued in office over an
almost uninterrupted period of seventy years.

The elder Richard Smith lived at first in Charlotte Street
at the corner of Queen Square; he afterwards moved to a
house in College Green near St. Augustine's Church, on the
site of the present Royal Hotel, where he practised until he
died in 1796. He seems to have been a man of great ability
and industry, and bequeathed to his son a museum containing
nearly a thousand specimens, which were afterwards presented
by the son to the Infirmary, forming the nucleus of what is now
called Richard Smith's Museum.

The younger Richard Smith resembled his father in many
respects, especially in his love of collecting specimens. He
was particularly partial to monstrosities and freaks, and such

objects as the skeleton of a murderer or the enormous penis of a negro were to him veritable gems, to be obtained and preserved at all costs.

Mr. Augustin Prichard in his *Reminiscences* describes Richard Smith as he remembered him. He was then senior surgeon to the Infirmary, and very old and thoroughly incapable; so much so, that when he died a law limiting the tenure of office to twenty years was passed. He was universally known as "Dick Smith," and, wrapped in a rough camlet cloak, used to drive about in a gig, with a white dog running underneath. He was a Freemason, very high up in the craft, and was a *beau idéal* chairman at the jovial suppers the brethren were in the habit of giving.

He commenced practice in 1795, and lived at first in 17 College Street, in a house having a back entrance in Lamb Street. In 1803 he went to live at 7 College Green, where he remained until he died in 1843. His death took place very suddenly while he was sitting in a chair in the committee-room of the Philosophical Institution. He was one of the original members of the Medical Reading Society, founded in 1804, which still exists in a flourishing state, and is now approaching its centenary.

He seems to have taken a morbid delight in adding to his museum any specimens relating to murder trials, and no effort was spared on his part to bring the unfortunate prisoner safely to the gallows, and afterwards to secure the body for dissection and the skeleton for the museum. Full particulars of several such trials have been preserved by him in manuscript volumes, which contain many curious details and illustrate in a ghastly manner the craze which then existed for capital punishment.

Among his collection is the articulated skeleton of John Horwood, a man who was hanged in 1821 at the gaol on the Cut for the murder of his sweetheart. Many of my hearers who have been students at the Infirmary are familiar with the old volume in the Museum, bound in human skin, so carefully preserved by Richard Smith, and containing such a detailed account of the trial and execution of this man.

The body of the murderer having been ordered, as a part of the sentence, to be given over to the surgeons of the Infirmary for dissection, Richard Smith went himself in a coach to the gaol and brought away the body to the Infirmary, wrapped up in an old cloak.   It was actually placed on the table in the operation room and allowed to remain there for four days, while Richard Smith gave popular anatomical demonstrations to any citizens of Bristol who chose to attend.   No less than eighty persons were attracted on the first day alone to this gruesome spectacle, and on the succeeding days there were also very full audiences, while finally the students of the house were allowed to finish the dissection of the body in the dissecting-room which then adjoined the dead-house.   The skeleton was afterwards articulated and now hangs in the Infirmary museum, while the skin underwent a process of tanning and now serves as a binding for the volume which contains a record of the proceedings.

This handing of the bodies of murderers to the surgeons of the Infirmary for dissection seems to have been a long-established custom in Bristol, for in 1741, when Captain Goodere was executed for the murder of his brother on the high seas, his body was removed to the Infirmary, where it was placed in the operation room, and, in the presence of as many spectators as the room would hold, a surgeon stuck a scalpel into the breast.   In this state it was exposed to the popular gaze until the evening, and then given over to the friends for burial.

Another instance of the same kind occurred in 1802, when two young women, named Charlotte Bobbett and Maria Davis, were hanged for infanticide.   Their bodies were given over to the surgeons of the Infirmary for dissection, and after execution at St. Michael's Hill gallows they were conveyed to the Infirmary in an open cart, followed by an immense mob. The surgeons were in attendance to receive them, and after the bodies had been stripped and laid out on the table of the committee room a crucial incision was made in the chest of each by Mr. Godfrey Lowe, the senior surgeon, in the presence of as many of the rabble as were able to crush into the room.

On the following day, at the request of the Mayor and Aldermen, who were present, the brain of one of the girls was dissected and lectured on by Richard Smith, then the junior surgeon. The articulated skeletons of these young women now hang in the Infirmary museum, and particulars of the trial are fully recorded in a separate manuscript volume.

CLASSES OF PRACTITIONERS.

The members of the profession last century were divided into four classes; viz., physicians, surgeons, barber-surgeons, and apothecaries. In 1754 there were in Bristol 5 physicians, 19 surgeons, 13 barber-surgeons, and 29 apothecaries, making a total of 66. In 1793 there were no more barber-surgeons, but the number of apothecaries had risen from 29 to 35, and the surgeons from 19 to 20, while the number of physicians seems to have remained about the same as before.

PHYSICIANS.

The physicians held their heads very high. They were some of the best educated men of that day. They all had a good knowledge of the classics, and many of them went to foreign universities for a part of their professional training. They were very particular in their dress and deportment, and were easily to be distinguished from the common herd. Thus of Dr. Wm. Logan, one of the first physicians to the Infirmary, we read: "He was a strict observer of professional costume, and never stirred abroad or was visible at home, unless in full dress, that is to say, his head covered by the immense flowing wig of George II.'s time, a red roquelaire hanging from his shoulders to his heels, his wrist graced by a gold-headed cane, and his side furnished with a long French rapier."

Of Dr. Ludlow, physician to the Infirmary in 1774, we read: "He was distinguished from the common mass by an imposing exterior. He moved in a measured step and affected a meditative abstraction of countenance, with a pomposity of diction and manner which could not but keep the vulgar at a respectable distance. His peruke alone was enough in itself to command respect, for it was ornamented with regular and formidable tiers of curls to the number of one hundred and ten, and was known as 'The Royal George,' in allusion to the great line-of-battle ship, then the pride of the navy."

So also of Dr. John Wright, physician in 1771, we read: "His practice was extensive and laborious, so that latterly he was obliged to keep a horse, which was rather unusual for an M.D. in his day. An observer told Richard Smith that he was passing Stoke's Croft one very wet day when Dr. Wright turned the corner; he had on a large white dishevelled wig, over which hung a huge flapped Quaker's hat. With one hand he held up an umbrella, and with the other the bridle of a little pony upon which he rode; from his shoulders his red roquelaire was spread over the hind quarters of the animal, reaching almost to the ground, and forming altogether a caricature so droll that everybody turned round to look at him."

It was customary for the surgeons of the Infirmary also to wear a wig and the red cloak known as the roquelaire, also to carry a gold-headed cane. This fashion prevailed for about forty years after the foundation of the charity in 1735; but when Mr. Noble was elected in 1776, he refused to comply with the custom, in consequence of which the other surgeons agreed to wear out the cloaks in their possession and then to allow the custom to drop. Few of the faculty of the city wore them when Richard Smith first remembered the house in 1787, but Dr. Plomer wore his until 1795, and Dr. Wright until 1798.

Dr. Middleton, who was elected to the Infirmary in 1737, was the first physician who kept his carriage in Bristol. It was a great lumbering thing without springs, with two small glasses in the doors. The horses never went beyond a foot pace, in fact it was a sort of genteel waggon.

Physicians were called in chiefly when the sick person was *in extremis;* in fact, as they then complained, "they came only to administer musk and to close the eyes of the patient!" The practice of giving musk began to decline about the year 1790. Richard Smith could remember when it might be smelled in the street as you passed the house of a dying person, as very few who could afford to pay for it were allowed to depart without having it administered.

When Dr. John Paul was physician to the Infirmary, from 1772 to 1775, the surgeons of the day called him "their good friend Sangrado," since the minute he was in attendance one of them was sent for to make use of his lancet. Mr. Metford used to say that he had bled thirty patients a day at the Infirmary by Dr. Paul's order, and that he was occasionally in the admission-room when Dr. Paul was taking in, and that the first question he asked of every male patient was, "Are you a Bristol man?" If the reply was in the affirmative, he regularly wrote in his book "V. S. ad ℥xx" by way of beginning. Mr. Metford requested to know why, without further enquiry into their complaints, he ordered them to lose so much blood. "Because, sir," said Dr. Paul, "if he is a Bristol man, I know that he sits of an evening smoking tobacco and drinking your abominable fat ale; the first thing to be done therefore is to let some of that run out, and then we shall see what else is the matter."

SURGEONS.

The surgeons seem to have been largely occupied in bleeding patients at the request of the physicians, but they performed all the operations that were done at that day, the chie of which was to cut for the stone. In an old newspaper, called the *Bristol Weekly Intelligencer*, we find the following paragraphs:—

1742. "Last week two boys were cut for the stone by Mr. Thornhill, both of which are in a fair way of recovery."

May, 1750. "Within these few weeks past four boys have been cut for the stone in the Bristol Infirmary by Mr. Thornhill, and are all recovered. We hear he has more patients preparing for the same operation."

And in January, 1751. "Last week the operation for the double hare-lip was performed at the Bristol Infirmary. At the same charity, a man, aged 70, and two boys were cut for the stone, all which have had the most favourable symptoms and are in a fair way of recovery."

We see that surgeons understood the art of advertising even in those days, and it is not left to these degenerate times to discover a method of bringing an operator's name before the admiring gaze of the public.

The Wm. Thornhill alluded to above was one of the original surgeons of the Infirmary. Richard Smith describes him as a man of much genius and ability, but wanting in attention and assiduity—in fact, he was so remiss in his attendance that he more than once fell under the censure of the house visitors, and finally an incident occurred which I will relate, as it is told by Richard Smith, inasmuch as it exemplifies the way they then looked upon questions of payment in the matter of hospitals.

In 1754 a boy had been wounded in the leg by a gentleman who was shooting, and was brought as a patient to the Infirmary, where he was under the care of Mr. Thornhill, who seems to have neglected to see him. The gentleman, being very anxious respecting the lad, called at Thornhill's house, begged that he would see the boy, and by way of quickening his attention gave him a fee, which the surgeon put in his pocket. This coming to the ear of the house visitors, they considered it their duty to notice it in an official manner, first as an instance of dereliction of duty, and next as militating against one of the first and fundamental rules of the charity whose great feature is gratuitous assistance. Mr. Thornhill's friends advised an immediate resignation in order to prevent the intended report of the transaction, but he clung to the office, promised and retracted, heaping delay upon delay, in the hope that he might soften his accusers; but they were inflexible. At last he gave notice that he would resign in eight months. While this proposition was before the house visitors the secret leaked out, the city was soon in motion, others canvassed for the expected vacancy, and at last the nuisance became so intolerable that the subscribers proceeded to an election, and forced him from his seat in November, 1754. Mr. Thornhill nevertheless refused to consider that his functions were at an end, and the subscribers saw with astonishment six surgeons jostling each other and quarrelling about the proprietorship of the unfortunate patients. The fact was, Thornhill was determined not to be turned out, and therefore held the situation until June 2nd, 1755, the time which he had chalked out for himself; then he bade good-bye to the charity, the committee of which had the politeness afterwards to depute Dr. Bonython and Mr. Page to wait on him with "the thanks of their meeting for the care he had taken of the house from the beginning, and for his many services to it." When in practice he resided for some time in a large corner house, turning from the end of College Green to St. Augustine's Back, and afterwards in a house next St. Werburgh's Church, now the site of the Commercial Rooms. He was a handsome, well-grown man, and took care to show his person to advantage by constantly wearing an entire suit of black velvet and an elegant steel-handled rapier. He was well read, and polished in his manner. He kept a well-appointed equipage, an almost unprecedented luxury in those days, and lived altogether in a much better style than any surgeon in Bristol for many years after him or before him.

Richard Smith gives us a description of another surgeon to the Infirmary, Mr. John Townsend, who held office for twenty-five years from 1755 to 1780. His entire devotion to business procured him so much practice that in 1778 he set up his carriage, a matter of some consequence in those days, there having been only two surgeons before him who did so; viz., his master, Mr. Thornhill, and Mr. Peter Wells. He entered into contract with one Thomas Jones, who agreed to find him a day coachman and a night coachman, a vehicle and a pair of horses, for £100 per annum—a price which may well make us envious in these days, although we must remember that £100 then was probably equal to double that sum now. His drivers had no sinecure places, being in use almost perpetually. He resided in Broad Street, having a side door inside a house passage; this was then considered a great desideratum, as all venereal patients were in the habit of sneaking into a surgery after dusk, privately, and the greatest care was taken to conceal them. Mr. Townsend's surgery was in itself calculated to strike terror into all beholders. It was fitted up with glass cases, and there were exhibited in great display an iron screw ambé, for the reduction of dislocated shoulders; all the endless

"apparatus major" for cutting for the stone, with an endless
variety of blunt gorgets and dilating forceps, old actual cauteries,
and in fact all the farriery of Scultetus, Hildanus, and Am-
broise Paré.   One might easily have fancied oneself in the
torture room of a Spanish Inquisition, and surrounded with
the instruments of "The Question."   Mr. Townsend prided
himself not a little upon the possession and display of these
chirurgical treasures, for he considered, and it was so then to
a certain extent, that the minds of the vulgar measured by
them the abilities of the possessor.   Chatterton, whom nothing
of this sort escaped, used to come there occasionally to see
Richard Smith, who was indentured to Mr. Townsend, and
when he afterwards introduced them both into a satire, speaks
of Townsend as—

> "A thing of flatulence and noise,
> Whose surgery's nothing but a heap of toys."

Nothing could be more uncouth than Townsend's manner
towards his patients, public and private, for he made no
distinction.   He overawed them all by his taciturnity and the
sternness of his brow.   In his person and appearance he greatly
resembled Dr. Johnson.   His costume never varied; he wore a
large unpowdered wig, with a cocked hat, an entire suit of
dark snuff-coloured cloth, worsted stockings, square-topped
shoes, and small silver knee and shoe buckles; his waistcoat
had two large flaps hanging half-way down his thighs, and in
his coat he had always four pockets, generally filled with
a tow bag and instrument cases.   He was so great an
economist of time that he had fitted up in the front of
his carriage a spreading board with tin cases for ointments,
a spatula, and a drawer for white and brown tow.   He could
be seen, as he rode along, engaged in pulling and spreading of
pledgets.

He was once walking down Broad Street during an illu-
mination, and observed a boy breaking every window which
had not a light.   He asked him how he dared to injure people's
property in that way.   "Oh," said the boy, "all for the good of
trade; I am a glazier!"   "All for the good of trade is it?"

said Townsend, lifting up his cane and breaking the boy's head: "there then, you rascal, get that mended for the good of my trade; I am a surgeon."

BARBER-SURGEONS.

It is well known that at one time surgeons were united with barbers, and belonged to the United Worshipful Society of Barber Surgeons. This Society had for its Hall in Bristol, during last century, a large room in the West India Coffee House, in the Market Place, near the Exchange. This room was known as "The Surgeons' Hall," and it was here that the first meeting of the governors of the Infirmary was held, in 1737, to elect their first Faculty. In the year 1745 the surgeons were emancipated from the barbers, and were obliged to leave all their joint stock in the hands of the latter, and this Hall among the rest.

Mr. Thornhill served his time to a barber-surgeon, known as "Old Rosewell," who, to the day of his death, had at his door in All Saints' Lane the insignia of his trade; viz., a staff, a porringer, and a red garter. This mode of education was then so universal and regular, that in a controversy which took place in 1754 it was asserted as a recommendation to Mr. James Ford "that he was regularly educated in this city in a barber's shop."

When being bled, a patient would grasp a staff or pole, which the barber-surgeon always kept handy. To this staff was tied the tape used in bandaging the patient's arm. When not in use, the pole was hung outside as a sign of the trade followed within. Later, the identical pole used by the customers was not exhibited as a sign, but, instead, a painted pole was placed at the doorway. At first barber-surgeons' poles were painted red and white, while those of mere barbers were required to be white and blue. This law was enforced in England up to 1729.

The newspapers of the day designate Mr. Rosewell as "an eminent surgeon, with a fair character." Thornhill learned here, after the custom of the day, to shave, bleed, and draw teeth; his master being so celebrated that on a Sunday morning there were swarms of persons to be bled, for which each paid from sixpence to a shilling.

An advertisement in *Felix Farley's Journal* for March 9th, 1754, reads: " Henry Haines, barber, Redcliff Pit, shaves each person for two pence, cuts hair for three half-pence, and bleeds for sixpence. All customers who are bled he treats with two quarts of good ale, and those whom he shaves or cuts their hair with a pint each."

The last remnant of barber-surgery dropped with " Old Parsley," who lived next door to the Guildhall in Broad Street as late as the year 1807. This man dressed more wigs, drew more teeth, and spilled more blood than any man in Bristol. At his window and by the side of his door hung immense double strings of teeth. He regularly brought his patients to the door, either for the sake of a good light or for notoriety.

APOTHECARIES.

Most of the general practice of the city was then done by the apothecaries, who were a most important body of men. They dispensed their own medicines, and many of them, in addition, kept open shops for the sale of drugs. At the foundation of the Infirmary a resident apothecary was appointed to do the dispensing and to live on the premises, and inasmuch as he was the only resident officer he must have acted in addition as a kind of house surgeon. He was an unmarried man, and he had the magnificent salary of £30 per annum; but it seems to have been an appointment much sought after, and it evidently was a position of considerable importance. At many of the large London hospitals, the office of apothecary continued until quite recently, and even in my student days at Guy's Hospital Mr. James Stocker filled this office, the duties of which were very varied and dignified.

LECTURES.

There was no medical school in Bristol until 1833, but lectures on various subjects, such as Anatomy, Physiology, and Surgery, were given from time to time by members of the Infirmary staff and others, and full particulars of these courses of lectures may be found in Mr. John Latimer's *Annals*, chiefly drawn from Richard Smith's " Memoirs."

Mr. Frank Bowles gave anatomical instruction to students of the Infirmary gratuitously. This was before he became surgeon to the institution, and the work was carried on under great difficulties. The principal difficulty then, as now, was to obtain subjects for dissection. The students (Richard Smith among the foremost) played the part of resurrection men, and procured subjects in succession. In doing this they more than once got themselves into awkward scrapes, and one night Robert Lax and Richard Smith were actually shot at while engaged in abstracting a body from the Infirmary burial ground in Johnny Ball Lane.

They used to substitute old sacks filled with rubbish for the contents of the coffins, which were then buried in due form. They procured a key of the dead-house, and provided themselves with turn-screws, hammers, wrenching-irons, and everything likely to be wanted. The nurses and undertakers were allowed to take the ordinary course of laying out the subject and securing the coffin. Funerals were ordered generally for five o'clock, and during the hour or two preceding that time they used to steal into the dead-house, remove any of the corpse they wanted, even the whole body at times, and then made all fast and in the same order as before. Thus no suspicion was excited and the danger of an examination of the coffin rendered less probable. So eagerly was this pursued that there was scarcely a subject, unless immediately removed by the friends, which did not afford the students a demonstration, either of brain, or thorax, or abdomen, or the anatomy of an operation. In order to keep their secret of having a false key, they borrowed the real one occasionally from the old woman who kept the gate, and silenced her with a shilling now and then. Mr. Bowles was always their demonstrator; but as he was not a surgeon of the house, and as, moreover, there existed at that time a jealousy of him, it was necessary to smuggle him privately into the dead-house. This miserable place, which was in fact a mere coal-hole, lighted by a foot-square iron grating, was under ground, and had an opening into Lower

Maudlin Street. There the students spent hours in the ardent pursuit of anatomical knowledge, for there happened at that time to be a set of students who lost few opportunities for instruction.

In 1769 a complaint was made against the whole body of students at the Infirmary for removing the corpse from a coffin and substituting for burial a quantity of sand and wood. Being summoned to attend the Committee, and proving refractory, they were allowed a week to consider of it, being informed that if in that time due concessions were not made, a general Board would be summoned to settle the affair. The young gentlemen had to cry *peccavimus*, and an order was made that the key of the dead-house should always be in the custody of the apothecary.

One of the curious stories told by Richard Smith on this subject is the following :—

About the year 1750 a notorious vagabond, called Long Jack, having destroyed himself, a verdict of *felo-de-se* was pronounced against him. He was, in consequence, buried at the cross-roads leading to Kingswood. Mr. Abraham Ludlow formed with Mr. Page a scheme for the removal of the body, and Richard Smith accompanied them. A servant was behind leading a horse, with the resurrection implements. The subject was safely removed, and when the hole was filled up, the object of the expedition was fastened in a sack and laid across the horse. By this time, however, it was so late that the great portal of Castle Gate was closed, and no one could come through without leave of the porter.

This induced them to attempt driving the horse through the side avenue, intended only for foot passengers. In effecting this the body fell to the ground, and the porter, hearing a noise, came with his lantern, and was not a little alarmed to see the legs of a man at the mouth of the sack. He was, however, persuaded to hold his tongue, and the cavalcade reached Mr. Ludlow's house in safety. The body was placed upon a table in the back parlour, and the parties retired to rest themselves after their labours. But they had forgotten to lock the door, and in the morning when the servant girl opened the window she perceived the body of Long Jack, whom she very well knew.   Horror-struck at the frightful appearance of a miserable-looking wretch with his throat cut, she ran screaming into the street, and Mr. Ludlow, awakened by the noise, had but just time to prevent the intrusion of the bystanders into his house.   A buzz soon spread through the parish, and by evening it was so generally known, that some alarm was excited by the threats of some fellows to come in to know the truth. Mr. Ludlow, in consequence, resolved on replacing the body with all possible expedition.   In the night, therefore, they contrived to deposit Long Jack at the place from whence they had carried him away.   It was fortunate for them that they did so, for the next day a mob of fellows went to the spot to see if he were actually there or not, and vowed vengeance against all concerned in his removal in case they should not find him.   A few strokes of the pickaxe having removed all their doubts as to his being there, they soon dispersed, and except an occasional joke from his professional brethren, Mr. Ludlow heard no more of the matter.

The following anecdote was related to Richard Smith by Mr. Godfrey Lowe.   It occurred in 1761 :—

A Kingswood lad died in the Infirmary of fractured skull, and Mr. Castleman, who was surgeon to the institution, had secured the specimen before the body was delivered in a coffin to the friends for interment.   In the middle of the night there was a violent knocking at the door of the Infirmary, and the apothecary, who was known by no other name than " Neddy Bridges," thrusting his head and night-cap out of window, half asleep, yawned out, " What d'ye want ? "   " Want ! " said a hoarse rough voice, " want ! damn thee ! why I da want my zun's head, and I 'll ha' en too, or else I 'll ha' thine ! "   Bridges endeavoured in vain to pacify him, and make him come on the morrow, but the fellow became outrageous, and continued to vociferate, " Gee I my zun's head ; gee I my zun's head, or else I 'll zend a stwoan drough thine and pull the Furmery about thy ears ! "   Bridges, finding the matter becoming serious, was obliged to tell him that he must speak to Mr. Castleman, who lived hard by in Duke Street.   Away went the man, and began to thunder away at that gentleman's, who, speedily throwing up the window, enquired, "Who's there?" "Who's there? Why, I be here!" "Well, who are you?" "Who be I? What! dostn't know me? Why, I be Jack's vather, and thee'st got his head; and if thee dostn't ge'en to me I'll ha' thine, and there's zomeut for year nest;" and with that he hurls a great stick up and knocks to pieces a pane of glass. Castleman, as he well might, feeling very much alarmed, told the man that it was at the Infirmary, and if he would step there he would come to him and get it. "Oh!" said the fellow, "thick's the geam, is it? Measter Bridges zends I to thee, and thee zends I to he! I'll tell thee what, if thee dostn't gee I my zun's head in vive minutes, I'll smash every window thee'st got!" Seeing that all manœuvring was useless, Mr. Castleman went to his surgery, and wrapping the cranium in a towel, with no very pleasant feelings unbolted the street door, and delivered it into the hands of the collier, who had on the instant thrust himself into the hall. The fellow, that he might not be deceived, deliberately unfolded the cloth, and having exposed the countenance, said, "Aye, aye, thick's Jack, and till's well vor thee that thee'st gid en to me, for if thee hadsn't, we'd a come and had thy house down to-morrow." Mr. Castleman, half-naked, shivering with the cold, and extremely anxious to get his guest outside the door, civilly wished him a good-night. "Damn thy good-night!" said the collier: "what bizness had'st thee to cut poor Jack's head off? I got a despurt good mind now to gee thee a dowse in the chops, and then thee't know better another time;" at the same moment he grinned horribly a ghastly smile, and shook a tremendous fist at him. Mr. Castleman was too prudent to come between such a dragon and his wrath, and with as much composure as he could muster, begged his excuse for the trouble he had given him, and hoped that they should part friends. "Vrend, indeed!" said the fellow, "damn sitch a vrend as thee, or any o' the like o' thee!" and then, clapping the bundle with his "zun's head" under his arm, he stalked into the court, and went off grumbling to Kingswood, leaving Mr. Castleman to receive the congratulations of his wife, who was trembling at the head of the stairs, at his being delivered from so troublesome a customer.

Another curious story about the Infirmary, related by Richard Smith, is the following :—

One of the Infirmary surgeons, named Mr. John Ford, was in the habit of lounging in a poulterer's shop where there was a remarkably pretty girl. A passer-by remarked " how improper it was for a man of his rank and years to be dangling after a girl." " Pooh ! " said another, " that is not his errand ; why he goes there about the used poultices, they are sold to the poulterers by the Infirmary." This getting about, no one would buy poultry, and the shop was almost ruined. At length the matter was carried to such a height that the following affidavit appeared in the public newspapers (see *Pine's Gazette*, January, 1773) :—

" Whereas it hath been currently reported in and about the city that the poulterers residing here have frequently purchased or received from the Infirmary divers quantities of poultices there made use of, for the purpose of feeding their poultry ; whereby a great number of dealers and others have been led to think it hath been their general practice, and have declined further dealings with them. We, whose names are hereunder written, in justice to ourselves and families, and to clear as much as lies in our power our character and reputation from such a foul and infamous charge, think it proper to declare that we nor either of us, did ever, by ourselves servants or others, purchase or receive from the Infirmary, or any other place whatever, any poultice or other unwholesome thing, for the purpose of feeding or fattening our poultry. But it had been and shall continue to be our practice to feed them with the very best barley, barley-meal and other wholesome corn food, and with milk and clean water ; and we hereby call on the author of this report and the propagators thereof to prove the contrary, by themselves or any other person.

Sworn at the city of Bristol,	Signed
the 12th day of Jan., 1773,	CHRISTOPHER KEMPSTER,
before me	WILLIAM PRITCHARD,
NATHANIEL FRY,	+ The Mark of
Mayor.	MARTHA JONES."

Time would fail me to quote at any considerable length from the entertaining reminiscences and stories recorded by Richard Smith in these volumes. They bring vividly before us the

22

everyday life of members of our profession in Bristol in the
last century. They have been recorded with extraordinary
diligence, and the mere labour of writing and arranging the
memoirs must have been no light matter. It is to be regretted
that they are not more accessible to members of this Society :
perhaps some day we may be able to have copies made for the
Bristol Medical Library; but at present they are jealously
guarded by the Committee of the Infirmary, who were kind
enough, however, to consent to my application to be allowed
to read them and make extracts from them.

THE VARIETIES OF UTERINE NEOPLASMS
AND THEIR RELATIVE FREQUENCY.

BY

W. ROGER WILLIAMS, F.R.C.S. Eng.

UTERINE tumours are of great interest to the surgeon and
pathologist, as well for the frequency of their occurrence as
for the important surgical procedures now often undertaken
for their removal. It was very different half a century ago,
when but little was known of the pathology of these tumours,
and their surgical treatment was limited to the occasional
removal of specimens that projected into the vagina.

In this essay, I propose briefly to set forth some results of a
statistical investigation of uterine neoplasms; and then to make
passing reference to the bearing of the facts thus revealed on
the question of pathogenesis.

The great frequency of uterine tumours is shown by the
following data :—

Of 13,824 patients of both sexes, with primary neoplasms,
consecutively under treatment at four large London hospitals,
I have ascertained that 2,649 were of uterine origin, or 19.2

per cent.; while next in order of frequency came the
mammæ with 17.5 per cent.; then the skin with 9.4 per cent.;
and far removed from the last, the stomach with only 2.6
per cent.

Similarly of 13,971 neoplasms analysed by Gurlt, the
patients being under treatment at the chief Vienna hospitals,
4,115 originated from the uterus, or 29 per cent.; next in order
came the skin with 12 per cent., the mammæ with 11 per cent.,
and the stomach with 8 per cent.

With regard to the sex of the patients in my list, 9,227 were
females: in 28.7 per cent. of these women the uterus was the
organ affected; the mammæ in 26 per cent., the ovaries in 8.7
per cent., and the stomach in only 1.4 per cent.

In striking contrast with the foregoing, I find that of 4,597
neoplasms in males only 25, or .5 per cent. were of the mammæ.

Of my 13,824 neoplasms, 7,297 were cancers: of the latter
4,628 occurred in persons of the female sex, the uterus being
the seat of origin in 1,571, or in 34 per cent., the mammæ in
40.3 per cent., the skin in 4.1 per cent., and the stomach in
2·8 per cent.

Of Gurlt's 13,971 neoplasms, 9,898 were cancers: 7,020 of
the latter occurred in persons of the female sex, the uterus
being affected in 3,449, or in 49 per cent., the mammæ in 20
per cent., and the stomach in 7 per cent.

For comparison with the above clinical data, I append some
of the results deducible from the chief mortality statistics.

From the Registrar-General's analysis of the cancer mortality of England and Wales for the year 1897, I find that
among females the uterus, etc., was the seat of the disease in
23.5 per cent., the mammæ in 15.5 per cent., the stomach in
13.3 per cent., and the liver in 13.2 per cent.: similar returns
have been published for the years 1888 and 1868; they show
the following percentages: uterus 34.7, mammæ 21.2, and
stomach 10.9.

From the reports of the Registrar for Ireland, for the years
1887–89, it appears that among women the stomach was the
part affected in 22.4 per cent., mammæ in 21.5 per cent., and
uterus in 14.1 per cent.

The Frankfort-on-Main mortality returns for the 30 years, 1860–89, show that the uterus was the seat of the disease in 27.5 per cent. of the female cancer mortality, the stomach in 18.5 per cent., and the mammæ in 11.3 per cent.

It will be gathered from the foregoing that these mortality statistics differ from the clinical data, chiefly in that they indicate greater frequency of the disease in the stomach, etc.

Schroeder's analysis of 19,666 cases of cancer in women shows that 33.3 per cent. were uterine; and of 8,746 similar cases tabulated by Simpson, 34.3 per cent. were of the uterus.

Of the 9,227 females with neoplasms in my list, in 2,649 (28.7 per cent.) the uterus was the part affected. In these cases the relative frequency of the occurrence of the different varieties of uterine tumour is shown by the subjoined table:

ANALYSIS OF 2,649 CONSECUTIVE CASES OF UTERINE NEOPLASMS.

Cancer	1,571
Sarcoma	2
Myoma	883
Polypus (non-myomatous) ...	191
Cystoma	2
Total	2,649

Of Gurlt's 4,115 uterine neoplasms, 3,449 were cancers, 8 sarcomas, 481 myomas, 175 polypoid pseudoplasms, and 2 were papillomas.

Throughout the organism in general, malignant neoplasms occur, in females, with greater relative frequency than non-malignant ones, the ratio being—according to my estimate— 55 per cent. of the former to 45 per cent. of the latter. In the uterus the proportionate numbers are 59.38 per cent. of the former to 40.62 per cent. of the latter.

In order to show the relative frequency of the chief uterine neoplastic manifestations in comparison with those of the female organism in general, and with those of the female mammæ, ovaries, skin and stomach (in females), I have compiled the subjoined table:—

TABLE SHOWING THE RELATIVE FREQUENCY OF FEMALE
NEOPLASMS IN GENERAL, AS COMPARED WITH UTERINE,
MAMMARY, CUTANEOUS, GASTRIC, AND OVARIAN NEOPLASMS.

KIND OF NEOPLASM.	Female Neoplasms in General per cent.	Uterine Neoplasms per cent.	Female Breast Neoplasms per cent.	Skin Neoplasms in Females per cent.	Gastric Neoplasms in Females per cent.	Ovarian Neoplasms per cent.
Cancer	48.7	59.30	77.7	34.1	100	3.36
Sarcoma	6.3	.08	3.9	1.8	nil.	2.98
Non-Malignant Neoplasms	33.4	40.54	15.7	29.1	nil.	.12
Cysts	11.6	.08	2.7	35.0	nil.	93.54

This shows that the proneness of the different organs to
evolve the various neoplasms is extraordinarily variable. Thus,
while in some organs certain neoplasms hardly ever arise, these
same organs nevertheless often originate other neoplasms,
although the latter are of the rarest occurrence in yet other
organs.

Thus, although the proneness of the uterus to originate
cancer, as compared with its proneness to originate other neoplasms, is above the average for females in general, yet it is
much surpassed in this respect by the stomach and mammæ;
the liability of the skin is, however, much less, while that of the
ovaries is quite insignificant.

On the other hand, so great is the relative frequency of
cancer of the stomach, as compared with its liability to other
neoplasms and cysts, that for practical purposes the very existence of these latter may be ignored.

Although the liability of all these organs to sarcoma is much
below the average, yet *inter se* the relative frequency of its
occurrence presents considerable variations: in the uterus and
stomach, for instance, sarcoma is remarkably rare; whereas in
the female breast, ovaries, and skin it is relatively not so very
uncommon.

The most striking feature in the neoplastic pathogeny of the
uterus, however, is its great relative proneness to non-malignant
growths; with this the almost complete immunity of the stomach
and ovaries from such growths contrasts markedly.

Again, while the relative proneness of the uterus and stomach to originate cysts is infinitesimal, yet tumours of this kind arise in the ovaries with such preponderating frequency as to reduce the ratio of all other ovarian tumours to insignificant proportions.

In every part of the body, where neoplasms arise, we meet with similar phenomena.

These extraordinary differences in morbid proclivity are among the most remarkable facts in the whole range of neoplastic pathogeny; and no doubt the solution of the problem of the origin of neoplasms concentres in them.

It seems to me impossible to account for such vagaries, otherwise than as the result of biological peculiarities inherent to the various tissues of the affected parts. No doubt in every such locality there must be corresponding morphological changes, although the microscope has hitherto failed adequately to reveal them. In this connection some recent observations of Ribbert are of importance. He has shown that cancer is most prone to arise from epithelia in which active mitotic changes are normally always present, or in which such changes manifest themselves under certain conditions (as in the mammæ); whereas in organs whose epithelia seldom exhibit mitoses, such as the salivary glands, lachrymal glands, thyroid, thymus, male mammæ, etc., cancers seldom arise. These observations give direct anatomical support to the doctrine I have long advocated on other grounds; *viz.*, that cancers are most prone to arise in localities where cells still capable of growth and development most abound.

From the fact that no part of the body—not even the mamma — undergoes so many remarkable post-embryonic developmental changes as the uterus—which moreover also possesses unique reparative powers—we may infer that it is unusually rich in cells, still retaining much of their embryonic capabilities. The behaviour of the uterus, as compared with the tube, under the stimulus of pregnancy, strikingly illustrates these remarks. When a fertilised ovum lodges in the uterine cavity, the walls of the latter grow so rapidly, that they readily adapt themselves to the requirements of the nascent embryo; but when the ovum is arrested in the Fallopian tube and develops there—although at first the tubal structures grow so as to accommodate it—yet, as the embryo augments, the increase of these structures fails to keep pace with it, so that the tube is eventually ruptured.

It is probably owing to inherent peculiarities of this kind, that the uterus is so much more prone to originate neoplasms than other parts of the body. In like manner, the great proclivity of certain regions of the uterus to similar outbreaks, and the comparative immunity of other regions, may probably be explained. At any rate, it is evident that the influence of locality in determining the genesis, structure, and qualities of uterine neoplasms is very great.

A CASE OF NEURITIC MUSCULAR ATROPHY ("PERONEAL" TYPE).

BY

J. E. SHAW, M.B. Ed.,

Professor of Medicine at University College, Bristol;
Physician to the Bristol Royal Infirmary.

To render fully intelligible the complete significance of the illustrations, a brief abstract of the notes upon this case must be given:—

E. G., aged 22, single, formerly a domestic servant, was admitted to the Bristol Royal Infirmary on March 2nd, 1899.

Family History.—Father is of a nervous disposition; one sister is also nervous, and another suffered for a long time in childhood from a malady which caused "trembling" and difficulty in walking (chorea?), but no known case of a similar character has occurred in the family.

Previous History.—At 5 years of age had a long attack of rheumatic fever, and has had frequent attacks of less severity since. About Christmas, 1893, she observed that her legs were beginning to get weak; three months later she suffered from pain which she distinguished from "rheumatism." and which passed from the right natis down the outer and posterior part of the thigh to the calf. At Whitsuntide, 1894, having further failed in her powers of walking and of getting upstairs, and having noticed that her right foot dragged upon the ground occasionally, she finally gave up her occupation as a domestic servant. She attended the Bath United Hospital, first as an out-patient and afterwards as an in-patient, until November of the same year. While in that institution she observed that her hands were beginning to waste. In the following year she was a patient at the Bath Mineral Water Hospital for nine weeks, without receiving appreciable benefit. During the last four years the complaint has continued to make slow progress.

PRESENT CONDITION.

Nervous System: Motor.—There is a great loss of motor power in the legs and thighs; patient can just walk alone, heeling over from side to side in the attempt to lift each foot successively off the ground; notwithstanding, the toes of the right foot always, and those of the left foot occasionally, drag upon the floor; the gait is not high-stepping, on account of the weakness of the thigh muscles. There is no impairment of the action of the sphincters. The hands and fore-arms are extremely feeble, and the fingers cannot be completely extended or closed—the patient manages, however, to use a spoon and fork. The upper arms are slightly affected: the shoulders, neck, and back not at all. There is defective action of the right side of the face, and the tongue on being protruded deviated strongly to the right. (See Fig. 1.)

Sensory.—There is decided (but not total) anæsthesia of all forms in both feet, most marked in the right foot; a less degree of anæsthesia

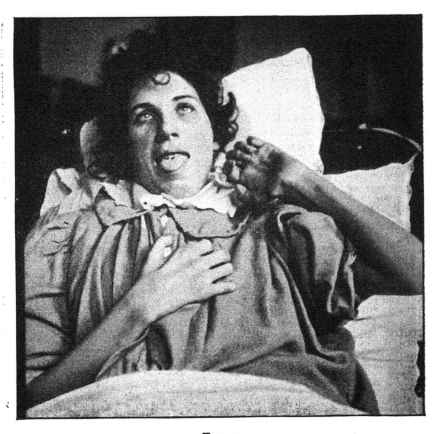

FIG. 1.

of the legs, particularly of the anterior surfaces; slight anæsthesia, superficial to the vasti interni. The hands also are distinctly anæsthetic to all forms of sensation, but less so than the feet. The fore-arms are slightly anæsthetic, the upper arms apparently not so at all. There is no anæsthesia of the face.

Reflexes.—Knee-jerks, plantar reflexes, ankle- and rectus-clonus are all completely absent.

Trophic.—The extensor brevis digitorum of each foot is quite atrophied, and apparently also the interossei and plantar muscles, although of this it is impossible to be certain. There is considerable atrophy of the muscles on the anterior surface of the legs, leading to marked foot-drop (see Fig. 2); the muscles on the posterior aspect of the legs are also atrophied, although not excessively so; the muscles on the anterior and inner surfaces of the thighs are also wasted. In the hands the whole of the intrinsic muscles appear to be completely atrophied; the muscles in the fore-arms, including the supinator longus, are also much diminished in bulk, the extensors particularly so: the upper-arm muscles are but slightly affected, and the shoulder muscles not at all so. There is no fibrillary tremor.

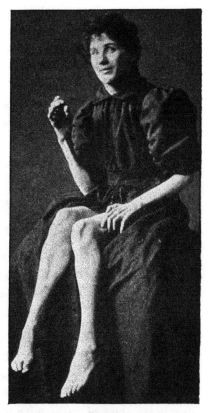

FIG. 2.

Electrical Reaction.—There is no response to the interrupted current in either foot, leg, or thigh, except in the vastus externus, which reacts slightly to a strong current. Electro-sensibility is much impaired, though not destroyed, in these same regions. Similarly there is no response in the hand and fore-arm muscles; the biceps acts slightly, the deltoid and pectoralis major normally. Electro-sensibility in the hands and fore-arms is slightly diminished.

The other systems presented no phenomena of importance. Six weeks after admission patient suffered an exacerbation of her condition. She complained of pains down her legs and arms, which upon investigation were found to be seated in the nerve-trunks. These continued for three or four days, and were followed by increased feebleness of the extremities, increased lateral deviation of the tongue, and some difficulty of articulation and deglutition. From this condition she made some improvement, but three weeks later had another attack of the same nature: this left her so feeble that she could not stand alone, or turn herself in bed, or feed herself; her speech was almost unintelligible from defective lingual and palatal action, mucus accumulated in her pharynx, and occasional regurgitation through the

nares occurred upon swallowing liquids. From this second exacerbation she had recovered to a considerable degree when she returned
to her home a week or two later.

The case is interesting and perhaps somewhat unusual,
inasmuch as while on the one hand it resembled in many
respects a case of ordinary progressive muscular atrophy, with
bulbar symptoms becoming developed as the case progressed, on
the other hand the sensory phenomena, the condition of the
reflexes and of the electrical reaction show indisputably that
the lesion was not exclusively myopathic or even situated
in the nerve-centres, but was partly, if not wholly, seated
in the peripheral nerves. Possibly the case was an example
of the combined form of which Sir William Gowers speaks,
but the complete absence of Faradic response in the considerable volume of calf-muscles which still existed (see Fig. 2)
is in itself a proof that the process was not exclusively seated
in the muscles.

IRREDUCIBLE INTUSSUSCEPTION:

WITH NOTES ON A FATAL CASE.

BY

G. L. KERR PRINGLE, M.D. Ed.,
Surgeon to the Bridgwater Infirmary.

To obtain a correct knowledge of the best methods of procedure
in surgery, it is necessary that we should acknowledge our
failures as well as our successes, however distasteful that may
be to us. Irreducible intussusception is one of the most
desperate class of cases with which we have to deal in surgery,
and all measures which we may adopt must be drastic.

Mr. D'Arcy Power,[1] in his Hunterian lectures on intussusception, considers that the outlook for irreducible cases treated
by enterectomy is distinctly favourable. He says that Braun's[2]

[1] *Brit. M. J.*, 1897, i. 514; *Some Points in the Anatomy, Pathology, and
Surgery of Intussusception*, 1898.

[2] *Verhandl. d. deutsch. Gesellsch. f. Chir.*, 1885, xiv. pt. 2, 491.

statistics, published in 1885, gave 1 recovery, and Rydygier,[1] in his addendum up to 1895, has 25 recoveries; to these may be added 10 more, Banks,[2] Pick,[3] Cripps, Heaton,[4] and others having had successful cases.[5]   Thus we see that during the last fifteen years, owing to improved technic, etc., there has been a considerable reduction in the mortality.

At the present time five different methods have been suggested and carried out for the treatment of the irreducible bowel. These are :—i. To remove or excise the whole invagination, and to unite the two ends of the divided bowel in some manner or other. ii. To remove or excise the invagination and establish an artificial anus. iii. To leave the invagination and establish an artificial anus above it. iv. To short circuit the bowel and leave the invagination alone. v. To suture the entering piece of intestine to the ensheathing tube at its neck by a continuous suture, and then opening the ensheathing tube and extracting the intussusception, excising it within the sheath.

The first method is certainly the ideal one, but, unfortunately, patients are seldom in a condition to stand the extra shock caused by the time occupied in carrying out the anastomosis. Murphy's button considerably shortens the time, but it cannot well be used in all cases, such as the large intestine, as the presence of the appendices epiploicæ renders the two surfaces uneven and irregular. Of other methods, the end-to-end anastomosis by suture in the hands of an expert surgeon, backed up by assistants conversant with the surgeon's particular methods, is the most satisfactory. The temporary anastomosis forceps recently introduced by Laplace[6] of Philadelphia should considerably shorten the time occupied in suturing, for not only do they hold the parts well together, but they give the surgeon a command over the bowel which previously he has not had.

The second method appears to be the most feasible, and was

---

[1] *Verhandl. d. deutsch. Gesellsch. f. Chir.*, 1895, xxiv. pt. 2, 446.

[2] *Brit. M. J.*, 1896, ii. 1197.   [3] *Quart. M. J.*, 1896–97, v. 121.

[4] *Brit. M. J.*, 1899, i. 958.

[5] Since above was written, Nicoll of Glasgow reports another successful case, *Brit. M. J.*, 1899, ii. 1094.

[6] *Ann. Surg.*, 1899, xxix. 297.

the one carried out in the subjoined case, but it is not applicable
in those enteric cases where the obstruction is high up, as the
patient will gradually sink from starvation.

Method No. 3 is the simplest, but here the patient is almost
bound to have a resulting fæcal fistula, while the bowel below is
in a state of gangrene till the intussusception is passed.

No. 4 likewise leaves the bowel to take care of itself, and the
chances of peritonitis and gangrene are probable.

The fifth method, proposed by Rydygier[1] and carried out
with modifications by Barker,[2] Greig Smith,[3] and Leszczynski,[4]
has one great advantage, because there is not so much bowel
removed, but this method is useless when the invaginated bowel
is attached to the returning layer by adhesions for any great
distance. It is also probable that leakage would occur, as a
considerable portion of the ensheathing tube is occupied by
the puckered-up mesentery.

The case which came under my notice is as follows:—

On August 10th I saw Mrs. W., in consultation with Dr. Wilberforce
Thompson, who gave me the following history: The patient, a well-
preserved woman of 50 years, had thirty years ago a local peritonitis
which laid her up for a week. Six or seven months ago she had a sharp
attack of colic which lasted some hours. She is inclined to be con-
stipated; menstruation has not ceased, and at the present time she is
unwell. Two mornings ago Dr. Thompson was sent for, the patient
complaining of severe colicky pains in the region of the descending
colon. She was given an opiate. Subsequently she vomited twice.
She was kept under opium all day; bowels confined; temperature
slightly raised; pulse, 70.
   The following morning she was still suffering pain; bowels still
confined. Opium continued. On seeing her, Dr. Thompson found the
pain was slightly less, but the temperature had risen to 99.6°, and the
pulse was 102. Pain is more in the region of the transverse colon.
The abdomen is distended, and on each side below the level of the
umbilicus there is a firm mass, dull on percussion; the rest of the
abdomen is tympanitic. Examination *per rectum* revealed that the uterus
was retroverted and the pelvic contents pressed down; the fundus of
the uterus could not be felt bi-manually. A soap-and-water enema,
with long tube, was given, which brought away four small scybala with
blood-stained mucus. At 11 a.m. I saw her, and found her lying with
knees drawn up, facial expression fair, temperature 99.6°, pulse 114;
the abdomen distended and very painful to touch, a dull area just
below the umbilicus on each side, flanks resonant; no vomiting, no
hiccough. Patient passing wind by the mouth, but not by the anus.

[1] *Loc. cit.*, 439.

[2] *Lancet*, 1892, i. 79.   [3] *Abdominal Surgery*, 5th Ed., 1896, vol. ii. p. 675.

[4] Quoted by Rydygier, *loc. cit.*

The symptoms being obscure and her environment unsatisfactory, she was removed to the Bridgwater Infirmary, where she was placed under ether. Nothing further could be made out on examining the abdomen, except that it was questionable whether the two masses felt were not connected. The hydrostatic douche was then tried with a long tube for some considerable time, but neither the tube nor the water would pass into the colon. The abdomen was then prepared and laparotomy performed, with the assistance of Dr. Thompson. An incision two inches in length was made to the right of the linea alba, which was subsequently enlarged to four inches, a large mass of bowel presented, coiled upon itself, having the appearance of a volvulus, as the bowel formed a complete circle, but on closer examination proved to be an intussusception of the small intestine, the sausage-shaped circular tumour being about eight inches in circumference: reduction was tried without success, and manipulations had to be stopped, as the subserous coat was commencing to tear. The bowel was dull and congested. Resection of the invagination was then carried out. Considerable trouble was experienced with the mesentery, which was all screwed up and very much congested.

Anastomosis was the next step, but no Murphy buttons were available, only those of Ball and Hey being to hand. On considering the weak state the patient was in and the time she had been under the anæsthetic (before the abdomen was opened), we decided to postpone the suturing to a later date, so both ends of the gut were brought out and stitched to the abdominal wall, and the wound closed as far as possible with some deep sutures.

She did very well for the first three or four days, but after that began to fail, the bowel acting constantly. Rectal feeding was most unsatisfactory, both suppositories and enemata being tried. She gradually got weaker, and died on the thirteenth day. At no time was her condition such as to allow of a second operation.

On examination after death the free end of bowel was found to be situated less than three feet from the pylorus; there was some localised peritonitis round the wound.

On examining the specimen subsequently, it was found that the valvulæ conniventes were large and numerous, showing that the invagination had taken place high up in the small intestine, and that the patient's chance of recovery was very doubtful.

The condition occurred about fifty hours before operation ; adhesions had taken place, and the bowel was dull and much congested. To have carried out the method of Rydygier and Greig Smith would have been very difficult, if not impossible, as the entering piece of intestine was so much smaller and more puckered than the ensheathing portion.

If we had recognised at the time of operation that the obstruction was so near the stomach, immediate anastomosis would have been risked, but all the symptoms were against a high lesion. There had been no vomiting for two days, no hiccough ; in fact, the signs and symptoms were by no means diagnostic of intussusception, for the bleeding *per rectum* was so slight that it might have been caused by the long tube, and, also, the patient was menstruating. The usual sausage-shaped tumour could not be felt on palpation, but in its place a double mass.

On considering the case, there is no doubt that had a

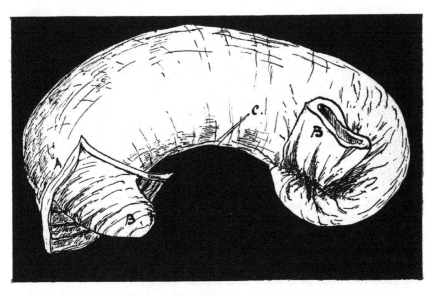

A. Intussuscipiens.　　**B.** Intussusceptum.　　**C.** Cut edge of Mesentery.

Murphy button been available it would have been the best method, on account of its rapidity.

Undoubtedly too much time was occupied in trying by irrigation to relieve the obstruction, but one is loath to operate if other means will avail.

Progress of the Medical Sciences.

MEDICINE.

The observations of Dr. Meinhard Pfaundler on **lumbar puncture in children**[1] are interesting. From experiments on

[1] *München. med. Wchnschr.*, 1898, xlv. 1393 ; abstract in *Neurol. Centralbl.*, 1899, xviii. 507.

the pressure-conditions in the subarachnoid space, he finds that variations in the pressure have some diagnostic importance. In tuberculous meningitis not only is the pressure raised, but the pressure-curve is characteristic, as it rises during the "stage of irritation" until "the stage of pressure" and falls from the beginning of the "stage of paralysis" until death. The localisation of the exudate also influences the height of the pressure. If the pressure is found normal in a case in which there is no disturbance of the heart's action, any cerebral or meningeal affection is unlikely.

With regard to the chemical characters of the fluid removed, he finds that in the different stages of tuberculous meningitis a characteristic curve can be obtained for the amount of albumin present, and that the quantity increases with the duration of the case until death.

By means of "fractional centrifugalisation" he could nearly always demonstrate the presence of the tubercle bacillus in tuberculous meningitis, and distinguish sharply between two diplococci, which he indicates as of Weichselbaum's and Heubner's types respectively, in cases of epidemic cerebro-spinal meningitis.

As a therapeutic measure he found lumbar puncture of some palliative value in cases of high intracranial pressure, giving some relief to the patient. In 200 lumbar punctures in children he has scarcely once seen evil consequences of a serious nature.

* * * *

Dr. Hermann Pfister[1] has made an exhaustive study of the condition of the pupils and eye-reflexes in infants. His observations were made on 300 children. He holds that it is not certainly established that the reaction of the pupil to light is always present in the newborn, and particularly in the prematurely born; it failed in one child for two weeks, and in another, a prematurely born child, for eight to ten days: in the latter, the consensual light reaction at first distinctly present, had disappeared on further testing. The diameter of the pupil increases from an average of 1.5 mm. at the end of the first month to 3.2 mm. for the seventh to the twelfth year. There is no difference in this respect between boys and girls. The magnitude of the light reaction increases from .9 mm. at the first month to 1.9 mm. at the sixth to the twelfth year, but does not show the same regularity of increase as the pupil diameter. The average amplitude is greater in girls than in boys. Diseases, unless they directly cause nervous symptoms, do not affect the light reaction.

Hippus occurred three times in the 300 children, once in a child aged two weeks as a precursor of hemorrhagic encephalitis.

Reflex closure of the eyelids was absent or uncertain in the

[1] *Arch. f. Kinderh.*, 1899, xxvi. 11; abstract in *Neurol. Centralbl.*, 1899, xviii. 172.

first month, often present in the second month, almost constant in the third, and after that never failed. Dilatation of the pupil to sensory irritation (pain), difficult to ascertain in children, was never certain in the first month, and in the second month only once positive. From the third to the sixth month it increased in frequency, so that there were only a small number of negative results. Dilatation of pupil to loud noises could only be proved in some cases, and was first obtained after the tenth week.

*　　　*　　　-　　　*

Drs. E. Weil and Rouvillois [1] report the case of a girl aged 10, who after a severe fright suffered from pains in the head, passing disturbance of speech, and thirty-three days after the fright from paralysis, affecting first the right side, then the whole body. The paralysis gradually passed off, but left stiffness of the right arm and leg, with a tremor resembling that of **paralysis agitans**. Other usual characteristic signs of paralysis agitans which were present were the maintenance of the trunk in a position bent forwards, flexed position of the arms, and difficulty in locomotion. The rate of the tremor corresponded to that of paralysis agitans, and the diagnosis of that disease was made. The patient's condition remained unaltered during the year that she was under observation. The authors could only find six cases of paralysis agitans in children in the literature of the disease, and these cases were not beyond dispute.

-　　　-　　　*　　　*

The occurrence of **nervous diseases in children** after an attack of one of the **acute specific fevers of childhood** is well known. Perhaps this connection is especially frequent in disseminated sclerosis: many cases are on record in which the disease began in this way. Dr. Haushalter[2] describes three cases of muscular atrophy in children, in one of which the disease began immediately after measles; the patient was 7 years old, and the disease took the facio-scapulo-humeral type, the first symptoms appearing at the age of 5 years. There was no other case in the family. The reaction of degeneration was obtained in the face muscles.

Prof. Allen Starr[3] reports three cases of Friedreich's disease, in two of which the symptoms of ataxy were excited by an attack of measles: all the patients were children of 13 to 16 years of age; they presented the typical group of symptoms, but in one of them the knee-jerks were exaggerated. He believes that too much stress has been laid on heredity as an etiological factor of the disease, and lays the chief blame on the infectious

[1] *Rev. mens. d. Mal. de l'Enf.*, Juin, 1899; abstract in *Neurol. Centralbl.*, 1899, xviii. 938.

[2] *Rev. de Méd.*, 1898, xviii. 445; abstract in *Neurol. Centralbl.*, 1899, xviii. 179.

[3] *J. Nerv. & Ment. Dis.*, 1898, xxv. 194.

diseases of children. He regards the pathological basis of Friedreich's disease as not confined to the lesions in the spinal cord, but, as in the case of disseminated sclerosis, comprising diffuse changes in the whole nervous system, and as evidence refers to the weakness of mind and affection of the eye-muscles present in his cases.

Dr. Dreisch[1] reports three cases in which, after an attack of measles, he observed paresis of the oculo-motor muscles and paralysis of accommodation, which, however, soon passed away completely. He compares these paralyses with the similar ones observed after diphtheria and other infectious diseases, and attributes them to the toxic products of the hypothetical measles bacillus.

Dr. L. Michaëlis[2] gives from Prof. Senator's clinic the account of a child, aged 13, who was confined to bed for eight days in February with an attack of influenza. On attempting to stand up it was found that walking was impossible from spasm of adductors of thighs, stiffness, and trembling of the legs. When examined in the following May there was spastic paresis of both legs, with increase of the knee-jerks, and clonic spasms of the muscles; there were no disturbances of sensation, or of the bladder or rectum. Recovery was perfect.

*　　　*　　　*　　　*

Dr. von Schultze,[3] on the causes of acute poliomyelitis, draws attention to the remarkable similarity of the initial symptoms of poliomyelitis, encephalitis, and labyrinthine otitis in children, and is of opinion that first of all a special form of acute meningitis occurs, which passes on either to the anterior spinal arteries or to certain parts of the cerebrum or to the cochlea and labyrinth. The causes of this meningitis, which can occasionally be demonstrated, are unknown. In a case of acute poliomyelitis lately observed, the author found in the fluid from a lumbar-puncture Weichselbaum's diplococcus as the sole organism present. He thinks that acute poliomyelitis can be produced by different micro-organisms, but how they get into the cerebro-spinal fluid is still doubtful. Besides infection through the nasal mucous membrane, an otitis media preceding labyrinthine otitis is most probable.

*　　　*　　　*　　　*

Dr. C. Thiry,[4] in a study of general paresis in the young (under 20 years) based on sixty-seven cases published since

---

[1] München. med. Wchnschr., 1898, xlv. 627 ; abstract in Neurol. Centralbl., 1899, xviii. 173.

[2] Deutsche med. Wchnschr., 1899, xxv. 108 , abstract in Neurol. Centralbl., 1899, xviii. 507.

[3] Deutsche med. Wchnschr., 1898, Nos. 23, 39 ; abstract in Neurol. Centralbl., 1899, xviii. 175.

[4] " Thèse de Paris," 1898, Gaz. hebd. de Méd., 1898, n. s. iii. 529 ; abstract in J. Nerv. & Ment. Dis., 1899, xxvi. 196.

23

1877, says that in a majority of the cases a neuropathic family history is to be found. Syphilis plays an important part, its effects upon the general nutrition predisposing to degeneration of the nervous tissues. Both the cerebral and spinal symptoms closely resemble those found in the adult. The general course of the disease is so characteristic, even in children, that no mistakes need be made in diagnosis. Remissions do not occur, and the prognosis is most grave. Antisyphilitic treatment is unavailing.

Dr. Purves Stewart[1] gives a short summary of the symptomatology of **general paralysis of the insane occurring during childhood and adolescence.** He states that the age of onset varies from the ninth year onwards, the commonest being from 13 to 16. Both boys and girls are about equally liable. There is a history of inherited syphilis in 90 per cent. of cases: the ordinary objective signs of congenital syphilis in the teeth, bones, and eyes are very rarely present in these patients, the syphilitic poison seeming to expend itself on the nervous system. In a few cases a history of a fall or head injury preceding the onset of symptoms and perhaps precipitating it was given. The mental symptoms consist of a simple progressive dementia in a child of previously normal intelligence. The child becomes forgetful, dull, and apathetic, with occasional bursts of passion. Grandiose ideas are as a rule absent, mild delusions and hallucinations may exist. Physically, the general development is arrested; the genital organs remain infantile in type; the catamenia do not come on or cease. Fits or " congestive attacks " are common, and may be the first symptom. These may be typical epileptic fits, or attacks of " general trembling," or of speechlessness, or of loss of consciousness without convulsions. Optic atrophy is not uncommon; the pupil-symptoms resemble those found in adults. Fibrillary tremors of the face, lips, and tongue are usually present when the disease is well established; the speech becomes typically slurring and slovenly, and the handwriting resembles that of the adult general paralytic. General analgesia has been found in a number of cases. Motor symptoms and the knee-jerks vary as in adult cases. Unsteadiness of the upper extremities on voluntary movement may resemble the " intention tremor " of disseminated sclerosis. The superficial reflexes remain normal, and the sphincters are unaffected, though the latter may become uncontrolled with the progressive advance of mental dulness. The duration of the disease has varied from six months to eight and a half years. The morbid anatomy does not differ essentially from that of the adult variety of the disease.

The recognition that a form of **dementia closely resembling general paresis** may occur in the young is becoming generally admitted. Drs. Toulouse and Marchand[2] point out that many

---

[1] *Brain*, 1898, xxi. 39.
[2] *Soc. méd. d. Hôp.*, 1899, Juin 23; abstract in *J. Nerv. & Ment. Dis.*, 1899, xxvi. 571.

cases of paresis occurring in the very young are mistaken for cases of idiocy. In a case reported the progressive dementia began after a period of normal development. There were inequality of pupils, speech disturbances, rapid emaciation, and epileptiform attacks. *Post-mortem* cerebral atrophy, adherent meninges, proliferation of neuroglia, and other changes held to be typical of general paralysis were found.

Dr. August Hoch reports[1] two typical cases of general paralysis in two sisters, commencing at the age of 10 and 15 respectively, and Drs. van Deventer and Benders[2] two cases, one beginning at the age of 9 and the other at 11 years.

Dr. Grannelli[3] gives the case of a child who, at the age of 7, after a severe attack of scarlatina with nephritis, showed signs of beginning dementia. Her disposition changed, and she developed a general fine tremor. Later she had an epileptiform attack, and subsequently became a more or less typical case of general paralysis. The father was alcoholic and infected the mother (who developed tabes dorsalis at 44) with syphilis three or four years before the birth of the child.

J. MICHELL CLARKE.

SURGERY.

In the *Bristol Medico-Chirurgical Journal* for 1895,[4] I gave a summary of some remarkable results of **extensive operations for cancer of the breast,** as advocated and practised especially by Watson Cheyne, Halsted, and Meyer. As two of these surgeons have brought their statistics up to date, and given us the results of their further experience; and as some new pathological evidence has been adduced, it may be useful to review the subject afresh.

The pathological evidence is mainly embodied in a very important and exhaustive paper on the dissemination of cancer of the breast, by Mr. Stiles,[5] which is an eloquent substantiation of the radical operations they have urged on the profession. He criticises the opinion that so largely prevailed in the discussion which followed Mr. Marmaduke Sheild's paper read at the Royal Medical and Chirurgical Society last year,[6] by pointing out that the ultimate prognosis for patients free from recurrence three years after the old operation cannot be as good as when the same immunity has followed a modern extensive operation, since in the latter case the risk is largely limited to internal recurrence.

To begin with Mr. Cheyne's statistics. He gives the present condition, as far as he can ascertain it, of the 61 cases reported [7]

[1] *J. Nerv. & Ment. Dis.*, 1897, xxiv. 67.
[2] *Psychiat. en Neurol. Bl.*, 1898, ii. 118; abstract in *Neurol. Centralbl.*, 1899, xviii. 855.
[3] *Riv. quindicin. di psicol.* [etc.], 1898, ii. 213; abstract in *J. Nerv. & Ment. Dis.*, 1899, xxvi. 196.
[4] xiii. 29.   [5] *Brit. M. J.*, 1899, i. 1452.
[6] *Ibid.*, 1898, i. 300, 557.   [7] *Lancet*, 1896, i. 397 *et seq.*

by him more than three years ago, which then covered a period of six years. In 21 of these three years or more had elapsed since operation, and 12 of them (57 per cent.) had remained free from recurrence, 1 having died of an independent illness three years and five months after operation. Of these 11 patients 9 are reported as being still well, 1 was alive and well a year ago (seven years after operation), but has since been lost sight of, and 1 has had a recurrence of the disease. If a patient operated upon more than nine years ago (and who was not included among the 21 cases), and who was recently seen with no signs of recurrence, be added to the number, the percentage of successes remains practically the same as before. Of the 40 cases under the three-year limit, 27 had shown no sign of recurrence when the last paper was written, and 18 of these are still alive and well, while 1 died without sign of recurrence. Mr. Cheyne points to these figures as a corroboration of Volkmann's well-known dictum, since of 11 patients reported well three to six years after operation, only 1 has recurred in the succeeding three years, while of 20 who had survived the operation a year at his last writing 17 still remain well, thus showing, as he believes, the great chance of freedom from recurrence which patients obtain who pass one year without a return of the disease after a radical operation. To his original 61 cases, Mr. Cheyne adds 38 fresh ones in which one to three years have elapsed since operation, and 26 of these remain well.

Dr. Halsted[1] gives the following statistics of the cases operated upon at the Johns Hopkins Hospital by his method up to April, 1898. They are 133 in number. There have been 13 (9 per cent.) "local" and 22 (16 per cent.) "regionary" recurrences. Of 76 cases operated upon three or more years ago, 31 (40 per cent.) are living and well; 10 died more than three years after operation, and 1 as late as five and a half years after. 35 cases (46 per cent.) died within three years of the operation.

In his recent paper Mr. Cheyne calls special attention to certain points, which may be taken categorically, and discussed in the light of clinical and pathological knowledge.

Exploration in Doubtful Cases.—He strongly deprecates an incision into the tumour in such a case, and asserts again that the cancer cells may escape and infect the wound afterwards made for removal of the breast. He says he has more than once seen a diffuse cancerous infection, especially when glands have burst during removal, and in spite of the greatest care in clearing out all the escaped material. Hence he recommends that the suspected swelling should be "excised along with an area of apparently healthy tissue around," and only cut into away from the site of operation; that it should not be touched by the surgeon's fingers; and that all instruments employed should be

[1] *Ann. Surg.*, 1898, xxviii. 557.

discarded. To guard against the risk of contamination from lymphatic channels cut across, Mr. Cheyne, after stopping the bleeding, stuffs the wound with a small sponge and stitches it closely up, and then disinfects his hands and the patient's skin as thoroughly . as in the first instance, before proceeding to remove the breast. Dr. Halsted recommends the same scrupulous avoidance of an incision into a suspected tumour.

Skin Incisions.—Mr. Cheyne believes that in the free removal of the skin—quite independently of the question of closure of the wound afterwards—lies one of the chief reasons why he has so seldom had local recurrences; and he gives a useful series of diagrams representing the incisions he employs in different positions of the growth—the skin over the breast always being removed, and when the growth is excentral the incision being planned to keep wide of it. Then the skin is undermined all round (leaving just enough fat with it to ensure its vitality) as far as the clavicle above, beyond the middle of the sternum internally, down to the origin of the abdominal muscles below, and out to the edge of the latissimus dorsi—and not till these limits are reached are the muscular fibres exposed. By this undermining (sometimes still further extended for the purpose) it appears that the edges of even these large wounds can be brought together as a rule, but when this cannot be done the unclosed part is skin-grafted at once. Dr. Halsted[1] says: "We remove rather more skin than we did originally, and in all cases we graft the wound immediately." As bearing on the importance of such free removal of skin and fat, I may quote Mr. Stiles's observations.[2] He describes the suspensory ligaments of Cooper as being tooth-like processes of breast-tissue ending in fibrinous prolongations into which the parenchyma is prolonged—these processes branching and joining to form a reticular network, while from the circumference of the gland similar processes radiate between the lobules of the circummammary fat: and in both cases lymphatic vessels are carried with them which are directly continuous with those in the skin and subcutaneous tissue of the whole mammary area. Mr. Stiles has often demonstrated the presence of disseminated foci of disease upon the exposed surface of the parts removed, and he has found cancerous lymphatic emboli towards the inner margin of the breast when the primary tumour was situated in the outer hemisphere, and *vice versâ*. At other times cancerous foci are found beneath the skin, or in the corium, which can sometimes be shown to be at the end of a paravascular lymphatic in a ligament of Cooper. In this connection Mr. Stiles states that it is not always easy to say whether a cancerous embolus is in the paravascular lymphatic or in a small vein itself, and he quotes Goldmann as having demonstrated that blood-vessels, especially small veins, are more frequently and more extensively invaded (from without) than has been hitherto supposed. More rarely

[1] *Loc. cit.*   [2] *Loc. cit.*

the arteries are invaded, and he suggests that possibly the sudden formation and extensive distribution of lenticular dissemination in the skin may sometimes be due to arterial embolism. Goldmann also declares that the lactiferous ducts may be invaded and give rise to a condition indistinguishable from duct cancer.

Pectoral Muscle.—There is no longer any difference of opinion as to the necessity of removing the pectoral fasciæ, but the controversy with regard to the treatment of the muscles themselves is still unsettled. Rotter[1] examined the pectoral muscle after removal of the breast in 40 cases, and found that the branches which perforate the pectoralis major into the retromammary fat, and into the breast itself (branches of the internal mammary, superior thoracic, and long thoracic arteries) were accompanied by efferent lymphatic vessels from the breast. He also found that one or two small glands were constantly present alongside the trunk of the superior thoracic artery, while in half the specimens examined others were situated in the angles of bifurcation of its branches, not far from the perforating branches; and in a few instances one was discovered in the substance of the pectoralis in relation to one of the same arteries. In rather more than a third of the carcinomatous breasts examined he found small cancerous nodules upon the posterior surface and in the substance of the pectoralis major, adjacent to the superior thoracic artery. It is worthy of notice that out of the 15 preparations in which the retropectoral glands were diseased, only 5 showed direct invasion of the muscle of the tumour—a layer of retromammary fat separating the two in the other 10 cases; while, on the other hand, of the 18 cases in which there was no evidence of retropectoral infection the tumour in the breast was adherent to the muscle in 5 cases. Rotter draws the following conclusions from these observations :—(1) That when the pectoral muscle is directly invaded by the tumour it is not infected throughout but through the main paravascular lymphatics. (2) That at an early stage, before any adhesion has taken place between the breast and the underlying pectoral fascia, cancer cells may be conveyed through the muscle to the glands in the retropectoral fascia, and this in about one-third of the cases. (3) That these efferent lymphatics only pass through the sternal portion of the muscle, and that the clavicular portion need not be removed unless large cancerous infraclavicular glands have become adherent to it. Dr. Halsted removes both pectoral muscles before exposing the subclavian vein; whence the axilla is stripped of its contents from within outward and from above downward. Cheyne removes the lower part, "say half of the muscle," in all cases—that is to say, all the muscle which lies behind the cancer from a little above the cancer down to its lower edge; and he only takes away the whole of the muscle, or even the whole of its pectoral origin,

[1] Quoted by Stiles *loc. cit.*

when there is evident disease of the muscle itself. He asserts that when the lower half of the pectoralis major has been taken away it is quite easy to completely expose the axilla, and that the removal of the pectoralis minor is quite unnecessary for that purpose. The fasciæ covering both sides of the two pectoral muscles should be removed as a matter of routine. In clearing out the axilla the fat and glands are dissected off as much as possible *en masse*, with the superficial fibres of the serratus magnus muscle, and the fascia over the latissimus dorsi, up to the level of the vessels; then the fat is dissected off the front of the vessels and nerves, opening and stripping the sheath; and finally the space behind them is cleared. Stiles recommends removing the branches of the axillary vein which come to it from the chest, on account of their lymphatic accompaniments.

The Supraclavicular Glands.—Two questions arise here: whether and when it is necessary to clear out the posterior triangle of the neck; and how far supraclavicular gland infection is a contra-indication to operation. Cheyne points out that the lymphatic course which passes upwards behind the axillary vessels to the glands in the posterior triangle of the neck is decidedly the less frequent one for cancerous infection: hence his rule is—assuming that there is no palpable enlargement— not to clear out the posterior triangle unless he finds enlarged glands in the fat running up behind the vessels. He adds that, as a matter of experience, he has hardly ever seen a recurrence in the supraclavicular glands. On the other hand, Dr. Halsted's rule is to "operate on the neck in every case." In 67 such operations cancer was found microscopically in 23 cases (34 per cent.), while in 14 more its absence had not yet been exhaustively ascertained. Fourteen of these operations were performed for palpable glands after the original breast removal, and 4 of the patients are living and free from recurrence: 2 more than four years, and the other 2 three and a half and three years after the primary operation. Dr. Bloodgood[1] is reported to have done as many as three operations for glandular involvement in the neck in two instances, and "apparently" saved both patients.

Dr. Cushing[1] cleaned out the anterior mediastinum on one side for recurrent cancer in three instances; but the results are not stated. Dr. Halsted's comment, however, is that in the near future he expects the anterior mediastinum to be cleared out at some of the primary operations. He hopes that we shall not abandon as hopeless all cases in which there is supraclavicular gland infection. Mr. Cheyne is much more pessimistic. He doubts the expediency of operation when there is marked enlargement of cervical glands in front of or beneath the sternomastoid; but if there is enlargement of gland "in the posterior part of the posterior triangle" he does not think it necessarily a contra-indication, provided the patient is in a state to stand a prolonged operation. Time and further experience can alone

---

[1] Quoted by Halsted, *loc. cit.*

determine the best routine practice in this respect. Mr. Cheyne's last word may fittingly close this review of the subject: "I may add my firm conviction that *the patient's chance lies in the first operation.*" Secondary operations, as we all sorrowfully have to admit, are seldom successful.

To the pathological side of breast cancers, Dr. Halsted[1] contributes an interesting account of certain **adeno-carcinomata**, of which he has met 5 or 6 in less than 150 cases of cancers of the breast. These adeno-carcinomata (which are minutely described and figured) resembled on section the carcinomata, without any villous or papillomatous tendency: in some cases fine, worm-like cylinders of epithelium could be expressed from the cut surface; all infiltrated the surrounding tissues just as the other carcinomata do. Microscopically the power of the epithelium to make ring-like combinations was very conspicuous. Clinically they seem to be characterised by a tendency to exuberance and fungation, and sometimes to distinct pedunculation; and when fungating, a serous fluid can sometimes be squeezed from the tumour: the glands in the axilla, although enlarged, seem never to show any evidence microscopically of malignant infection, but always of endothelial proliferation; and they seem to exhibit a relatively low malignancy.

In some a change was evident from adeno-carcinoma to the purer carcinoma; and one case is reported of a true scirrhus starting in the wall of a cyst, which surrounded a little field of intracanalicular papillomatous adeno-carcinoma, which in certain parts resembled the variety of adeno-carcinoma just described, but more closely recalls the duct-cancers.

There would seem, therefore, to be several transitional varieties between the pure carcinoma and the pure adeno-carcinoma. Clinically it will be well to bear in mind this occasional and less malignant variety of breast-cancer.

W. M. BARCLAY.

LARYNGOLOGY AND RHINOLOGY.

Dr. Dundas Grant[2] drew attention to a very important matter, at the Portsmouth meeting of the British Medical Association, when he pointed out that amongst many **causes of headache** nasal and aural disease must be remembered. As regards the forms of nasal disease that may give rise to headache, adenoid vegetations in the naso-pharynx and |hypertrophy of the middle turbinated body are the most frequent. Then come disease of the accessory sinuses, antrum of Highmore, frontal, sphenoidal, and ethmoidal. Operative measures for the cure of the nasal mischief cured the headache.

Hajek[3] alludes to the same matter, and says that the headache

---

[1] *Loc. cit.*   [2] *J. Laryngol.*, 1899, xiv. 452.
[3] *München. med. Wchnschr*, 1899, xlvi. 336.

may depend directly on the nasal disease and disappears with its cure, or the nasal condition predisposes to headache. Apart from ulcerative conditions of the nose, disease of the accessory sinuses and hypertrophic changes of the nasal mucous membrane come under consideration. In disease of the sinuses it may be of a neuralgic nature or of an indefinite character (frontal, vertical, feeling of pressure or of numbness) or hemicrania. The pain in acute empyema of the antrum or frontal sinus may be in the infra-orbital, superior dental or supra-orbital nerve. It varies in intensity at different times. It is more apt to be neuralgic in disease of the frontal sinus than in that of the antrum, and in the acute stage of frontal sinus mischief it is intense. It may be absent in chronic empyema of the antrum, and also, but less frequently, in that of the frontal sinus. It is aggravated by coryza, mental or physical disturbance, and abuse of alcohol. Simple hypertrophy of the turbinated bodies is rarely a cause of headache; but where the septum is also deflected or thickened so that pressure can take place, then patients complain of heaviness in the head and pressure at the root of the nose.

* * * *

A discussion on the diagnosis and treatment of **chronic empyema of the frontal sinus** took place at the same meeting.[1] The discussion was opened by Mr. Charters Symonds, of London, and Dr. E. J. Moure, of Bordeaux.

Mr. Charters Symonds divided the cases into three groups:— (i.) Those in which there is purulent discharge from the nose, with, as a rule, formation of polypi. (ii.) Those in which there is distension of the sinus without nasal discharge. (iii.) Those in which there is distension of sinus, together with nasal discharge of pus. Attention was chiefly given to the diagnosis of the first class of cases, as the class most frequently coming before the rhinologist. He laid stress upon the fact that, whenever pus was seen amongst or around polypi, suppuration of one or more of the sinuses was indicated. He considered the pus to be the cause of the polypi, and to explain the frequent recurrence of polypi when the pus itself had not been traced to its origin. Where the polypi were numerous, it was impossible to say from which sinus the pus was coming, but he held that where they were very numerous, and there was much pus, with a foul odour, the maxillary antrum was certainly involved, with or without the frontal sinus. In the pure frontal cases the polypi were less numerous, the granulations fewer, and the pus as a rule inodorous; in these cases also there was no pain.

Dr. Moure said that although habitually associated with empyema of the antrum, it occurs alone. Probable signs were: unilateral discharge of pus, seen on rhinoscopic examination after the antrum has been thoroughly cleaned by irrigation; growths in the upper part of the infundibulum, in the direction of the naso-frontal canal, with dilatation of this canal, giving free access to the sinus; supra-orbital pains, spontaneous or on pressure. As certain signs he mentioned temporary or permanent swelling over the frontal sinus, or the presence of a fistula in that region; the flowing away of pus after irrigation, when that is possible in the frontal sinus; darkness on transillumination as compared with the opposite side. Absence of the sinus, fortunately rare, also gives rise to this sign.

The differential diagnosis between frontal empyema and that of the anterior ethmoidal cells may be difficult, but injection and transillumination will generally solve the difficulty. Ethmoidal growths are usually situated further back than those coming from the frontal sinus.

As regards treatment, there was a balance of opinion in favour of intranasal methods, and removal of the anterior portion of the middle turbinated body was held to be often of much value. Breaking into the sinus from the nose was considered not to be devoid of risk, and for bad cases an external operation and securing free drainage into the nose is necessary.

Dr. Milligan,[1] writing on the same subject, lays much stress upon the presence of pain when pressure is made just under the supra-orbital arch over the floor of the sinus and in a direction upwards and inwards, as a diagnostic sign. Transillumination is of value; and when pus is seen to proceed from the region of the infundibulum and there is opacity over the area of the frontal sinus, the presumption is certainly in favour of the presence of a frontal empyema. An accurate diagnosis is very difficult to arrive at, and opening and inspecting the sinus is often the only way of verifying it.

*   *   *   *

Mr. A. J. Brady[2] relates a case of **muco-purulent catarrh of the antrum of Highmore** simulating post-nasal catarrh, in which there was no discharge from the anterior nares after inversion of the head, nor was any to be seen in this situation. Posterior rhinoscopy revealed a thin rope of muco-pus issuing below the posterior end of the right middle turbinal, and extending above the right Eustachian cushion on to the post-pharyngeal wall. The antrum was opened and found to contain pus and polypoid tissue. The reason assigned for the direction of the flow of muco-pus backwards into the naso-pharynx is either some local abnormality, or more probably the thickness of the discharge which clings to the membrane uninfluenced by gravitation. Ciliary motion may have something to do with its backward course.

*   *   *   *

[1] *J. Laryngol.*, 1899, xiv. 568.   [2] *Ibid.*, 565.

Villy, writing on vomiting and cardiac failure in connection with **diphtheria**[1] states his objections to the "paralysis theory." In the present state of our knowledge it is almost impossible to prove or disprove the existence of cardiac paralysis of nervous origin, but he brings forward a good deal of clinical and pathological evidence to establish the following points as a summary of the pathological changes found. Out of 15 cases, the stomach showed fatty degeneration of the glandular epithelium in all, an excess of leucocytes in the mucous and submucous layers in all, hemorrhages in the mucous membrane in 8. The heart showed fatty degeneration in 14 cases, granular changes in the fibres and indistinctness or loss of their striation in 15 cases, hemorrhages in 7 cases. *Ante-mortem* clot was found in its cavities 8 times. The day of disease on which death occurred ranged from the 3rd to 40th. The degenerative changes of the heart and stomach, therefore, begin early in the disease and persist for a prolonged period.

From the clinical evidence it may be deduced that: (1) Signs of heart-failure are much more common than are paralyses in other parts, and have an earlier date of onset; (2) They are such as may be ascribed to muscular failure; (3) When vomiting occurs, heart-failure generally follows; (4) The date of vomiting and heart-failure is distinctly anterior to that of paralysis in other parts.

From the pathological data it appears that: (1) Evidence of degeneration and inflammation of the mucous membrane of the stomach is constantly present, and is often accompanied by hemorrhages; (2) The heart-muscle is constantly found to be in a degenerated condition; hemorrhages are commonly present.

* * * *

Goodale[2] examined 16 cases of **acute tonsillitis** which had been inflamed for three or four days, and which were of non-diphtheritic origin. Sections of the excised glands show a diffuse inflammation of the parenchyma of the organ, appearing in the form of an increased proliferation of lymphoid cells, and of the endothelioid cells of the reticulum, due probably to the absorption of toxin formed in the crypts. While bacteria are rarely demonstrable in the tonsillar tissue in cases characterised by purely proliferative lesions, yet at times infection of the follicles occurs, giving rise to circumscribed suppuration and the formation of abscesses, which eventually discharge into the crypts.

Barclay J. Baron.

THERAPEUTICS.

Enteroclysis or irrigation of the large intestine in the treatment of summer diarrhœa in children does not seem, if one may

[1] *Med. Chron.*, 3rd Ser., 1899, i.　　[2] *J. Boston Soc. M. Sc.*, 1898–99 iii. 63.

judge from the amount of literature published on the question in this country, to have been received with the favour that has been accorded to it in America or on the Continent. The most modern text-books published in England mention it, but not in that enthusiastic tone adopted by physicians in the United States. For instance, in the sixth edition of Goodhart [1] the matter is dismissed in eight lines, and Dawson Williams,[2] though advocating it, speaks of the use of "clysters" in summer diarrhœa, and not of irrigation of the bowel, using only a pint of water, which is retained for half an hour. The excellent results which are recorded by American physicians, as well as my own experience, induce me to recommend it strongly in most cases of diarrhœa in children, whether the attack is one of so-called " summer diarrhœa " or due to other causes.

It was at first thought that this line of treatment would be only applicable for those children not severely attacked, and so not collapsed, but experience of the beneficial effects it produces now warrants it in all cases; in fact, the weaker the child, provided it is not moribund, the greater is the indication for enteroclysis.[3] Before all things, it is necessary to remove the toxic matters in the intestines, and no surer or quicker way is obtainable than by washing out the large bowel. Not only is the intestine cleaned, but peristalsis is encouraged, and the warmth of the water stimulates the failing vitality, the fluid, as is well known, supplying fresh liquid to the circulation. It is claimed that cerebral thrombosis, due to the drain upon the blood, is prevented by this means.

By some physicians **lavage of the stomach,** which can very easily be done in quite young children, is recommended as a preliminary to washing out the bowel; but, except in cases where there is much vomiting, it is not necessary, and many cases do quite well when it is omitted. Should it be considered advisable, the child should be placed on its back and a No. 20 French size indiarubber catheter, connected with a tube and funnel, passed down the œsophagus. Normal saline solution is then poured in and withdrawn in the usual manner till the fluid comes away clear. Care must be taken in small children not to over-distend the stomach or insert the fluid at more than a very moderate pressure, as the fluid cannot escape by the side of the tube as it does from the bowel. Jacobi[4] recommends a disinfectant being added to the fluid, such as thymol, 1 in 3,000, or resorcin, 1 in 1000, but this is not necessary. The temperature of the saline solution should be 98.6° F.: but if there is fever it may be below that temperature; if much collapse, above. He also says that pure boiled water should not be employed, as it causes " osmosis of the body fluids into the stomach, sometimes to such an extent as to visibly increase the amount returning from

[1] *Diseases of Children,* 1899, p 63.
[2] *Medical Diseases of Infancy and Childhood,* 1898, p. 426.
[3] Lockhart Gillespie, *A Manual of Modern Gastric Methods,* 1899, p. 141.
[4] *Therap Gaz.,* 1899, xxiii. 505.

the stomach," which, of course, in any stage of this disease is undesirable. This procedure need seldom be done more than once, whereas irrigation of the bowel may be performed oftener, and in many cases must be.

To **perform enteroclysis** a soft rubber No. 14 English catheter, attached to a fountain syringe, or tube and funnel, is passed just within the sphincter and normal saline solution allowed to run in. In my cases we have always used a tube and funnel, as the pressure can be regulated to a nicety, and we generally raise the funnel about two feet. Jacobi[1] recommends four to twenty inches; Holt[2] as much as four feet, which, though high, does not appear to have done any harm. Lichty[3] says there is no fear of rupture of the bowel, since the rectum will expel the water after a certain pressure is obtained. As the sigmoid flexure becomes distended the catheter may be inserted further, the folds of that part of the bowel becoming opened. How far the fluid will reach will depend on the pressure, but little difficulty will be found in reaching the ileo-cæcal valve or even higher. Records of it reaching the stomach must be received with caution, if not scepticism. Ssokolow[4] points out that over-distension of the rectum will lead to expulsive efforts and prevent the fluid reaching higher parts, and he was able in 103 patients out of 200 experimented on to pass water through the valve. Lavage of the small intestine is not however desired, as the peristalsis produced by the evacuation of the fluid will stimulate the small intestine to expel its contents. When about a pint or thirty ounces has been passed into the bowel of an eighteen months child, Kerley[5] advises that the solution should be allowed to run in and out at the same time, but the tube should not be passed in more than nine inches. I have employed a double catheter in irrigation, stopping up the escape one till I wished to allow the escape to begin. Hubbard[6] breaks the connection with the funnel and catheter when the baby begins to strain, and allows the outflow to pass through the catheter.

The **fluids employed** are: normal saline solution, salt solution 1 in 7,000 (Jacobi), boric acid .5 per cent. (Dawson Williams and Ashby), boiled water (Mercier), HCl solution 1 per cent. (Grimm), sulpho-naphthol (Hubbard); but the first mentioned appears to work quite satisfactorily. Starch solution is recommended if there is much inflammation, and Thomson[7] says that American authors advise leaving in the bowel 15 to 20 grains of tannic acid to render inert soluble peptones. The amount of fluid used is generally about two quarts, but as the excess escapes even larger quantities than that may be used.

[1] *Loc. cit.*   [2] *Therap. Gaz.*, 1899, xxiii. 512.   [3] *Med. News*, 1898, lxxii. 496.
[4] *Jahrb. f. Kinderh* , 1894, xxxviii. 186 ; abstract in *Am. J. M. Sc.*, 1895, cix. 481
[5] *N. York M. J.*, 1898, lxviii. 145.
[6] *Arch. Pediat* , 1899, xvi. 263.
[7] *Clinical Examination and Treatment of Sick Children*, 1898, p. 281.

Irrigation should be the first means of attack, being employed as soon as the patient is seen, and may be repeated every two hours till all toxic material is removed from the bowel. No purgatives need be given, no astringents, and sedatives such as opium are contra-indicated, as they prevent the peristaltic action of the small intestine which is necessary to push on the materials there. In fact, as Jennings[1] says, "with the thorough use of water internally and externally, opium and other sedative and astringent drugs will rarely be necessary;" while Holt[2] says it is "of more value than anything else we can do for these cases," and Graham[3] describes it as "an absolute necessity," and declares that "many cases are undoubtedly lost through a failure to appreciate their usefulness." In the face of such strong statements as these, it is remarkable how little English physicians appear to have adopted this line of treatment, which is at the same time effective and simple.

BERTRAM M. H. ROGERS.

Reviews of Books.

Dictionary of Medical Terms (English—French). By H. DE MÉRIC. Pp. vi., 394. London: Baillière, Tindall and Cox. 1899.

The average Englishman's knowledge of the French language, consisting for the most part of an imperfect acquaintance with a few classical authors, is of little value to him in the practice of medicine. We remember well when a few years ago attending a child with croup how great we found the difficulty in explaining to the French parents the use of a steam-kettle. M. de Méric has come to the rescue of those who suffer embarrassment in speaking or reading medical French. This English-French dictionary includes many terms derived from the cognate sciences as well as those belonging to medicine proper, and is especially rich in the matter of surgical terms. An exceedingly useful book has been added to our lexicographical store.

George Harley, F.R.S. Edited by Mrs. ALEC TWEEDIE. Pp. xii., 360. London: The Scientific Press, Limited. 1899.

The life of Dr. George Harley was no ordinary one; he was a pioneer in various branches of scientific work. The story of his life and work is told by his daughter, and a most interest-

---

[1] *Therap. Gaz.*, 1899, xxiii. 589.
[2] *Loc. cit.*　　[3] *Therap. Gaz.*, 1899, xxiii. 517.

ing volume has thus been given to the world. Her hero appears naturally as a wonderful man, learned in a variety of subjects— *nihil tetigit quod non ornavit*—nevertheless he was a somewhat disappointed man, inasmuch as " success and failure lie not in what a person has done, but in what he hoped to do." As a physician he was twice a partial success, as a man of science he was always in the front : he had, however, many difficulties to overcome ; ill health overtook him when still quite young, and all his hopes in life were blasted by a severe attack of glaucoma, which necessitated complete retirement from work for a period of over two years. He was a man of many sides, and " hobbies were his solace and his joy." These hobbies are the points by which he will be usually remembered, but they must not make us forget the solid foundation of scientific knowledge on which his work was built.

As a charming companion, a mine of curious information on many out-of-the-way subjects, an excellent story-teller, and a ready speaker, he had a personality which greatly endeared him to a large circle of friends and patients : to those, and to others, the book is one which will give much pleasure, inasmuch as it can be characterised as a biographical and literary success.

***

A Junior Course of Practical Zoology. By the late A. Milnes
   Marshall, M.D., F.R.S., and the late C. Herbert Hurst,
   Ph.D. Fifth Edition. Revised by F. W. Gamble.
   Pp. xxxv., 486. London : Smith, Elder, & Co. 1899.

Owing to the early death of Dr. Hurst, following as it did so comparatively shortly after that of Dr. Milnes Marshall, the task of bringing out the fifth edition of this well-known and valuable work has fallen to Mr. Gamble. No new figures have been added, and, as is mentioned in the preface, the alterations in this latest edition are mainly in the introductory chapters on technique, which have been recast. A word of special praise should be given to the index, which is admirable in its completeness.

***

Kirkes' Hand-Book of Physiology. By W. D. Halliburton,
   M.D., F.R.S. Fifteenth Edition. Pp. xx., 872. London :
   John Murray. 1899.

Because it is especially distinguished by the fact that it treats of histology as well as physiology proper, and because the book is popular with the student, a new edition has become necessary after many short intervals, the last only a little over two years. The fourteenth edition was practically a new book, retaining the old form and scope of the previous work ; the fifteenth incorporates all the important facts which have been since discovered, but with little alteration otherwise. The illustrations throughout the book are exceedingly good, and more especially those on the nervous system.

A Clinical Text-Book of Medical Diagnosis. By OSWALD VIERORDT, M.D. Authorized translation by FRANCIS H. STUART, M.D. Fourth American Edition, from the Fifth German. Pp. 603. London: The Rebman Publishing Co. (Ltd.). Philadelphia: W. B. Saunders. 1898.

A veritable mine of information on all points in medical diagnosis, this book is one of the best which has yet been written on the subject. To become an accomplished diagnostician is the aim of every physician: the particular purpose of this work is to furnish the physician with the material by which he may attain his object. "The foundation of a correct diagnosis must rest upon a careful examination of the individual organs, and then a study of the whole organism, the totality of the picture of the disease." We are somewhat surprised to find that the centrifuge is not mentioned for the examination of blood.

It is impossible within any ordinary limits to give an adequate idea of the merits of this volume, which should be not only in the hands of every clinical clerk, but should also be the cherished and oft-used possession of every one upon whom rests the responsibility of medically treating sick persons.

Encyclopædia Medica. Under the General Editorship of CHALMERS WATSON, M.B. Vol. I.—*Abdomen to Bone*. Pp. vi., 579. Edinburgh: William Green & Sons. 1899.

The fifty articles of this volume are written by almost as many well-known physicians and surgeons of Edinburgh, Manchester, London, Birmingham, Bristol, Aberdeen, Leeds, Dundee, Dublin, Rome, Strathpeffer, and Montreal. The whole work is intended to be a complete and authoritative library, covering the entire field of general medicine and surgery, midwifery, diseases of children, eye, ear, and throat, public health, tropical diseases, &c., and it is expected that this encyclopædia "will become the generally accepted work of general reference by the profession." These are the days of encyclopædias: it is difficult for the busy practitioner to form a complete reference library in any other way than by providing himself with some such work as this or a combination of them.

There is neither introduction nor preface to this volume, but we learn from a circular which was issued before the publication of the work that it will be complete in twelve volumes, which will be published quarterly, and "it is intended to keep it up to date by the issue from time to time, and at a small cost, of a supplementary volume, and along with it a simple and original device in the shape of gummed printed marginal notes."

As regards the articles themselves, it is difficult to select any for especial criticism : there must be some inequality as regards the different subjects—*e.g.*, the whole subject of antipyretics is dismissed in about three pages, whereas blackwater fever occupies ten. Anthelmintics are dismissed in less than a page, and chloroform is not mentioned as a vermifuge. The article on Balneology, by Dr. Fortescue Fox, is very full, comprising some twenty-seven pages, but we are not surprised to observe that our local Spa has not yet earned a right to the distinction of a reference. The articles on Alcohol, Alcoholic Insanity, and Alcoholism are full ones. They are written by Dr. William Ewart and Dr. George Wilson; they extend to thirty-one pages, and are an excellent epitome of the use and abuse of alcohol in health and disease. Mr. Stanley Boyd gives thirty-two pages on Aneurysm, and Dr. Dreschfeld an additional seven pages on Abdominal Aneurysm; a third article on Aneurysm and Dilatation of the Thoracic Aorta, by Dr. Graham Steell, extends to ten pages, so that we have in all nearly fifty pages on the important subject of aneurysm, which, much to our surpise, is not elucidated by a single diagram or illustration of any kind. The article on the Physiology and Clinical Investigation of Blood is by Dr. T. H. Milroy, who gives a condensed epitome in twenty pages of everything needful to the understanding of the varieties of anæmia described by Dr. G. Lovell Gulland.

Dr. James Swain writes on Injuries of the Abdomen, and deals in an interesting way with injuries to the various abdominal viscera and the methods of treating such injuries. He also writes on Traumatic Peritonitis and on Abdominal Abscess.

The important subject of Anæsthesia is considered in four sections. Dr. Dudley Buxton writes on the Physiology of Anæsthetics, and on Minor Anæsthetics, while Chloroform and Ether are written on respectively by Dr. Alexander Ogston and Mr. Pridgin Teale ; the latter writes with all his well-known enthusiasm on the subject of ether and its superiority over chloroform, but he apparently still uses it without the preliminary administration of nitrous oxide, for he makes no mention of this, but refers the reader to the chapter on Minor Anæsthetics for any account of this now universal preliminary to the administration of ether.

The article on Appendix Vermiformis is by Mr. F. J. Shepherd, of Montreal, who deals with the subject of appendicitis in an eminently judicial spirit. He says very truly that in acute cases it is always better to operate if one is in doubt, for early operations are comparatively safe, and he

24

has never repented having operated too early, but has been sorry in many cases that operation had been postponed until too late.

The article on Auditory Nerve and Labyrinth is by Dr. Dundas Grant, who writes with his usual clearness on the various tests for nerve-deafness, as well as on the different varieties of the affection. The first volume ends with an important chapter on Diseases of Bone, by Mr. Alexis Thomson, who gives an excellent account of the bacterial forms of bone-disease, such as tubercle and syphilis, and a brief account of the tumours of bone; other diseases of bone, such as rickets, scurvy, &c., are to be dealt with under their special headings.

Dr. Chalmers Watson is to be congratulated on having secured the help of so many eminent men in his colossal undertaking. The "literature" appended to some of the articles strikes us as meagre. The book is very sparsely illustrated. Achondroplasia has one not very informing process-block; there are three illustrations of anæsthetic apparatus; a diagram in each of the articles on Antipyretics and Aphasia; some small woodcuts illustrating ligature of arteries and artificial limbs; an excellent plate of urinary calculi, and a coloured picture of normal blood.

A System of Medicine. By Many Writers. Edited by Thomas Clifford Allbutt, M.D., F.R.S. Vol. VI. Pp. x., 944. London: Macmillan and Co., Limited. 1899.

Nearly half of this volume deals with the diseases of the circulatory system, continued from the fifth. Dr. G. Newton Pitt gives a very complete account of the right-sided valvular diseases, and Sir R. Douglas Powell of angina pectoris. His well-known division of angina into the two varieties, the vaso-motor and the graver form, including both the secondary and the primary cardiac angina, is now usually accepted as authoritative. Dr. Frederick T. Roberts follows with nearly a hundred pages on diseases of the mediastinum and thymus gland, with intrathoracic growths and tumours.

The article on Thrombosis by Professor Welch, of Baltimore, occupies some seventy pages, and is quite a noteworthy addition to the literature of the subject; that on Embolism is a little shorter, but is also a complete and very comprehensive monograph; it is of interest that "in the great majority of cases, fat-embolism is entirely innocuous . . . it is only in the comparatively rare instances of extensive fat-embolism that effects of any consequence are produced" (pp. 258-9). A short article on Phlebitis is by Mr. H. H. Clutton; and that on Arterial Degenerations and Diseases is by Dr. F. W. Mott. The veteran Professor Sir W. T. Gairdner writes an article of ninety pages on Aneurysm of the Aorta, in which he states that "we have in iodide of potassium a remedy which ought to be carefully and deliberately employed in most, if not in all, cases of aneurysm of the aorta." A short account, by Dr. H. D. Rolleston, of Aneurysms of Arteries in the Abdomen and of Diseases of the Lymphatic Vessels concludes this portion of the volume.

Four chapters on Diseases of the Muscles include myositis, myotonia congenita, idiopathic muscular atrophy and hypertrophy, and facial hemi-atrophy and hemihypertrophy. Then follows a chapter on the General Pathology of the Nervous System by Dr. W. Bevan Lewis, giving a succinct description of the modern conception of the neuron and the neuronic system, and pointing out "that the morphological unity of the neuron and the doctrine of contiguity rather than continuity of related neurons, favour a strict limitation of degenerative changes, arising in a nerve chain, to the individual neuron affected." Dr. Sherrington describes Tremor, " Tendon - Phenomenon," and Spasm, of which the physiological basis "is a compound reaction from two integrated tissues of the body—the nervous and the muscular." These two factors are considered in detail as a preliminary to the clinical and pathological section by Dr. Seymour J. Sharkey. Chapters follow on Trophoneuroses, including the Neurotrophic Affections of Bones and Joints; the Neurotrophic Diseases of Soft Tissues; Adiposis Dolorosa; Raynaud's Disease; and Erythromelalgia. These chapters are very complete, and introduce a great variety of interesting topics relating to the pathology of many obscure affections.

Further chapters on diseases of the nervous system and of the spine conclude the sixth volume of a work which well repays careful study, and which is rapidly approaching completion.

A Manual of Diseases of the Nervous System. By Sir W. R. Gowers, M.D., F.R.S. Third Edition. Vol. I.—*Diseases of the Nerves and Spinal Cord.* Pp. xvi., 692. London : J. & A. Churchill. 1899.

Sir W. R. Gowers's *Manual of Diseases of the Nervous System* is so well known and widely appreciated, that this third edition of his first volume will be read with much interest. At the same time in the case of a book that is so well recognised as a standard and trustworthy authority on the subject and as a model of clear exposition it is superfluous to do more than indicate the differences from the previous editions. Dr. James Taylor is associated with Sir W. R. Gowers as joint-editor of this volume. As was inevitable the book is enlarged, and is well abreast of the advances made in the neurology of the nerves and spinal cord since the last edition. A new chapter is added which gives an excellent summary of the changes made during the last few years in our conceptions of the constitution of the

Nervous System and their bearing on its physiology and pathology. The section on Neuritis has been extended; and there are separate sections on Beri-beri and Herpetic Neuritis. In tabes dorsalis a positive history of syphilis or of a hard chancre was obtained in 77 per cent. of private patients, and it is stated that in less than 10 per cent. can syphilis be excluded with confidence. There is a good account of sclerosis of the cord from toxic blood states, which includes Pellagra, and is illustrated by some excellent figures. The account of the muscular dystrophies and idiopathic muscular atrophies is very full and good; the peroneal form of amyotrophy, with its tendency to affect more than one member of a family, has for a sub-title "Neuritic Muscular Atrophy," and the evidence for regarding the disease as due to a "peripheral neuritis, motor or total, of extremely chronic course and peculiar origin" is discussed.

Enough has been said to show that the book, whilst retaining those features which have made it such an admirable guide to practitioners and students in the past, contains in this new edition much added matter of value. We must not omit to mention the appendix dealing with the muscle spindles.

Sanatoria for Consumptives. By F. Rufenacht Walters, M.D. Pp. xviii., 374. London: Swan Sonnenschein & Co., Lim. 1899.

This book comprises "a critical and detailed description, together with an exposition, of the open-air or hygienic treatment of phthisis," with an introduction by Sir Douglas Powell, who points out that "the chief object of the author is to advocate the establishment in this country of public institutions of the convalescent hospital class, and of sanatoria designed for the reception of cases of tuberculosis from amongst those who are more or less well-to-do." The usefulness of such institutions "extends far beyond the immediate purpose for which they are proposed," inasmuch as "lessons in self-management are learned by those who sojourn for a time in such sanatoria . . . and these persons when they pass again into the general community become centres of instruction in domestic hygiene." The author remarks that "up to recent times England had probably done more to reduce phthisical mortality than any other country; but she is now being outstripped in the race by several others" where "public opinion . . . both lay and medical, is overwhelmingly in favour of the sanatorium system."

This is one of the first attempts to present a general review of the subject in English; the first 82 pages give a general *résumé* of considerations regarding climates, sites for sanatoria, construction, cleansing, disinfection, diet, and general management. An enquirer naturally turns for information to the chapter on results, and it is claimed that the percentage of improvement from sanatorium treatment in different parts of the world varies from 50 to 90 as compared with only 20 to 30 in the Brompton Hospital. It is very difficult to draw any conclusions from statistics compiled by various persons adopting different standards, in a disease subject to so much spontaneous variation as phthisis; but the general average shows a well-marked difference in favour of sanatorium rather than any kind of climatic treatment.

A review of the various sanatoria of the world occupies some 280 pages: these have been compiled with care, and appear to be fairly accurate. It is shown that there is a great need for the increase and extension of such institutions in this country, inasmuch as "Professor v. Leyden estimates that if each consumptive has three months' treatment, there should be one bed for every 1000 inhabitants."

The author concludes his interesting survey with the following paragraph :—" The establishment of various societies for the suppression of tuberculosis, one of them under most distinguished patronage, is but one of many signs that Great Britain is at last waking from her satisfied slumbers, and preparing to again take her place in the van of the nations. Our country's sanitary past has been great and fruitful; and there is every reason to hope that with growing consciousness of the possibility of destroying this dread scourge of humanity, by the abolition of town smoke, the improvement of our dwellings, the better ventilation of rooms and streets, the admission of sunshine into our midst, the inculcation of more rational habits of life, the destruction of sputa, the erection of sanatoria, and in many other ways, she will gradually prepare for herself a still more great and glorious future."

The bibliography extends to nine closely printed pages.

The Surgical Anatomy of the Lymphatic Glands. By Cecil H. Leaf, M.B. Pp. 72. Westminster [London] : Archibald Constable & Co. 1898.

The object of the author has been to indicate, by a series of diagrams with descriptive text, the position of the main groups of lymphatic glands in the human body, and to show the important bearing of this in surgical practice.

In his introductory remarks he draws attention to the great value of passing an excessive quantity of formalin solution (one in seven of water) under a very high pressure into the cadaver, to prepare it for the dissection of the lymphatic vessels. The solution escaping into the tissues hardens and dries up the fat in which the lymphatic vessels are embedded, and also hardens the walls of the vessels themselves, rendering their subsequent dissection easy. Using this method, Mr. Leaf demonstrated in one instance an afferent lymphatic vessel partly terminating in an inguinal gland and partly, by a branch, in a vein; and in another instance an efferent lymphatic from an inguinal gland terminated directly in a vein. These observations are of great interest, and it is important to determine if such communications between lymphatics and veins are common throughout the body.

The positions of the lymphatic glands, in all parts, are clearly shown in eighteen full-page illustrations. These are coloured, and from the point of view of clearness leave nothing to be desired. In the text the author gives a concise description of the position of the glands, taking them in groups.

The book well fulfils the aim of its author, and we cordially recommend its study to those interested in this branch of anatomy. We should like to see in another edition some of the blemishes removed, which are either the fault of the proof reader or the result of a slip-shod style. Instances are to be seen in the sixth line of page 25, in line five of page 30, and in line fourteen of page 41.

A Manual of Surgical Treatment. By W. Watson Cheyne, M.B., F.R.S., and F. F. Burghard, M.D. Part I. Pp. xiv., 285. London: Longmans, Green and Co. 1899.

A thorough knowledge of the nature of a disease we have to treat is essential, but our great aim is always to treat the patient in the best possible way. It is so easy to read of the treatment of a case in a text-book of surgery, but it is very difficult when we have to treat a case to determine which of several methods—all recommended by competent surgeons— shall be employed, or even whether there is any real evidence to show that any method of treatment is of value. It is not so much to assist us in deciding which plan of treatment to choose that the authors have written this work, as to give us the full details of the methods which they would themselves employ. This is very important. When we are engaged in active practice we need minute directions to which the mere student would pay but little heed.

In this volume those subjects are considered which would occupy the early chapters of a text-book of surgery—Inflammation, Abscess, Syphilis, Tumours, &c., &c. Dr. Silk contributes a very able article on the administration of anæsthetics. As an instance of the way in which information is given as to details, we would refer to the directions for the electrolysis of nævi. In the treatment of wounds we have a very trustworthy guide to antiseptic surgery. Many of the chapters are like those by Mr. Watson Cheyne in Treves's *System of Surgery*, only the question of treatment receives so much more attention and the details of the methods advised are given at length.

We heartily commend this book, and feel sure that the possession of the work in its complete form of six volumes will be of very great value to the busy general practitioner, as

well as a help to the surgical specialist. The book is dedicated
to Lord Lister, and there could not be a more fitting dedication,
for, as all who know Mr. Watson Cheyne's work will readily
believe, the methods recommended by the author are just those
which the application of the great Listerian principles would
suggest.

Atlas and Epitome of Operative Surgery. By Dr. Otto
Zuckerkandl. Edited by J. Chalmers DaCosta, M.D.
Pp. 395. London: The Rebman Publishing Co. (Ltd.)
Philadelphia: W. B. Saunders. 1898.

Intended as an elementary guide for students, this work,
though written in a clear style and in most respects embodying
the present knowledge of its subject, would have been more
valuable if the description of some of the operations had been
less scanty: its pages abound with illustrations, of which the
coloured plates are very clear and well executed; some of the
woodcuts however might, in a later edition, be improved or
omitted. Some English names appear in the text, but our
vanity is a little upset by the omission of many which we think
are of world renown.

We do not often now use the old sliding artery forceps as
mentioned under amputations; their place has been taken by
the more convenient catch forceps, which are applied to the
vessel much more easily: the buried suture ought to have been
noticed in this chapter. We are so imbued with the usefulness of
the aneurysm needle in ligation of vessels, that we think it might
be mentioned in describing these operations. In performing the
operation of temporary division of the lower jaw, it would be well
to impress on the student the importance of drilling the holes
for the metallic sutures before the jaw is sawn through. The
mode of introducing the sutures for holding each half of a
Murphy button in place in the divided intestine is certainly not
the best; the sutures ought to be shown as going over the raw
edge of the bowel. We should like to see in the pages devoted
to catheterisation some instructions concerning the disinfection
of the surroundings of the meatus, and also of the catheter, as
want of this attention leads sometimes to disaster. The portion
of the work devoted to plastic surgery is excellent, and the
illustrations here are all that could be desired.

The Surgical Complications and Sequels of Typhoid Fever. By
William W. Keen, M.D. Pp. 386. London: The
Rebman Publishing Co., Ltd. 1898.

This book is a monument of patient and laborious research.
It contains in the form of an appendix a reprint of the author's
" Toner Lecture " delivered in 1876, " On the Surgical Compli-

cations and Sequels of the Continued Fevers," and in addition it contains the substance of a lecture delivered by the author in 1896, or just twenty years after the former lecture, embracing the literature on the subject which had accumulated during the interval—an important interval for such a topic, inasmuch as it introduced the discovery of the typhoid bacillus of Eberth, and the development of modern surgery in respect to opening the abdomen for the relief of perforations and other lesions arising in the course of typhoid fever. The author, in conjunction with Dr. Thompson S. Westcott, has collected no less than 1700 cases, which practically include nearly all the cases recorded in the last fifty years, and he expresses his obligation to the gentlemen in charge of the library of the Surgeon General's Office, U.S.A., for placing at his disposal "the treasures of that unrivalled collection. . . . The enlightened and liberal management of that library has made the whole world debtors to America," and such books as the one before us would be impossible without such an institution.

Dr. Keen commences with a good account of the pathology of typhoid fever, sufficiently full to show its bearing from the surgical side; thus such subjects as the viability of the typhoid bacilli both outside and inside the human body, and their wide diffusion in various organs and tissues of the body, are fully considered. He next describes in full detail the various surgical complications, such as affections of the bones, joints, blood-vessels and other organs, gangrene, abscesses, and, chief of all, perforations of the intestine and gall-bladder. In the case of perforations of the intestine, he gives a table of 83 operations, collected by Dr. Westcott for this work. Of these 83 cases, 16 recovered, or 19.36 per cent. of cures and 80.64 per cent. of deaths. When this is contrasted with Murchison's figures of 90 to 95 per cent. of deaths after perforation without operation, we may (as Dr. Keen remarks) well take courage for the future.

This book will certainly be the standard work on the subject for some years to come. It has evidently been prepared with great care and attention to detail, and should be studied by all surgeons who are liable to be called upon to treat complications occurring during or after typhoid fever.

An Experimental Research into Surgical Shock. By GEORGE W. CRILE, M.D. Pp. 160. Philadelphia: J. B. Lippincot Company. [1899.]

A brief enumeration of the theories on the subject of surgical shock forms the introduction to this essay, which was awarded the Cartwright Prize for 1897. Then, after a description of the apparatus used, over one hundred and thirty experiments, carried out for the most part on dogs, are detailed. In these experiments cannulas were fixed into various arteries, and the blood pressure estimated after injuries of every conceivable description were inflicted on almost every tissue and organ of the body. Following on the record of the experiments is a summary of the results of these injuries on the various parts affected. Some well-known facts as to the causes, prevention, and treatment of shock are then narrated. The final conclusion arrived at is that surgical shock is mainly due to impairment or break-down of the vaso-motor mechanism. The book repre-- sents a vast amount of labour, which is chronicled in a very elaborate and graphic manner by means of a large number of diagrams and charts.

A Manual of Bacteriology. By RICHARD T. HEWLETT, M.D. Pp. viii., 439. London: J. & A. Churchill. 1898.

There are several novel features in this book which will commend it to the student of bacteriology and to the clinician. The early chapters are devoted to the description of laboratory work, preparation of media, and the methods of cultivating and staining bacteria. There then follow detailed descriptions of the several varieties of pathogenic organisms. At the end of each chapter there is added a series of paragraphs on clinical diagnosis in which very full details are given of the methods to be pursued in taking cultures from the patient, and of the best ways of preparing and examining these cultures. The directions given are clear and concise, and we regard this new departure as one of great practical value.

It is satisfactory, too, to find space devoted to the bacteriology of such diseases as variola, conjunctivitis, diarrhœa, noma, otitis media, ozœna, rheumatoid arthritis, and syphilis. Chapters are also given to the hyphomycetes, the blastomycetes, and the protozoa. Under the first named group are described the ringworm and thrush parasites, together with minute directions for the preparation of cultures and microscopic specimens of these organisms. Mention is made of the pathogenic nature of certain of the blastomycetes and of their relationship to new growths. Recent investigations of Sanfelice in Italy, and of Russell and Plimmer in this country, would point to the cancer organism being included in this group; but we note that malignant disease is dealt with under the heading of diseases of uncertain etiology.

The information in the appendix relating to the nature and preparation of antitoxins and vaccines is full and abreast of present knowledge. The book is excellent throughout; the only alteration which we could have wished for is a fuller description of the microscopic appearances of the various organisms. For instance, the Klebs-Löffler bacillus is described as " a small delicate bacillus with rounded ends," a description which is not calculated to facilitate the recognition of many or indeed the majority of forms met with.

An American Text-Book of Gynecology. Edited by J. M.
BALDY, M.D. Second Edition. Pp. xxii., 17-718.
London: The Rebman Publishing Co. (Ltd.). Phila-
delphia: W. B. Saunders. 1898.

Of the manner of preparation and the subject matter of the
first edition of this work we have previously spoken in terms of
praise, and the appearance of the present edition bears testimony
to a general appreciation which is well bestowed.

Although the work has been rearranged to some extent,
there is no need to criticise it in detail. The main alterations
consist in fuller treatment of the chapters on the bladder, urethra
and ureters, hysterectomy, and plastic operations. The teach-
ings of its pages are thoroughly sound and well abreast of the
times, and we can confidently recommend the book as a guide
to the routine work of the gynæcologist. The illustrations as a
whole are good; but there are still some, such as Figs. 26 and
27, which might without loss be omitted in a future issue.

A Treatise on the Science and Practice of Midwifery. By W. S.
PLAYFAIR, M.D. Ninth Edition. Two volumes. Pp. xviii.,
446; xv., 454. London: Smith, Elder, & Co. 1898.

Evidence of the popularity of this standard work is proved
by the fact that yet another edition is added to those which
have already appeared. Its popularity is easily understood.
It is written in a very taking style, is well illustrated, and is
sufficiently dogmatic to be impressive to the student. The last
edition brings it into line with the latest research work done on
the subject, and contains many new and valuable facts.

The description of the structure and function of the placenta
is based upon the recent work done by Dr. Eden, and gives
several interesting and important observations carried out by
him. The subject is handled in a masterly manner. The
management of labour and its complications is dealt with as in
previous editions, and needs little comment: the author's well-
known sound teaching and correct deductions leave little scope
for the critic.

Two extremely interesting additions are introduced: one
is the account of the death of the Princess Charlotte—a most
impressive picture of the dangers of labour unduly prolonged
by reluctance of the attendants to interfere. The other
is an excellent criticism of a paper by Dr. Japp Sinclair, who
ascribed the present surgical aspect of gynæcology largely to
defective operative midwifery practice. Dr. Playfair brings
some excellent arguments to show that Dr. Sinclair's views are
at least exaggerated.

We notice that Dr. Playfair omits to mention the use of
veratrum viride in eclampsia, and rather discourages forced

delivery in these cases. His views on the latter subject are powerfully opposed by several first-class authorities, and the use of the drug named has been shown to be valuable.

There is one point to which we would take exception: Dr. Playfair advises that uterine irrigation should be carried out by means of a Higginson's syringe. We regard this as a most unfortunate piece of advice, as that instrument is likely to inject air, is difficult to clean, and necessitates the use of two hands; it is an inefficient, dirty, and dangerous instrument, fit only for the original purpose for which it was devised. Gravitation is the only sound method of uterine irrigation. Hayes's tube, which Dr. Playfair also recommends for intra-uterine injections, has the great defect of having no provision for the passage of the outflowing current from the uterus.

An American Text-Book of the Diseases of Children. By AMERICAN TEACHERS. Edited by LOUIS STARR, M.D., assisted by THOMPSON S. WESTCOTT, M.D. Second Edition. Pp. xvi., 604, 605–1244. London: The Rebman Publishing Co. (Ltd.). Philadelphia: W. B. Saunders. 1898.

Four years ago we had the pleasure of reviewing this excellent text-book on the diseases of children, when the first edition made its appearance. We have now before us the second edition, revised and enlarged. The old problem, whether a book containing twelve hundred pages should be published in one volume or two, appears to have been exercising the minds of the publishers, for this new edition, unlike its predecessor, appears in the latter form. Personally we have hitherto been in favour of the single volume wherever it was possible, but the far easier handling of the two volumes has in this instance at any rate almost converted us.

We remember, we trust now with regret, the reception, vigorous if curt as far as language was concerned, which we were from time to time apt to give to so-called *new* editions of medical books, when, with a belief born of inexperience that the newest treatment must of necessity be the best, we rushed to expend our hard-earned guineas, alas! only to find that our "new edition" contained nothing in addition to the old one, except perchance a few improvements in punctuation, a slight enlargement in the index, a fresh preface and a *later date*. The handsome work before us, however, is a "new edition" in the real sense of the word. The articles on typhoid fever, rubella, chicken pox, tuberculous meningitis, hydrocephalus, and scurvy have been entirely rewritten, whilst new articles appear on modified milk, lithæmia, and orthopædics, and more or less revision has been given to the chapters on infant feeding, measles, diphtheria, and cretinism. We are sorry to see, however, that the section on exercise and massage has been omitted from the new volumes, especially as we seem just now to be realising more than ever the value of physical exercise and the great importance of exercising and developing *all* the muscles of the body, and learning more and more about the use of massage, that great agent in "depriving rest of its evils."

In a book like that under consideration classification always presents a certain amount of difficulty, especially where diseases medical and surgical are considered in the same work. In this matter there has been some improvement, though the classification in the present volumes is by no means perfect. Tuberculosis and malaria have been quite rightly removed from their old places, and included in the section on infectious diseases; but we are puzzled to understand by what process of reasoning tracheotomy and intubation of the larynx are called "diseases of the respiratory system." We had hitherto looked upon them as methods either of relief or cure.

After these few adverse remarks, we feel that we should not be doing justice to this thoroughly trustworthy text-book if we did not call attention to one section that did not appear in the first edition. We allude to the admirable contribution on orthopædics by Dr. James E. Moore. It is contained in twenty-eight pages of text, well up to date, which are illustrated by some exceptionally good figures, of which we specially commend those representing congenital torticollis, early hip-joint disease, rachitic spine, and a little patient supporting his weight in the position so characteristic in dorsal Pott's disease. A large number of full-page plates, many of which are beautifully coloured, and a full and good index, complete two volumes which would make a valuable as well as handsome addition to the library of any medical practitioner.

A Treatise on "Unripe" Cataract. By WILLIAM A. M'KEOWN, M.D. Pp. 202. London: H. K. Lewis. 1898.

Dr. M'Keown draws attention to the length of time which is allowed to elapse before cataracts are pronounced to be ripe enough for operation. The difficulty of evacuating the lens cortex, after the nucleus has been removed, which always exists in immature and sometimes even in ripe cataracts, has especially engaged the attention of the author for many years, and has led him to devise methods for doing away with the necessity for this weary waiting. He denounces removal of the lens in its capsule, and any artificial maturation of it by massage, and regards extraction with iridectomy, or his method of injection and irrigation, as alone admissible. The various measures previous to and during operation are described in full. They do not appear to differ materially from the ordinarily accepted methods. He states, however, that cocaine is decomposed by boiling, and therefore he uses the solid hydrochlorate. He advocates in certain instances one of two special procedures. (1) Injection of a 1 per cent. saline solution inside the lens capsule by means of a fine syringe. The idea is to loosen the cortex, but it involves risk of rupturing the lens capsule and seems to have no very distinct advantage to recommend it. (2) Irrigation by introducing the point of a specially made nozzle into the lens capsule after the nucleus has been evacuated. The nozzle is connected by an indiarubber tube with a flask of saline solution held at a requisite elevation by a specially trained nurse. Statistics of 155 cases are given, and it must be said that the results are certainly good, and prove that in his hands the methods are harmless. It is, however, impossible to gather from his description the extent of immaturity of the lenses in question. Every detail of the procedure recommended is abundantly illustrated by the most beautifully executed drawings.

Atlas and Abstract of the Diseases of the Larynx. By Dr. L. Grünwald. Edited by Charles P. Grayson, M.D. London: The Rebman Publishing Co. (Ltd.). Philadelphia: W. B. Saunders. 1898.

This little volume is by no means an atlas of the diseases of the larynx pure and simple, but, as the American editor happily and very truly says in his preface, "it exemplifies a happy blending of the didactic and clinical;" for the remarkably faithful 107 coloured figures of the laryngoscopic and histological appearances of various conditions are associated with nearly 100 pages, having a concise and clear summary of the main points to be noted and their import. The full-page plates are accompanied with very full descriptions. To advanced students and practitioners the work will prove an extremely useful handbook.

A Primer of Psychology and Mental Disease. By C. B. Burr, M.D. Second Edition. Pp. ix., 116. Philadelphia: The F. A. Davis Company. 1898.

We seriously question whether it is requisite to give instruction in so peculiarly an abstract study as that of psychology to nurses and attendants, for whom this book has been written. So far, however, as this portion of the book is concerned, it matters perhaps but little whether the crude intelligence of the average nurse or attendant attacks it or not; on the whole, we should prefer a state of ignorance to that of mystification.

But when teaching on clinical insanity is attempted to this class of student, it is obvious that only well-considered and carefully-expressed statements should be made. As an instance of the failure to appreciate this, we may cite the assertion made at page 37, "In Mania there is no tendency to suicide." We can find nothing which serves to exclude puerperal mania, and, indeed, the only mention made of this condition is under the section of causation. Such an omission is serious. Again, under the head of what the author pleases to call "melancholia simple," acute and delusional forms are described, and the tendency to suicide is said to be strong. It is surely unwise not to qualify a statement which tends to oppress the nurse with needless responsibility in all degrees of melancholia alike. On the other hand we are informed that in melancholia with stupor there is not, as a rule, a tendency to suicide; this assertion betrays as much lack of caution as the previous one shows excess of it. The author speaks of dementia after mania and melancholia as a condition of temporary impairment : it is not wise to use this term loosely; dementia as properly understood implies an irrecoverable reduction in mind. Under the section, epileptic dementia, we meet with the truly surprising remark that just before, *during* (the italics are ours), or immediately following epileptic convulsions there are apt to be great mental confusion, irritability, and impulsiveness; this is as happily expressed as the statement in the next paragraph, that "epileptic patients are apt to be untidy, especially during convulsions"! Later on we learn that an objection to rest in bed is the danger of suicide.

It is not needful to quote further excerpts from this book; the author has not realised the great difficulties attending the production of a manual suitable for the nursing staff of an asylum, or grasped the necessity for sound and indisputable, even though brief, statements, and this want of careful purpose has gravely blemished a work which in many parts contains useful enough matter.

Atlas of Legal Medicine. By Dr. E. von Hofmann. Edited by Frederick Peterson, M.D., assisted by Aloysius O. J. Kelly, M.D. London: The Rebman Publishing Co. (Ltd.). Philadelphia: W. B. Saunders. 1898.

Since the publication of this work in Vienna, Dr. E. von Hofmann, well known to medico-jurists, has joined the great majority, and the present translation and Englished edition of his work has appeared since his death.

The work is exactly what it purports to be; it consists of 56 plates in colours, and 193 illustrations in black and white. The letterpress descriptions given with the plates are good, sufficient, and to the point. The illustrations, with only one or two exceptions, are original, nor do they in any way repeat the usual stereotyped ones of the English books. They are excellently produced by process and in colour. Those in colour are worthy of all praise, and those that fail in any way owe their failure to the very great difficulty of the subject and not to the way in which the plate is produced. Plates 5—the respiratory organs and heart of a child at full term, 49—arsenical poisoning, and 54—*post-mortem* lividity, are particularly good. The plates illustrating the conditions of the hymen will prove most useful to the student who can have so little opportunity of practical knowledge on this point. The process plates of the ossification of the epiphyses of the lower extremities, (Figs. 79, 80), are most useful. We think that photographs of types of the insane and of idiots should have been given.

Instructive instances of the most important matters in medical jurisprudence are given. We trust our students will make good use of this excellent work.

The Animal as a Prime Mover. By R. H. Thurston. Pp. 297—338. Washington: Government Printing Office. 1898.—This is an essay, republished in separate form, from the Smithsonian Report for 1896. It deals with man from the point of view of a mechanic. The energy-value of the various food-stuffs is considered, then that of the various dietaries; and, subsequently, the various ways in which energy is dissipated from the body, such as muscular work. The vital machine is then compared and contrasted with other machines, and its efficacy discussed. Most of the facts brought forward are to be found in any standard work on physiology.

On the Study of the Hand for Indications of Local and General Disease. By Edward Blake, M.D. Pp. 53. London: Henry J. Glaisher. [1898.]—A considerable amount of interesting information is here given. The temperature, dryness, and moisture of the hand, its colour and texture, the varieties of nail development, the condition of the hand in various diseases, clubbed fingers, the varieties of perverted sensations, are all referred to in a manner that will bring home to the reader the utility of careful examination of the hands in the diagnosis of many diseases. Dr. Blake does not profess that this *brochure* touches much on the hand as a diagnostic factor in diseases of the nervous system, although he gives plates of the hand in acromegaly in the adult, in congenital cretinism, and in Mongol idiots, and he mentions the *main en griffe* of Duchenne. The shortening of the second phalanx of the little finger, with lateral displacement of the terminal phalanx, is interesting as being associated with certain forms of cretinism. Although fault may be found with the way in which this booklet is issued, it shows acute power of observation and cannot fail to be of use in clinical work.

Practical Uranalysis and Urinary Diagnosis. By Charles W. Purdy, M.D. Fourth Edition. Pp. xvi., 365. Philadelphia: The F. A. Davis Company. 1898.—The fact that is stated in the preface to this book, that three large editions of it have been exhausted in three years, and that it has been extensively adopted as a text-book in the United States, speaks for its value as a practical guide to the study of the urine.

This issue retains the essential features of the former editions, but has been thoroughly revised, and the chapters on the chemistry of the urine have been largely re-written, whilst a number of new illustrations have been added. It may be regarded as a trustworthy guide to the subject. We differ, however, from Dr. Purdy in his appreciation of the relative value of the clinical tests for albumin, and think the salicyl-sulphonic test might have been given. The book is well printed in excellent type, and the illustrations are good.

Observations on Cardio-Vascular Repair. By W. BEZLY THORNE, M.D. Pp. 26. London: J. & A. Churchill. 1898.— This paper, which was written for the 1898 meeting of the British Medical Association, deals with heart failure associated with arterial disease, and the therapeutic value of saline baths and exercises in such cases. Dr. Thorne adopts the view that defective metabolism of the body may cause disease of the arteries, and upon the vascular changes cardiac derangement may follow. Two skiagrams are given to show that the heart diminishes in size after resisted exercises. Although we believe, in some measure, in the therapeutic value of saline baths and exercises, the rapid diminution in the size of the heart does not appear to us to have been proved. We cannot see further evidence in these skiagrams. It appears to us that in the photograph in which the heart appears the smaller, there has been longer exposure to the X-rays.

On So-called Spasmodic Asthma. By ERNEST KINGSCOTE, M.B. Pp. 18. London: Henry J. Glaisher. 1899.—The author tells us that he is "engaged exclusively in the treatment of heart affections," and that he is "Physician in Ordinary to the Imperial Ottoman Embassy." We therefore conclude that the only maladies of the Sultan's official representatives in this country are cardiac—and this, to say the least, is extraordinary. Dr. Kingscote informs us that the effects of asthma "consist essentially in spasmodic contractions of the voluntary muscles of inspiration, and of the involuntary muscles which surround the bronchioles." Both these statements are misleading if not inaccurate. The next astonishing statement is, that "It is pretty generally conceded that the origin of asthma is to be found in the irritation of one or . . . many ramifications of the vagi; whether it be from . . . Meckel's ganglion . . . through the recurrent laryngeal . . . or through irritation of the . . . abdominal and pelvic viscera." From which it may be gathered that the author's knowledge of the anatomy and physiology of the vagus is not great. The author's "consideration of the amount of space taken up . . . by the enlarged heart" leads him to the conclusion that "the following may be instanced as direct effects of intermittent pressure." Of "the following" we may quote "brachial pain, due to perineuritis," "pain from perineuritis of the intercostals," "interference . . . through pressure on the thoracic duct," as not having a tittle of evidence in their favour. The main thesis of the paper is that a largely dilated heart, " say the size of a small football (not at all an unknown condition) . . . flops in the direction of gravity," and " can hammer " the vagus nerves on the bony spine and so cause asthma ! It has rarely been our misfortune to read such a tissue of unwarrantable inferences from clinical phenomena. The progress of medicine is retarded by such publications.

Golden Rules of Surgical Practice. By E. HURRY FENWICK. Fifth Edition. Pp. 71. Bristol: John Wright & Co. [1898.]— Many of these rules are undoubtedly valuable, and some are not to be found in ordinary text-books; but every now and again we find one of very doubtful worth, or which conveys very imperfect information. For instance, all the directions we find given for dealing with hemorrhage are, " Always tie both ends of a divided artery in a wound." This is most important; but, surely, we might have a few rules about venous bleeding and secondary hemorrhage. Again, we are told never to hesitate or delay in opening an abscess in the loin, due to rupture or injury of the kidney; but why hesitate or delay in opening any abscess in the loin? Then the author lays it down as a rule that we are not to open a collection of pus anywhere near a large artery without first using a stethoscope. The meaning of this rule is obscure. Probably the idea is that by excluding a *bruit* we may exclude the possibility that we have, not an abscess, but a ruptured or traumatic aneurysm to deal with; but we should not like to exclude this possibility because no *bruit* was present. Before we gave the book to a student we should like to have some rules removed and others more fully elaborated. But probably no surgeon would be quite satisfied with such a series of rules drawn up by any other surgeon, and there is certainly much useful information in this waistcoat-pocket booklet.

Drs. Harvey and Davidson's Syllabus of Materia Medica. By WILLIAM MARTINDALE. Tenth Edition. Pp. xvi., 64. London: H. K. Lewis. 1898.—This edition is rendered more valuable than its predecessors by having quantities and doses expressed in metric as well as in imperial measurement, thus going one step further in advance than the *British Pharmacopœia*. This small work is designed to assist students in getting up the subject of Materia Medica for examination, and to this end it is admirably adapted, being a classified epitome of the *B.P.*

The Treatment of Disease by Physical Methods. By THOMAS STRETCH DOWSE, M.D. Pp. xii., 412. Bristol: John Wright & Co. 1898.—This is a new edition of the author's work entitled *Lectures on Massage and Electricity in the Treatment of Disease*, and contains a fair account of the methods of massage and the use of electricity in the treatment of various diseases, but it lacks conciseness. Its bulk is due in large measure to mere padding; for

25

instance, there is an account of Latham's theories of the constitution of proteids, and a long *verbatim* report of several of Charcot's cases of hysteria. The book is full of such superfluous matter. One does not need sketchy and incomplete descriptions of every disease in which massage may be useful. By reason of this the work is far inferior to such a treatise as Murrell's on the same subject. Life is too short for one to read such a watered account of what after all is only one method of treatment.

The Erection of a Consumptive Sanatorium for the People. By Dr. NAHM. Translated by WILLIAM CALWELL, M.D. Pp. 52. Belfast: Mayne & Boyd. 1898.—The interest which has recently been aroused in England in the question of the open-air treatment of consumption makes it all the more needful that English physicians should be familiar with the practices which have existed in many health-resorts in Germany since the establishment of Brehmer's Curhaus at Görbersdorf in 1859. It seems now to be a fashionable doctrine that "we can create a local climate through the arrangement of the buildings," and hence that we should endeavour to carry out a climatic treatment of consumption in all countries, at any elevation and at any temperature. Surely the climatic question in the treatment of phthisis is dwindling down to something like vanishing point.

The Properties and Uses of Pure Glycerin. By M.D., M.R.C.S. Pp. 49. [1898.]—Some years ago, at a time when pure glycerine was not such a common commodity as at present, Price's Patent Candle Company issued a pamphlet intended to draw attention to the many applications of this useful substance to medicine and pharmacy. This has been re-written, and the origin, properties, and uses of glycerine are well reviewed in half-a-dozen brief chapters, concluding with a bibliography embracing the period 1854—1897.

The War with the Microbes. By E. A. DE SCHWEINITZ. Pp. 485—496. Washington: Government Printing Office. 1898.—Reprinted from the Smithsonian Report, this will serve a good purpose, as Dr. de Schweinitz gives a clear and popular account of the germ theory of disease and of the system of serum-therapeutics. Attention is first drawn to the living micro-organisms, and then to those chemical products known as ptomains, enzymes, and toxins, and the specific differences of these bodies are clearly explained. The nature and method of action of antitoxins are discussed, and the paper concludes with an enumeration of the useful purposes to which germ activity is now applied.

Golden Rules of Gynæcology. By S. JERVOIS AARONS, M.D. Pp. 63. Bristol: John Wright & Co. [1898.]—This is not a book to be recommended. Without the safeguard of experience, it is likely to be productive of more harm than good. Works of this kind are not needed. Students should not be allowed to acquire their knowledge after the methods here set forth, and to the expert and operating gynæcologist the book is an impertinence.

The Pocket Formulary for the Treatment of Disease in Children. By LUDWIG FREYBERGER, M.D. Pp. xv., 208. London: The Rebman Publishing Company, Limited. 1898.—There are included in this work many useful formulæ, but why the author has put the equivalents of the solid and not the liquid measures in the metric system does not appear to be very clear. The work is not merely a collection of prescriptions, but a sort of materia medica in brief, each drug having its properties, use, therapeutics, dose, and incompatibles clearly put. Useful hints are given how the taste of nauseous drugs may be disguised. It will be found a useful book.

Informes Rendidos por los Inspectores Sanitarios de Cuartel y por los de los Distritos al Consejo Superior de Salubridad, [1896], 1897. 2 vols. Mexico: Imprenta del Gobierno, en el ex-Arzobispado. 1898.—Previously to the year 1898 the city of Mexico, having a population of 350,000, was in a deplorably insanitary condition. There was no drainage, unless the open sewers in the town could be called so; the streets were polluted with every description of filth and garbage, and there was but little potable water. The natural consequence was that zymotic affections flourished unchecked, and the mortality from all causes reached the high figure of 58.6 per thousand. Of these the most formidable was typhus fever, which has been endemic in the city and neighbourhood since 1545, and in 1895 was responsible for nearly 2,000 deaths. Other diseases of the same class were proportionately fatal, notably smallpox and measles; but the former affection has not been so bad of late; because vaccination has been most effectually carried out, there being no conscientious objectors in Mexico. At last this heavy mortality attracted the attention of the authorities, and they determined to grapple with the difficulty: for this purpose the city was divided into eight wards, and a medical man and a sanitary inspector were appointed to make a house-to-house visitation in each and report to the Council of Health on the state of things in every district. They recommended *inter alia* that a system of underground drainage should be carried out in all parts, that a number of workmen should be regularly employed in keeping the streets in a proper sanitary condition, and that water should be brought from a distance, filtered, and distributed in pipes throughout the city.

Medico-Chirurgical Transactions. Vol. LXXXI. London: Longmans, Green and Co. 1898.—Such a deservedly high reputation belongs to the work of this society, that it is hardly necessary to do more than to say that this present volume contains many papers of great interest. Perhaps their chief characteristic is that they all deal with subjects of direct practical importance in medicine and surgery.

Transactions of the Medical Society of London. Vol. XXI. London: Harrison and Sons. 1898.—The present volume contains some interesting and important papers, among which we would especially notice Cases of Operation on Pancreatic Cysts, by Mr. Alban Doran, Dr. H. G. Rolleston, Mr. G. R. Turner, and Dr. J. D. Malcolm; also a paper on "Rectal Surgery," illustrated with numerous drawings, by Mr. Thomas Bryant. The reports on the discussions at the Society's meetings are, as usual, full and instructive.

Transactions of the Association of American Physicians. Vol. XIII. Philadelphia: Printed for the Association. 1898.— Medical subjects of present interest are dealt with in these papers, which uniformly maintain a high level of excellence, and represent a large amount of original work and observation. Exigencies of space forbid our discussion of individual papers, and we must be content with commending the book to the careful perusal of our readers. Many of the contributions are very well illustrated.

Transactions of the Michigan State Medical Society. Vol. XXII. Grand Rapids: Published by the Society. 1898.— The volume is an account of the thirty-third annual meeting of the Society, held at Detroit, and consequently contains papers and discussions on most branches of "medicine"— papers differing in merit, of necessity, but many of which can be read with interest and profit. The printing has not been carefully corrected. "Program" is an Americanism we do not mind accepting, as we already have "diagram," but not so with "French capitol" (p. 24), "hair lip" (p. 13), and "preperation" (p. 192). An amusing *lapsus* occurs on p. 13, where it is said of Celsus (who was not an American, or we should have thought less of it) that "in wounds of the intestines, he performed gastrorrhaphy."

Transactions of the South Carolina Medical Association. Charleston: Lucas & Richardson Co. 1898.—In the opinion of the President the general appearance of the *Transactions* could be greatly improved. That is so, and the proof-reading also; we noticed "Opthalmology" (pp. 3 and 7), "Diptheria" (p. 25), and "parisites" (p. 187). The book should have a cloth cover; and if the sheets must be wired, it should not be done through their sides. Among the many good papers in this record of the forty-eighth meeting we were specially attracted to one on "Serum Diagnosis of Typhoid Fever," by Dr. Robert Wilson, jun., who reflects the general opinion when he says that the Widal test is one the usefulness of which "no physician who lays claim to scientific attainment can afford to ignore."

The Transactions of the Edinburgh Obstetrical Society. Vol. XXIII. Edinburgh: Oliver and Boyd. 1898.—The valedictory address of Dr. Alexander Ballantyne, contained in this volume, makes a pleasing reference to Spencer Wells and to the general work of the Society during the present year. It is perhaps not unnatural that some remarks should have been made on professional secrecy, as the case of Kitson *v.* Playfair and Wife had recently been before the public, and the retiring president's words may be read with profit. Among the papers is one by Dr. John Moir, a veteran practitioner of 90 years, on the induction of premature labour, another by Dr. J. W. Ballantyne on a vitelline placenta in the human subject, and a description of a sireniform fœtus. The other communications are of great value.

Saint Thomas's Hospital Reports. Vol. XXVI. London: J. & A. Churchill. 1898.—Besides a number of papers dealing chiefly with cases of interest that have occurred in the hospital, there are the usual full reports of the medical and surgical sides and of the various special departments. A full abstract of cases of special importance is also given. Dr. Payne has a very interesting contribution on some old physicians of St. Thomas's Hospital, with portraits of Dr. Wharton and Dr. Mead. A new department for physical exercises has been added to the hospital, and should prove a very excellent departure, which might well be copied by other hospitals.

Tuberculosis. Vol. I., No. 1. October, 1899. London: 20 Hanover Square.—This modest-looking new journal, issued by the "National Association for the Prevention of Consumption and other forms of Tuberculosis," is destined to perform good service in disseminating the proceedings of the association. Sir Hermann Weber's views on the production and prevention of tuberculosis would alone give the journal every title to a friendly welcome.

Notes on Surgery for Nurses. By Joseph Bell, M.D. Fifth Edition. Pp. 194. Edinburgh: Oliver and Boyd. 1899.— The fifth edition of this useful book has been thoroughly revised, and will prove a valuable text-book for the nurses' library.

Case Paper. Designed by Drs. J. K. Couch and E. Le C. Lancaster. Bristol: John Wright & Co.—These papers are of the usual type, but with the advantage that they have at the back outline figures for all parts of the body. They are sold separately, or bound up in books of 250, indexed and numbered. For those who like forms for case-taking this one should be most convenient and useful.

Burdett's Hospitals and Charities. London: The Scientific Press (Limited). 1899.—This hardy annual is, as usual, brimful of useful information; but as we have said on previous occasions, we attach far more importance to the statistical tables

than the commentary upon them or the deductions drawn from
them.   Last year Sir Henry strongly advocated the payment of
medical men for their services at hospitals : this year the matter
is consigned to oblivion, and possibly wisely dropped ; but it is
replaced by the author's views on payments by patients, to
which he has been converted.   This is a feather in the cap of
Mr. Sidney Holland, of the London Hospital, who has always
supported this system ; but we should not be surprised if this
was next year replaced by some other plan for establishing our
hospitals on a more sound financial basis.   With regard to local
matters, we find no reference to the Bristol Hospital Sunday
Fund, which has been two years in existence on its present
basis.   We suggest to Sir Henry that he should apply for a
properly-audited balance-sheet of any institution included in his
annual, and that he should not be led away by the names of
titled people as patrons.

The International Directory of Booksellers and Bibliophile's
Manual.   Rochdale: James Clegg. 1899.—This is a carefully-
compiled work, containing in alphabetical order the names and
addresses of booksellers, publishers, book-collectors, etc., all
over the world.   There is other information, such as articles on
book-plates, copyright registry, sizes of books, etc.   The need
of such a book must be limited, but it will be found useful to
librarians and lovers of books.   The only relief from the
" seriousness " of the work is the " Book-Lover's Lexicon,"
wherein a few newly-coined words will be found.   The " book
borrower who carries off your choicest treasures and resents
any suggestion as to their return as the deadliest insult " may
be known to many of us, but there must be few who know
that such an one is correctly described as a " bibliopokomist."

Notes on Preparations for the Sick.

Bromidia.—BATTLE & Co., Saint Louis.—This hypnotic,
manufactured in Paris, is an excellent combination ready made
for those who cannot write a prescription or dispense one.   It
is composed of well-known drugs in convenient and palatable
combination, and it usually acts very efficiently in cases where
a chloral and bromide sedative is indicated.

Ferru-Cocoa.—FERRU-COCOA MANUFACTURING Co., London.
—A cocoa containing iron, kola nut, and malt is a combination
likely to be useful, not only to the anæmic girl, but to all varieties
of persons who require to be fit for any laborious occupation.

Soloids : Sodium Chloride; Sodium Chloride and Sodium Sulphate; Sodium Chloride Compound; Lead Subacetate; Lead and Opium.—BURROUGHS, WELLCOME & Co.—The sodium chloride preparations are intended for solution in sterilised water, and to be then used as intravenous injections. The advantages of having lead soloids in a portable form are obvious.

The "Alioné" Clothing.—ALIONÉ COMPANY, London.—These articles of clothing have been devised for the purpose of facilitating the dressing of infants and invalids without turning or disturbing them. The invalid night-dress can be opened at back, front, and sleeves.

The "Bella-Wattee Patent Teapot."—THE BELLA-WATTEE COMPANY, London.—This is so devised that, after a few minutes infusion, the leaves can be raised into the lid of the pot and there fixed quite clear of the liquid. The arrangement appears to be quite a success, and is well spoken of by those who have tried it.

MEETINGS OF SOCIETIES.

Bristol Medico-Chirurgical Society.

Annual Meeting, October 11th, 1899.

Dr. R. ROXBURGH, President, in the Chair.

The minutes of the last meeting having been read and confirmed, the President resigned the chair in favour of the President-elect, Mr. W. H. Harsant.

Mr. NELSON C. DOBSON moved, and Dr. J. E. SHAW seconded, a vote of thanks to the retiring president for the admirable manner in which he had conducted the presidential duties during his year of office. The resolution having been carried with acclamation, Dr. ROXBURGH replied.

The PRESIDENT then read his address, which will be found on pages 297—314, and at its conclusion Dr. A. J. HARRISON proposed, and Dr. SHINGLETON SMITH seconded, a vote of thanks to Mr. Harsant for his interesting address. This also was carried with acclamation.

The HON. SECRETARY (Mr. PAUL BUSH) read his Annual Report, which showed that there was a credit balance on the ordinary account of £85 : 19 : 6, as against £47 : 3 : 5 at the close of the previous session; and a balance in hand on the *Journal* account of £118 : 17 : 8, as against £103 : 9 : 4 for the year 1897. The large balance on the ordinary account was due to the receipt of £184 : 16 : 0 received for subscriptions, this sum being the largest amount ever received in one year.—The PRESIDENT moved, "That the report of the Hon. Secretary be adopted, and that he be thanked for his services." This was seconded by Mr. C. E. S. FLEMMING, and carried.

Dr. B. M. H. ROGERS, late Editorial Secretary of the *Journal*, read his report, which stated that in 1898 £224 : 16 : 11 had been received and £206 : 17 : 10 spent on the *Journal*, leaving a credit balance of £17 : 19 : 1.—Mr. A. W. PRICHARD proposed, "That the report be adopted, and that Dr. Rogers be thanked for his services." This was seconded by Mr. S. H. SWAYNE, and carried.

Mr. L. M. GRIFFITHS, on behalf of the Committee of the Bristol Medical Library, read a report which showed that, including 798 duplicates, the library of the Society contained 8,177 volumes. During the year 1,088 volumes were added, and 91 given to other libraries. The Society is in regular receipt of 188 periodicals. The names of donors and the attendances of the *Journal* Committee were read. The Bristol Medical Library, to which the members of the Society have access, contains 19,982 volumes and 224 current periodicals.—It was proposed by Mr. J. DACRE, and seconded by Mr. A. N. GODBY GIBBS, "That the report be adopted, and that Mr. Griffiths be thanked for his services." This was carried.

Dr. ROXBURGH proposed, and Mr. MUNRO SMITH seconded, Dr. D. S. Davies as President-elect. This was carried.

Dr. R. LANSDOWN proposed, and Dr. P. WATSON WILLIAMS seconded, the re-election of Mr. Bush as Hon. Secretary. This was carried.

Dr. SHINGLETON SMITH proposed, and Mr. L. M. GRIFFITHS seconded, that the six elected Members of the Committee be Dr. J. Michell Clarke, Mr. J. Dacre, Dr. B. M. H. Rogers, Mr. G. Munro Smith, Mr. James Taylor, and Dr. H. Waldo. This was carried.

Mr. BUSH proposed, and Dr. HARRISON seconded, that the representatives of the Society on the Committee of the Bristol Medical Library consist of Mr. L. M. Griffiths, Mr. G. Munro Smith, and Mr. J. Taylor. This was carried.

November 8th, 1899.

Mr. W. H. HARSANT, President, in the Chair.

The minutes of the last meeting were read and confirmed. Mr. L. W. Powell, Dr. A. S. Wohlmann, and Dr. J. Young were elected members of the Society.

Dr. W. H. C. NEWNHAM showed a specimen of ruptured tubal pregnancy from a woman aged 28. After taking some ecbolic medicine, procured from a chemist, vaginal hemorrhage commenced, and lasted for six days before the woman was brought to the General Hospital. The abdomen was opened and found full of bloodclot. Slight peritonitis was present. The operation was completed, but the patient never properly recovered from it, and died on the third day.— Dr. AUST LAWRENCE drew attention to the necessity of early diagnosis in these cases, and illustrated his remarks with certain cases. He asked Dr. Newnham's opinion on the drainage of the abdominal cavity, his own being against it if the case was seen early. He had known septic peritonitis to follow drainage, so that in future he would, after removal of the clot and such cleansing of the peritoneum as the patient's condition would allow, pour in saline fluid and suture up completely.—Mr. PAUL BUSH advocated rapid removal of the clot, as little manipulation and irrigation of the intestines as possible, and complete closure.—Dr. W. C. SWAYNE enquired if the abortion was the result of the medicine, as such drugs were, as a rule, only drastic purgatives. He advocated the use of normal saline fluid being left in the abdominal cavity.—The PRESIDENT referred to the necessity of early diagnosis, but admitted that in many cases this was very difficult. —Dr. NEWNHAM, in reply, said that in this case the symptoms were not so severe as they usually are in ruptured tubal pregnancies, and his belief was that the escape of blood was slow. He questioned whether blood could remain six days in the abdominal cavity without becoming infected from the intestines. He used saline irrigation, and did not drain, and in his opinion the drug was not the cause of the abortion.

Dr. T. FISHER read a paper on œdema of the eyelids, with intermittent albuminuria, in children. He had recently seen some debilitated children in whose urine he found traces of albumin at times. In some of them he obtained a history of œdematous eyelids, but in others was not able to do so. Transient albuminuria is found in dyspepsia and in other conditions in children, but it does not seem to affect their health in some cases.—Dr. H. WALDO asked Dr. Fisher's view of the prognosis in these cases.—Dr. B. M. H. ROGERS said swelling of the eyelids was by no means an uncommon thing with children quite apart from albuminuria, and that albumin was often present at times when there was no œdema or swelling of the eyelids.—Dr. F. H. EDGEWORTH asked if there were any signs of arterial degeneration in these cases, any casts or albumose in the urine.—Dr. G. PARKER said many cases of albuminuria were due to the circulation of toxins in the blood of children; the same conditions did not occur in adults. He referred to Henoch's purpura and Quincke's œdema, and other causes of œdema in children.—Dr. MARKHAM SKERRITT said he had seen albumose precede serum-albumin, and chronic renal disease develop subsequently. Had Dr. Fisher found albumose without serum-albumin?— Dr. MICHELL CLARKE did not think these cases very uncommon, particularly when the twelve o'clock urine was examined. A saline caused disappearance of the albumin. He doubted the existence of " physiological albuminuria," and considered examination of the vascular system very important.—Mr. C. H. WALKER said he had often been told in the eye department that swelling of the eyelids was present in children in the morning, but he thought it was often a maternal imagination. He found no changes in the fundus in these cases.—Dr. SHINGLETON SMITH thought intermittent albuminuria was a disease, and he did not accept the theory of physiological albuminuria.—Dr. FISHER, in reply, said he did not only rely on parents' statements, as he had seen the œdema himself. He had not tested for albumose or examined for casts, and in only one case had he found vascular changes. He did not believe crying produced œdema of the lids, though it did swelling.

Dr. MICHELL CLARKE read the notes of two sporadic cases of cerebro-spinal fever, aged 10 and 19 respectively. In the former the illness lasted eight days; in the latter only forty-eight hours, and in this case was ushered in by a general epileptiform convulsion. There were herpes labialis, high and irregular fever, delirium, and the usual symptoms of cerebro-spinal fever in each; in addition, a marked feature of the illness was the pronounced restlessness. Death was preceded by coma. Necropsy in each case showed the presence of a bright yellow exudation over the pia mater, especially over the convexity of the cerebral hemispheres and the dorso-lumbar region of the cord. Cultures from this exudation showed in each case the presence of Weichselbaum's diplococcus, and in the second case the pneumococcus also. The brain and cord from one case were also shown. He also described a case of posterior basic meningitis in a child, which, after an illness of eight weeks duration, ended in recovery. Retraction of the head was very marked in this case.—Dr. CECIL WILLIAMS recalled four cases of cerebro-spinal meningitis occurring during an epidemic of influenza in Wales in 1891.—Dr. H. WALDO thought hydrocephalus a valuable symptom, so that frequent measurements of the head should be made.—Dr. T. FISHER showed some sketches of cases of posterior basal meningitis, to show the retraction of the head. —The PRESIDENT thought it very difficult to differentiate between those due to middle-ear disease and simple basal meningitis. Would lumbar puncture assist?—Dr. CLARKE replied that the fever in septic cases would be higher, and there would be rigors; the whole case would, in short, be more severe. He thought it probable that lumbar puncture would assist the diagnosis. His patient had no hydrocephalus.

Dr. CECIL WILLLIAMS read a paper on some points on the artificial feeding of infants. After referring to the difference between human and cow's milk, he passed to the value of the various ingredients and the manner in which cow's milk may be treated to render it suitable for young children. He referred to the methods of preparing humanised milk, and the use of whey and proprietary foods. He classified the latter, and mentioned their value from different points of view.

BERTRAM M. H. ROGERS, *Reporter.*

J. PAUL BUSH, *Hon. Sec.*

The Library of the Bristol Medico-Chirurgical Society.

The following donations have been received since the publication of the List in September:

November 30th, 1899.

Clifton Shakspere Society (1)	1 volume.
Alban Doran (2)	1 ,,
Sir William Mac Cormac, Bart. (3)	1 ,,
Bertram M. H. Rogers, M.D. (4)	75 volumes.
R. Shingleton Smith, M.D. (5)	11 ,,
Surgeon-General, United States Army (6)... ... · ··	1 volume.

Charles W. Sutton (7) ... ...   1 volume.
Government of the Colony of Tasmania (8)   ...   2 volumes.
Council of University College, Bristol (9)... ....   1 volume.

Unbound periodicals have been received from Dr. R. Shingleton Smith.

THIRTY-FOURTH LIST OF BOOKS.

The titles of books mentioned in previous lists are not repeated.

The figures in brackets refer to the figures after the names of the donors, and show by whom the volumes were presented. The books to which no such figures are attached have either been bought from the Library Fund or received through the *Journal*.

Ashby and G. A. Wright, H. *The Diseases of Children* ... ... 4th Ed. 1899

Basham, W. R. ... *Renal Diseases*... ... ... (4) 1870

Bauhinus, C. ... *Theatrum Anatomicum, accessit Appendix* 1600

Beard and A. D. Rockwell, G. M. *Medical and Surgical Electricity* ... (4) 1871

Bennett, J. H. ... *The Principles and Practice of Medicine* (4) 4th Ed. 1865

Bentley, A. J. M. *The Maintenance of Health in Egypt* ... ... 3rd Ed. [N.D.]

Boott, F. ... ... *Memoir of John Armstrong : to which is added an Inquiry into the Facts connected with Malaria Fever.* 2 vols. ... ... (4) 1833–34

Bottone, S. R. ... *Radiography* 1898

Bryant, T. ... ... *On Villous Growths and the Common Affections of the Rectum* 1899

Bull, T. ... ... *The Sense Denied and Lost* ... ... (4) 1859

Carless, W. Rose and A. *A Manual of Surgery* ... ... 2nd Ed. 1899

Casserius *Placentinus, J. Tabulæ Anatomicæ* lxxiix. *D. Bucretius* xx. *supplevit* 1632

Catalogue (Index) of the Library of the Surgeon-General's Office, United States Army 2nd Ser., Vol. IV. (D—Emulsions) (6) 1899

Catlow, J. P. ... *Principles of Æsthetic Medicine* ... ... (4) 1867

Clarke, J. J. ... *Orthopædic Surgery*... 1899

Clever, W. ... ... *The Flower of Phisicke* 1590

Cohn, B. ... ... *Klinik der embolischen Gefässkrankheiten* ... ... (4) 1860

Columbus, R. ... *De Re Anatomica libri* xv. 1572

Cosgrave, E. M. ... *Experimental Proofs of the Role of Alcohol* 1899

Credland, W. R.... *The Manchester Public Free Li raries* ... ... (7) 1899

Davis, J. H. ... *Parturition* ... ... (4) 2nd Ed. 1865

Denis, P. S. ... *Recherches expérimentales sur le Sang humain* ... (4) 1830

Doran, A. ... ... *Shakespeare and the Medical Society* ... ... (2) 1899

Duns, J. ... ... *Memoir of Sir J. Y. Simpson, Bart.* 1873

Eccles, A. S. ... *Difficult Digestion due to Displacements*... 1899

Edinger, L. ... ... *Anatomy of the Central Nervous System of Man* (Tr. from 5th German Edition by W. S. Hall) 1899

Ellis, H. ... ... *Psychology of Sex.* 2 vols. 1897–1900

Encyclopædia Medica (Ed. by C. Watson). Vols. I., II. 1899

Féré, C. ... ..., *The Pathology of Emotions* (Tr. by R. Park) 1899

Fourier, C. ... ... *The Passions of the Human Soul* (Tr. by Rev. J. R. Morell) ... ... (4) 1852

Fox, W. T. ... ... *The Classification of Skin Diseases* ... ... (4) 1864

Gamgee, J. ... ... *The Cattle Plague* ... ... (4) 1866

Garnett, R. ... ... *Essays in Librarianship and Bibliography* 1899

Geoffroy-Saint-Hilaire, I. *Vie, Travaux et Doctrine scientifique d'Étienne Geoffroy-Saint-Hilaire* ... ... (4) 1847

Gerhardt, C. ... *Lehrbuch der Kinderkrankheiten* .. .. (4) 1861

Gillespie, A. L. ... *A Manual of Modern Gastric Methods* 1899

Gregory, G.... ... *Lectures on the Eruptive Fevers* ... ... (4) 1843.

Harrogate as a Health Resort ... ... (5) 1899

Hedley, W. S. ... *Therapeutic Electricity* 1899

Hickman, W. ... *Cancerous Disease of Bone* ... ... (4) 1865

Hippocrates, C. ... *Opera quae extant, Graece et Latine, scholiis illustrata à H. Mercuriali.* 2 vols. in 1 1588

Hobhouse, E. [Ed.] *Health Abroad*... 1899

Howard, T. ... ... *On the Teeth* ... ... (4) 5th Ed. 1853

Jamin, J. ... ... *Cours de Physique* (4) Tomes I, 3e Éd., 1871, II. III., 2e Éd. 1868-69

Kerbert, J. J. ... *Klinische Memoranda* ... ... (4) [1859]

Kölliker, A.... ... *Mikroskopische Anatomie* Bd. II. Erste hälfte (4) 1850

Leamington Spa, Royal : the Midland Health Resort ... ... (5) [N.D.].

Lebert, H. ... ... *Handbuch der allgemeinen Pathologie und Therapie* (4) 1865.

Liebig, J. ... ... *Animal Chemistry* (Ed. by W. Gregory) (4) 2nd Ed. 1843.

Mac Cormac, H. ... *Consumption*, ... (4) 2nd Ed. 1865.

Mac Cormac, Sir W. *The Hunterian Oration, 1899* ... ... (3) 1899

Macpherson, J. ... *Mental Affections* 1899

Madge, H. ... ... *The Diseases of the Fœtus in Utero* ... ... (4) 1854

Marsh, Sir H. ... *Clinical Lectures* (Ed. by J. S. Hughes) ... ... (4)[1867]

Mays, T. J. ... ... *Pulmonary Consumption*... ... ... (5) 1891

Méric, H. de ... *Dictionnaire des Termes de Médecine. Français-Anglais* 1899

Middleton, G. S.... *Clinical Records* ... ... (4) 1894

Miles, A. ... ... *Surgical Ward Work and Nursing* ... ... 2nd Ed. 1899

Monro, T. K. ... *Raynaud's Disease* 1899

Mullen, B. ... ... *Salford and the Inauguration of the Public Free Libraries Movement*... 1899

Murray, W.... ... *Rough Notes on Remedies* ... ... 3rd Ed. 1899

Neale, R. ... ... *The Medical Digest—Appendix, 1891–99* 1899

Newman, D. ... *Renal Cases* 1899

Pamphlets ... ... 7 vols. ... ... (4) [V.D.]

Physicist ... ... *Human Nature.* Part II. 1899

Pick, T. P. ... ... *Surgery* 1899

Piorry, P.-A. ... *De la Percussion médiate*... ... ... (4) 1828

Platt, J. E.... ... *Fractures and Dislocations of the Upper Extremity* ... 1899

Portsmouth, Southsea and Neighbourhood, Guide to (Ed. by H. T. Lilley) (5) 1899

Quain, R. ... ... *On some Defects in General Education* ... ... (4) 1870

Radcliffe, C. B. ... *Epilepsy and other Convulsive Affections* (4) 2nd Ed. 1858

Rayer, P. ... ... *Traité des Maladies des Reins.* 3 vols.... ... (4) 1839–41

Robinson, M. ... *A Guide to Urine Testing* 1899

Rockwell, G. M. eard and A. D. *Medical and Surgical Electricity* ... (4) 1871

Rose and A. Carless, W. *A Manual of Surgery* ... ... 2nd Ed. 1899.

Rutlidge, C. S. ... *Guide to Queensland* ... ... (1) [N.D.]

Sanitary Institute, The *Illustrated List of Exhibits to which Medals have been Awarded at their Exhibitions, 1889–98* ... 1899.

Seubert, M. C. W. *De Functionibus radicum arteriorum et posteriorum Nervorum Spinalium Commentatio* ... ... (4) 1833

Shaw's *Manual of the Vaccination Law* ... ... 7th Ed. 1899.

Smith, F. J.... ... *Differential Diagnosis with Clinical Memoranda* 1899

Snell, S. ... ... *On the Prevention of Eye Accidents Occurring in Trades* 1899

Spencer, W.... ... *Spencer's Disease* ... ... 1899.

Spigelius, A. ... *De Humani Corporis Fabrica libri decem* 1632

Steffen, A. ... ... *Klinik der Kinderkrankheiten* 2 vols.... ... (4) 1865–70

Stephanus, N. ... *Castigatio Epistolæ maledicæ quam L. de Bils scripsit ad T. Bartholinum* 1661

Stonham, C.... ... *A Manual of Surgery.* Vols. I., II. ... ... 1899.

Swieten, G. van... *The Commentaries upon the Aphorisms of Dr. H. Boerhaave* (Translated) (4) Vols. VI., 1757, IX. 1765

Tasmania, *Handbook of. Hints to Intending Settlers and Immigrants* (8) 1897

,, ,, *With list of Reference Works on the Resources of the Colony* .. .. (8) 1899.

Temple, W.... ... *Pro Mildapetti de Unica Methodo Defensione contra Diplodophilum Commentatio* 1584

Thomson, H. C. ... *An Introduction to Diseases of the Nervous System* ... 1899.

Thorne, W. B. ... *The Schott Methods of the Treatment of Chronic Diseases of the Heart* ... ... 3rd Ed. 1899.

Valleix, F.-L.-I... *Guide du Médecin Praticien* 5 vols. (4) 4e Éd. 1860–61

Ventilation, *Natural and Artificial Methods of*... 1899

Vesalius, A. ... *De Humani Corporis Fabrica libri septum* ... ... 1543.

,, ... *Suorum de Humani Corporis Fabrica Librorum Epitome* 1600

Virchow, R. [Ed.] *Handbuch der speciellen Pathologie und Therapie* Bd. I. ... ... (4) 1854

Walker, Jane H. *Open-Air Treatment of Consumption* ... ... 1899.

Walshe, W. H. ... *The Physical Diagnosis of Diseases of the Lungs*... (4) 1843

,, .. *Diseases of the Lungs and Heart* ... ... (4) 1851

Watson, J. K. ... *A Handbook for Nurses* ... . 1899.

Whytt, R. ... ... *Observations on those Disorders commonly called Nervous, Hypochondriac, or Hysteric* ... ...(4) 3rd Ed. 1867

Wilson, E. ... ... *Lectures on Dermatology* ... ... (4) 1875.

Wooton, E. ... ... *A Guide to the Medical Profession* (Ed. by L. F. Winslow) ... ... (4) [1882]

Wright, H. Ashby and G. A. *The Diseases of Children* ... ... 4th Ed. 1899.

TRANSACTIONS, REPORTS, JOURNALS, &c.

Advertiser's A B C, The ... ... (4) 1893.

American Public Health Association, Reports and Papers of the
Vol. XXIII. 1898.

Archives of Neurology from the Pathological Laboratory of the London County Asylums ... ... [N.D.]

Archives of the Roentgen Ray ... ...Vol. III. 1899.

Columbia University, Studies from the Department of Pathology of
     the College of Physicians and Surgeons   Vol. VI., Part 1 1898–99
Edinburgh Medical Journal   ...   ...Vols. XIV., Part 2, XV., Part 1   1869–70
Edinburgh Obstetrical Society, The Transactions of the   Vol. XXIV.   1899
Epidemiological Society of London, Transactions of the
                                       N.S., Vol. XVIII.   1899
Hospitals—
     Dublin Hospital Reports, The   ...   .Vols. III.—V.   1822–30
     Johns Hopkins Hospital Reports, The   Vols. VII., Nos. 5–9, 1899;
                                       VIII., Nos. 1, 2   1899
     London Hospital for Diseases of the Chest, City of—Pathological
         Report, 1887–88   ...   .   (5)   1889
Hospitals and Charities, Burdett's   1899
Journal of Mental Science, The   ...   Vols. IV.—VI., 1858–60 ;   VIII.—
     XII., 1863–67 ;   XIV.—XVIII., 1869–73 ;   XLII., XLIII., 1896–97;
     General Index   Vols. I.—XXIV., 1879; XXV.—XXXVIII.   [1893]
Medical Annual Synoptical Index, The, 1887–98   ...   .[1899]
Medical Society of London, Transactions of the   ..   ...   Vol. XXII.   1899
Medico-Chirurgical Transactions   ..   Vols. LXXIX., 1896 ; LXXXII.   1899
Mexico—Informes Rendidos por los Inspectores Sanitarios de Cuartel
     y los de los Distritos al Consejo Superior de Salubridad, 1898...   1899
Michigan State Medical Society, Transactions of the   ...   Vol. XXIII.   1899
New York, Transactions of the Medical Society of the State of   1899
Ohio State Medical Society, Transactions of the   1899
University College, Bristol—Calendar for the Session 1899–1900 ...   (9)   1899

Local Medical Notes.

BARNSTAPLE.

NORTH DEVON INFIRMARY.—Mr. Joseph Harper presided at the
annual meeting of those interested in this institution on August 15th.
The medical report showed that 622 patients had been admitted during
1898. The average daily number was 41 and the average stay was
twenty-three days. The financial statement showed that the expenditure amounted to £2,362, which is much above the ordinary income of
the infirmary. The friendly societies of Barnstaple have recently
collected over £200 for the local Infirmary and Dispensary.

BATH.

SEWERAGE.—A considerable amount of money has been spent upon
the proposed sewage scheme for Bath. Land has been purchased at
Salford, where it was proposed that the sewage should be intercepted
and chemically treated. The Local Government Board have recently
stated that they were not prepared to entertain any proposal as to a
partial scheme for sewage disposal, and consequently for the present
the matter is in abeyance. Apparently the only effective manner
of disposing of the sewage of Bath without sending it into the river is
for the authorities of that city to join in the Bristol scheme, and take

the sewage through a large drain to the Bristol Channel. The Bristol Authority has approached the Bath Corporation upon the matter.

PUBLIC HEALTH.—Dr. W. H. Symons has been re-appointed Medical Officer of Health for Bath, at a salary of £435 per annum.

BRENTRY.

ROYAL VICTORIA HOME.—Dr. W. Cotton has been appointed, *pro tem.*, Honorary Medical Officer.

BRIDGWATER.

PUBLIC HEALTH.—Mr. F. W. Stoddart has been re-appointed Borough Analyst.

BRISTOL.

THE CONVALESCENT HOME.—The visit of Her Majesty the Queen to open the Convalescent Home, which is for all time to maintain the memory of her sixty years of reign over her people, was, from the point of view of the many thousands who lined the route of procession, a small matter. What really interested the citizens of Bristol and the inhabitants of the neighbourhood was the presence of Her Majesty herself. This is hardly the place to enlarge on the loyalty of her subjects; but at the present time, when the Queen shows a greater interest, if possible, in the welfare of her people than she has ever shown, mention must be made of the enthusiastic reception she received from the moment she stepped out of the railway carriage to the time she entered it again. During the two hours she was in Bristol the roar of applause and cheers was continuous, and many a young child in years to come will remember the day when Queen Victoria was drawn by four horses through the streets of our ancient city. The weather, as it usually is when the Queen has any function to perform, was beautiful; in fact the day was just the one the Queen is said, and we believe truly, to like—crisp, sunny, and with a nip in the air, which does not please the fancy of many of her less robust subjects. At any rate, Sir Arthur Bigge telegraphed soon after Her Majesty's return to Windsor that not only was she much moved by her loyal reception by the city of Bristol, but that she was not unduly fatigued by the journey. When we consider Her Majesty's advanced age, many will wonder how she is able to bear, in the marvellous manner she does, the ordeals of such a reception and the fatigue of a journey of nearly two hundred miles by rail.

Of the civic ceremonies which took place at the Joint Station and the Council House little mention need be made in a medical periodical, except to record the graceful action of Her Majesty in dubbing the Lord Mayor a Knight, an honour which was exceedingly popular. At the Convalescent Home, Sir Herbert Ashman presented Sir Edward P. Wills, upon whom a K.C.B. has been recently so deservedly bestowed in recognition of his work in connection with the Institution. After a prayer from the Bishop of Bristol, and the singing of the hymn "Oh, King of kings" to the tune "Bishopgarth," an address was read to Her Majesty, who returned a written reply, and the President presented his daughter (from whom the Queen accepted a bouquet), Mr. J. Storrs Fry, Mr. Edward Robinson, Mr. P. H. Vaughan, the Rev. R. Glover, D.D., Mr. J. N. C. Pope, Mr. H. O. Wills, Sir Frederick Wills, Bart., Mr. F. J. Fry, Mr. Charles Thomas, Mr. P. F. Sparke Evans, Mr. W. L. Bernard, and the Matron (Miss Ellis).

The Queen's carriage was then drawn to the front entrance, and with an electric communication Her Majesty opened the door, the "jewelled electrical letter-weight" with which this part of the ceremony was performed being presented to her as a *souvenir*.

The procession then reformed and passed onwards to the station, which Her Majesty left soon after 4 p.m.

Reference must be made to the monster gathering of children on Durdham Down. Here, in a stand about a third of a mile in length, about 27,000 children were assembled, and, under the conductorship of Mr. Riseley, sang to Her Majesty two verses of the National Anthem. Those who were near inform us that the Queen was deeply touched at the sight, and the sounds of so many young voices. The shrill cheering could be heard a mile away. Since the ceremony, Her Majesty has telegraphed to enquire whether the children arrived safely at their homes, and it is a matter for sincere congratulation to those who so ably organised this wonderful gathering that not only was no child lost in the crowds, but that there was no accident of any sort, and among the immense number there were only four cases of fainting. Indeed, from what we can hear, the amount of work which the voluntary members of the St. John Ambulance Association had to do was inconsiderable. No serious accident has been reported, except one at St. Philip's Station late at night, when a lady was pushed under a train with fatal results. When we hear that the crowd has been calculated to have been composed of 700,000 persons, this speaks well for the good humour and patience of everyone.

MEDICAL SCHOOL DINNER.—The revival of the Medical School dinner reflects great credit on the organisers. It is now some years since the annual dinner was discontinued, and, if we can judge from the numbers who assembled at the Spa on November 16th, the new lease of life appears to be vigorous. Mr. Nelson C. Dobson took the chair, having on his right the guest of the evening, His Honour Judge Austin, and near them were seated most of the Professors of Bristol University College, both those connected with the Faculty of Medicine and of Arts. After dinner, the Chairman proposed in excellent taste the health of Her Majesty, and announced that a telegram had been sent to Windsor to say how gratified those assembled were to hear of Her Majesty's safe journey and that she was not over-fatigued by the ceremony of the 15th. The speech, however, of the evening was that made by the Rev. A. N. Blatchford in proposing "The Army, Navy, and Reserve Forces," which at a time like the present is sure to find a hearty response. Everyone—to use Kipling's expression —shouted "Rule Britannia" at the top of their voices, for Mr. Blatchford's oratory touched the patriotic *chordæ tendineæ*. Prof. Ryan, whose departure from Bristol at an early date robs us of our most amusing after-dinner speaker, indulged in his usual pleasantries, and was well received, while other speeches were made by Judge Austin, Dr. J. O. Symes, Mr. A. W. Prichard, Dr. A. J. Harrison, Mr. A. L. Flemming, Mr. Munro Smith, Dr. W. H. Daw of H.M.S. *Antelope*, and Mr. F. R. Cross. The Chairman's health was proposed by Dr. Shingleton Smith in felicitous terms, and Mr. Dobson replied. The gaiety of the evening was increased by several excellently-rendered songs, and the only criticism of an adverse nature we have to make was that the proceedings were rather too long, that a suspicion of rowdiness was noticed in one region of the room, and that the room was rather cold. We have no doubt that the School dinner will be an annual institution.

The point to which most speakers referred was the recent amalgamation of the clinical work of the Infirmary and Hospital, and the position of the Medical Faculty with regard to the University College, some claiming that the Medical School, as the elder, was the parent of the College, while others, though admitting the age of the Medical Department, argued that the University College was its mother. The physiological impossibility of the daughter being older than the mother did not seem to trouble those who claimed a maternal position for the Bristol University College.

CARDIFF.

PREVENTION OF CONSUMPTION.—At a well-attended meeting of the Cardiff Medical Society, held on October 13th, a resolution was unanimously carried approving of the formation of a local branch of the National Association for the Prevention of Tuberculosis. The Medical Officers of Health of Cardiff and Rhondda, in supporting the resolution, asked for the assistance of individual members of the medical society in addressing public meetings in Glamorgan and the adjoining counties. The Medical Officer of Health of Cardiff (Dr. Edward Walford) is issuing leaflets in connection with the steps being taken for the prevention of tuberculosis by the sanitary authority. In one of these it is stated that in Cardiff, out of a total number of about 2,500 deaths which occur annually from all causes, about 200 are due to phthisis. Instructions are given as to the precautions necesssary to prevent the spread of infection from a consumptive person to those about him. In another leaflet issued to dairymen, cowkeepers, and purveyors of milk, instructions are given as to the means of preventing the spread of tuberculosis among cattle.

INFIRMARY.—Dr. W. M. Stevens has been appointed Honorary Pathologist.

CHELTENHAM.

OBITUARY.—Mr. Lauriston Winterbotham died at his residence, Arundel House, on August 8th. The deceased, who was in his sixty-sixth year, was the son of the late Mr. John Winterbotham, and his brother, Mr. Alderman J. B. Winterbotham, is the deputy-mayor of Cheltenham. Mr. Winterbotham received his medical education at St. Bartholomew's Hospital, and qualified as M.R.C.S. Eng. and L.S.A. in 1858. He shortly afterwards commenced practice in Cheltenham, and was for several years surgeon to the General Hospital; upon his resigning this appointment, he was elected consulting surgeon to the institution. He was also consulting surgeon to the Dispensary for Diseases of Women and Children, and surgeon to the Cheltenham College. Mr. Winterbotham (who married a daughter of the late Mr. Solomon Leonard, of Clifton) has left a widow and three children to mourn his loss. The funeral took place on August 11th, at the Cheltenham Cemetery, in the presence of a large number of people.

CHEPSTOW.

OBITUARY.—Mr. Edward Pendrill King died on September 23rd, in his 66th year. He received his medical education at St. Bartholomew's Hospital, and took the qualifications of M.R.C.S. Eng. and L.S.A. in 1858 and 1859 respectively. The deceased held several public appointments, being formerly coroner for the manor of Chepstow, medical officer of health of Chepstow, and also medical officer of the Shire-newton District and the workhouse of the Chepstow Union. Mr. King was assistant-surgeon to the 1st Monmouthshire Rifle Volunteers.

He had been in failing health for some months past, and had recently resigned all his appointments. Mr. King will be much missed in Chepstow, where he was extremely popular.

DAWLISH.

HOSPITAL.—The recent fête organised on behalf of the Hospital has resulted in a sum of £236 being handed over to that institution.

DEVONPORT.

ROYAL ALBERT HOSPITAL.—Mr. J. J. N. Morris has been appointed Assistant Surgeon.

DORCHESTER.

LUNACY.—At the quarterly meeting of the Dorset County Council, held on August 1st, Lord Digby, the chairman of the Asylums Committee, referred to the great increase of pauper lunacy in the county, and stated that additional accommodation would shortly have to be provided, although the new asylum had only recently been opened.

EXETER.

TYPHOID FEVER.—At the meeting of the City Council, held on September 13th, it was stated that in the recent outbreak of typhoid fever at Exeter seventy out of eighty cases had been traced to the eating of uncooked cockles at Exmouth. The city analyst had examined the effluent from the mouth of the sewer at Exmouth, where the cockles were gathered, and he had found that it consisted of a mixture of sea-water and untreated sewage. It was stated that the sale of the cockles had been stopped at Exmouth, but that they were being sent to other towns. Mr. E. J. Domville proposed that the Devon County Council should be communicated with, in order that an application might be made to the Local Government Board to declare the whole of the estuary of the river Exe a stream within the meaning of the Rivers Pollution Act. After some discussion, the motion was carried. At the meeting of the City Council held on September 27th, a special report was presented by the senior District Medical Officer of the city upon the recent epidemic of typhoid fever. This stated that from July 1st to September 11th there were 85 cases of the disease notified, and of these 58 patients had partaken of raw cockles at or from Exmouth. Nine of the patients had only visited Exmouth, and one had partaken of other shell-fish than cockles. 67 cases had been treated at the sanatorium, with five deaths. One of the nurses there had contracted the disease. The cost of the epidemic would be between £1,500 and £2,000. During the discussion which followed the reading of the report some of the members said that they ought to be grateful to their medical officers for the steps which they had taken to cut short the epidemic.

WEST OF ENGLAND EYE INFIRMARY.—The annual meeting of this institution was held on October 27th. The medical report stated that 2,891 patients had been under treatment, of whom 2,517 had been discharged cured and relieved, so that on September 30th there remained 333 out-patients and 41 in-patients. The daily average number of in-patients had been 46. The financial statement showed that the ordinary income amounted to £1,494, and that there was a favourable balance of £179. The committee added that satisfactory progress is being made with the first section of the new building, which will be shortly completed, and an earnest appeal was made for £9,000 to continue the work.

FALMOUTH.

TYPHOID FEVER.—At the meeting of the Falmouth Corporation held on September 28th, the memorandum issued by Dr. G. S. Buchanan (of the Local Government Board) was considered. Dr. Buchanan advises that the residents should be cautioned to boil all water, and that the sewers should be flushed. He adds that there is a large number of defective house drains in Falmouth, and advises that all should be thoroughly supervised, and recommends the appointment of a second Sanitary Inspector without delay. The Corporation decided to follow the advice of Dr. Buchanan, who is still pursuing his enquiries into the sanitary condition of the town.

HALWELL.

A MUNIFICENT GIFT.—Mrs. Medley has promised to build, furnish, and endow a cottage hospital for Halwell, Devonshire. The building, which will contain four wards, is to be furnished by July next, the cost being about £2,220.

KINGSBRIDGE.

TYPHOID FEVER.—At the meeting of the Urban District Council, held on October 4th, the Medical Officer of Health (Dr. Webb) reported that there had been three cases of typhoid fever caused by eating cockles.

MAESTEG.

MEMORIAL TO A MEDICAL MAN.—The fund for providing a memorial to the late Dr. W. Hopkin Thomas has just been closed. The sum realised was about £700, and it has been decided that the memorial should take the form of a fountain with commemorative tablets.

PENRYN.

TYPHOID FEVER.—At the meeting of the East Kerrier Rural District Council, held on August 5th, the Medical Officer of Health reported that he had traced a case of typhoid fever to the patient having eaten cockles gathered from the mud of Penryn river. Last year he had traced three cases to the same cause.

PLYMOUTH.

PUBLIC DISPENSARY.—The annual meeting of those interested in the Plymouth Public Dispensary was held on October 18th. The report showed that during the year 3,670 patients had been treated, against 3,345 in the preceding year. In the provident department there were 112 admissions during the year—an increase of 29—and there were at present 696 names on the books. The expenditure amounted to £1,070, as against £987 for 1898. The gross receipts of the provident department were £132, against £128 in the previous year. The annual subscriptions were £367, as compared with £359 in 1898. The income from dividends amounted to £421, and Sir Massey Lopes had contributed £1,000 during the past two years. It has been decided to extend the accommodation of the Dispensary, and new buildings were being erected at a cost of £575. The chairman urged that this being the centenary year of the institution a strong appeal should be made to wipe off the debt of £219.

ST. GERMANS.

VACCINATION.—At the meeting of the Board of Guardians, held on August 2nd, it was stated that the vaccination fees for the past six months were four times the amount of those for the preceding half-year.

STROUD.

INFECTIOUS DISEASE HOSPITAL.—It is stated that the Stroud Joint Hospital Board have decided upon a site in the populous district known as Horns Road, for the erection of an infectious disease hospital. This proposal has already met with some opposition on the part of ratepayers.

SWANSEA.

GENERAL HOSPITAL.—Every alternate year for seventeen years past the Baroness Patti-Cederström (Madame Patti) has organised a concert in aid of the General Hospital and other charities in the town. Not only does she herself take part in the programme, but she induces other well-known artistes to volunteer their services, entertaining them at Craig-y-nos and bringing them by special train to Swansea. The last of this series of concerts was given on August 3rd, and is considered to have quite eclipsed any of its predecessors. About £600 was realised. Dr. D. E. Evans has been appointed Anæsthetist and Pathologist.

TAUNTON.

SEWERAGE.—At a special meeting of the Town Council, held on September 7th, it was decided to adopt the septic tank system of sewage disposal. The cost was estimated at about £22,000.

TAUNTON AND SOMERSET HOSPITAL.—£1,000 have been subscribed in Somerset as a memorial to the late Colonel Chard, V.C. It has been decided to erect a memorial bust and to endow a bed in the Taunton and Somerset Hospital for a Somersetshire-born soldier, his wife, widow, or child.

TAVISTOCK.

PUBLIC HEALTH. — Mr. E. C. Brodrick has been re-appointed Medical Officer of Health.

THORNBURY.

PUBLIC HEALTH.—Dr. F. T. Bond has been re-appointed Medical Officer of Health.

TIVERTON.

INFIRMARY.—The new wing, which has been erected to celebrate Her Majesty's Diamond Jubilee, was formally opened by Sir Stafford Northcote, M.P., on August 10th, in presence of a large gathering. The new building comprises two wards of two beds each for male and female patients, an operation-room, nurses' room, waiting-room, etc. The cost was about £1,550.

TORQUAY.

INCIPIENT CONSUMPTION HOSPITAL.—On the suggestion of the honorary medical staff, the committee of the Western Hospital for Incipient Consumption, some few months ago, made a special appeal to the public for funds, with the result that the hospital has been fitted with balconies and wind-screens for the adoption of the open-air treatment, the ventilation of the building has been improved, and the electric light installed.

OCKERDEN CONVALESCENT HOME.—Lady Helen Vincent re-opened this institution at Torquay on November 2nd. The Home was founded in 1890 by Miss M. Erle, who died last year, and it has now been given by her sister, Miss Eleanor Erle, for the use of patients from the Royal Devon and Exeter Hospital. With the gift of the Home, Miss Erle gave £400 to cover the cost of completely renovating the building.

TRURO.

ROYAL CORNWALL INFIRMARY.—The annual meeting of the friends of this institution was held on August 14th. The annual report showed that during 1898 there had been 416 in-patients admitted, as against 369 in the preceding year. The average duration of residence was 27 days, against 31 days in 1897. The average daily number of in-patients was 31. The out-patients numbered 650, an increase of 149 compared with the preceding year. The receipts amounted to about £2,100, as against £1,858 in 1897. The expenditure was £1,900, being nearly £100 more than last year.

WESTBURY.

PUBLIC HEALTH.—Mr. W. H. Reed has been appointed Medical Officer of Health.

YEOVIL.

WATER SUPPLY.—The new reservoir, constructed to hold 1,000,000 gallons, is now completed.

The College of Physicians of Philadelphia.

The next award of the Alvarenga Prize will be made on July 14th, 1900. Essays intended for competition may be upon any subject in medicine, and must be received by the Secretary of the College on or before May 1st, 1900. Further information may be obtained from the Secretary, Dr. Thomas R. Neilson.

SCRAPS

PICKED UP BY THE ASSISTANT-EDITOR.

Clinical Records (29).—A woman whose husband had been a sufferer for many years wrote to the proprietors of a well-advertised preparation: "My husband had suffered terribly for a long time from a distressing complaint. After taking four doses of your medicine he was in quite another world."

The Queen's Visit.—In one of the Bristol wards notice was given that the entertainment provided by the Lord Mayor's Fund would be given to all those who were alive at the time of the Queen's accession. A woman who applied for a ticket said that she was born in November, 1837. When she was told that she was not eligible, as the Queen's accession was in June of that year, she asked: "Do you mean to say that I was not alive then?" The presiding official, whose embryology was sound, gave her a ticket.

Obstetrics Home and Foreign (7).—In the collection entitled Sylva, or the Wood, p. 130, we read that "a few years ago, in this same village, the women in labour used to drinke the urine of their husbands, who were all the while stationed, as I have seen the cows in St. James's Park, straining themselves to give as much as they can."—Brand's *Popular Antiquities*, ed. Bohn, 1849, vol. ii., pp. 69, 70.

In ancient Mexico, a decoction of the root of a plant called *civapaethi*, which possessed some oxytocic properties, was given, but if the pains were too severe a small piece of the tail of an opossum, carefully rubbed down in water, had to be taken. However ridiculous this may seem, it is not more so than a prescription given by the court physician in Siam to a lady of high rank at the time of her confinement: "Rub together shavings of sapan wood, rhinoceros blood, tiger's milk (a fresh deposit found on certain leaves in the forest), and cast-off skins of spiders."—Engelmann's *Labor Among Primitive Peoples*, 1882, p. 135.

Medical Philology (XXXII.).—The word "disease," now almost monopolised as a medical term, had formerly a much wider signification, "with distinct reference to the etymological elements of the word." In its non-medical meaning it has had a longer life as a verb than as a substantive.

Illustrating its wide range of signification, two instances may be quoted from the particularly interesting uses of the word given by the *New English Dictionary*. Where the Authorised Version reads in *John* xvi. 33, "In the world ye shall have tribulation," Wyclif (1388) has "In the world 3e schulen haue disese," and in *Mark* v. 35 Tindale (1526) has "Thy doughter is deed; why deseasest thou the master eny further."

The *Catholicon* has "to Desese; *tedere*," with "to noye" in a cross-reference. Mr. Herrtage's note reads :

'*Desaise*, f. A sickenesse, a being ill at ease. *Desaisé*, out of temper, ill at ease.' Cotgrave. In the Version of the History of Lear and his daughters given in the *Gesta Romanorum*, p. 50, we are told how the eldest daughter, after keeping her father for less than a year, 'was so anoyed and *disessed* of hym and of his meanes' that she reduced the number of his attendants; and in chap. 45 we read of a law that the victor in battle should receive on the first day four honours, 'But the second day he shall suffre iiij. *diseases*, that is, he shall be taken as a theef, and shamfully ledde to the prison, and be dispoyled of Iubiter clothyng, and as a fole he shall be holden of all men; and so he shall have, thet went to the bataile, and had had the victorie.' E. E. Text Soc. ed. Herrtage, p. 176.

The Specialist and his Telegrams.—Perhaps it is because the specialist is a modern product that his bent is so strongly towards modern ways, and towards utilising for his own purposes the facilities offered by modern social methods. That he should be a man of many instruments is not surprising, and that these instruments should run largely to electricity is only in the nature of things; that his letters should be typed and his notes dictated to a shorthand writer may be taken for granted; and that he should be on the telephone, and have a registered telegraphic address are mere matters of course. This telegraphic address is of peculiar interest, for it enables the specialist to do what without it he would find difficult; namely, to announce his line of practice. No one would care to put on his door-plate, "Specialist in Heart Disease," but nothing is simpler than to stamp one's notepaper, "Telegrams—'Cardiac, London,'" which serves the same purpose. Moreover, this is just the sort of thing the public likes. There is something so "simple" and "common sense" about it. It really is becoming a serious matter to the well-to-do public, who of course never write letters but telegraph for everything, to have to decide what doctor to call in! But this telegraphic address business is the very thing. Why bother about knowing the names of all the specialists? If one knows one's own complaint that is quite enough; and every person of intelligence, of course, knows what is the matter with him, notwithstanding the fuss that pedantic doctors make about what they call diagnosis! All that one has to do when one feels "chippy" is to decide what sort of a man one wants, and then to send for him. Is it headache that we suffer from? "Headache, London," will fetch us just the specialist we want. Or, if we feel doubtful about our liver, "Liver, London," will do the trick. Who the man is, who, as they say of dogs, "answers to the name," what he has done, or even what his real name is, we do not know; perhaps we do not care. Why, indeed, should we trouble about all these details? It is the specialist that we want, and by this ingenious device we get him. Perhaps the specialist also gets what he wants, so that the accommodation is quite mutual. Which ought to be satisfactory to all parties—except those who have been too late in choosing their registered telegraphic address.—*The Hospital.*

Medicine as a Profession.—In an address delivered to the candidates for graduation of the Johns Hopkins University, Dr. Walter B. Platt said: "As a physician you will change many of the ideas you have previously held to be true. One of these is the view you have held of your fellow-men. Men will be found to be much worse than you ever dreamed and much better than you ever supposed; stronger in right purpose than you believed, and failing those nearest them at the critical moment. You will more than accomplish the desire of Adam and become as a god, knowing good from evil more than other men. You will see the human heart stark naked, and beautiful or hideous, as it is made. No robe or cassock can hide the dreadful deformity which you alone of human beings will sometimes see beneath it. No station or high office of great estate will afford the least protection or shelter from your gaze. You will find hearts as dry of human kindness as any rock smitten by Moses in the wilderness was of water, but others brimming over with a constant and endearing sympathy that makes you instant captive. Your ideas of what men usually call the power of religion will be rudely shaken, for you will see men of years devoted to the observance of the churches tremble at the far-off bugle call of the gray angel, while gigantic rascals hear the near rustle of his wings without a tremor . . . You will believe as much in the perfect virtue of many good women as in the almost total depravity of others. At times you will think that all men are liars, until you find those whose perfect truthfulness a thousand times outweighs those dark and devious ways. To know how good and how bad men and women are, you must practise medicine. . . . To feel that you hold the life of a man in the hollow of your hand, that his earthly career is at the ends of your fingers, that you are surely going to save him from death by your action, by your intelligence, and that his years will go on as if nothing had dragged him to the edge of a precipice and almost over; is not this a triumph greater than that of a soldier, who has taken instead of saved human life? Can you imagine any greater satisfaction than to do this, not once only but many times, not to speak of the pleasure of relieving pain or bringing peace and comfort where there was unhappiness and discomfort. Every physician should have in his office, for his own edification, the finest obtainable copies of the ' Prodigal Son,' to see if art can equal what he daily sees and hears. Have a statue of Venus in an opposite corner from one of Cupid, for you are a daily witness of the trouble which comes to young men and old who follow strange gods. . . . A physician ought to be a gentle Stoic, a bit of an Epicurean, and a true Christian gentleman. We read that Arthur, when he made a knight, said: ' Be ye a good knight, and so I pray to God, so ye may be, and if ye be of prowess and of worthiness, ye shall be a knight of the Table Round '; and we who are physicians say this to every one of you."—*Boston Medical and Surgical Journal.*

Medical Bibliography.—By the recent death of the *Index Medicus* all medical libraries and workers in medicine have had a severe loss. In our June number a method was suggested for carrying on the work. Other schemes are in the air. At the last meeting of the American Medical Association it was resolved, on the motion of Dr. Gould, to whom medical literature owes so much: " That the executive committee of the American Medical Association appoint a committee of three members of the Association to take general charge of the publication of the periodical, perfect plans for the same, and engage the services of an editor and of such editorial assistants as may be required, etc., to choose a publisher and make contracts with him for the printing, distribution, etc., of the work, all in such a manner that it shall continue the high standard of accuracy and bibliographic usefulness so well established by the previous editors; and That the treasurer of the Association be instructed to pay all bills endorsed by said committee in payment of the necessary expenses of such editing and publication, provided that these do not exceed an annual outlay of over $3000." (*Journal of the American Medical Association*, June 10, 1899.) Dr. Marcel Baudouin, that prolific worker in so many departments of medicine, thinks that France is especially fitted to take a leading part in establishing a successor to the *Index Médicus*, because the recently-founded Institut de Bibliographie has a great deal of the material ready to hand. (*Gazette médicale de Paris*, 10 Juin, 26 Août, 1899. See also *Medical and Surgical "Review of Reviews,"* July, 1899.) But whilst other people have been talking some persons in Vienna have been working, and several numbers of the *Index Medicus Novus* have been issued. That the interests of English readers will not be disregarded is evident from the circular which heralded the new venture, and of which I append a copy :—

" The necessity to have an organ of information of the whole medical literature of world is wellknowne percieved by all investigators and practioners all days more and more. Such work demands extreemely much toil, time and expenses, for there must be gathered the whole medical journal-literature of every country and even in all languishes, to give all times an resumption quite complete of the whole medical literature.

" Through the persuasion of prominent authorities and by cooperation of professioners, we resolved, to satisfy this pressing whishes, to produce such an underprize and so we founded the ' Index Medicus Novus.' — We must say that the sacrifices which are necessary to the work in each regard are more important as we thought in the beginn; but we will continue now the undertaken work because there is no doubt, that the whole medical world will have the greatest interest of it. Next time we will give also a specification of all medical-scientific-books coming just out, as all medical dissertations of the universities quite regular; so the ' Index Medicus Novus' will become a collection for consultation quite unsurpassed and as theer has been nothing likewise before it in the medical knowledge science.

" To have an easy and quiekly review of the great deal of the stuff we fixed to publish the ' Index Medicus Novus' twice mouthly to the 1. and 15., in mind to publish the literature of world who appeared in this short time as soon and complete as possible. Than we tryed to comprise the special compartments to have an easy review and we observe, that the division ' Naturalia' shows those essays which are composed by graduated phisicians or for the least acts of scientific, clinical questions and in the 'Academia' those recipients, which are discussed in the sessions of the academies of sciences on the jurisdiction for medical investi-gation. Those last named very important essays have been till now generally quite — unknown to the broader medical circles, because they are only published in the academical publications.

" Though all this performances we set the price for subscribition very low, to make it possible to each scientific searcher to buy the ' Index Medicus Novus.' So we hope con-fidently that the interested circles well assist (to this undertakement quite as important than scientific and exertions) by her participation and furtherance. We will not omit to say that our bureau translates in all languishes each essay wished by anyone.

" This number appears exeptionally as a double-number.

" We the honour to send you the ' Index Medicus Novus' and you can have, if you like it, still the numbers of the first quarter of the year.

" Saying that we will try to follow willingly to the wishes and incitations of learned-mans with great veneration

" the Redaction of

" INDEX MEDICUS NOVUS."

In order that an intending purchaser shall not go wrong, a detachable slip, worded in the form given below, is provided for the purpose of ordering the publication :

ORDRE.

To the redaction of "INDEX MEDICUS NOVUS"

Vienna, I. Tuchlauben 23.

I subscribe the "**Index Medicus Novus**" from the 1. Oct. ....till .... and send you the amount of

Frs. 5.— for 1 quarter of a year

„ 10.— „ ½ year

„ 20.— „ 1 year

Please to give a very clear adress

Date

The not disired is to strike through.

The ordre is to rip and send by the post in enveloppe to the redaction of "Index Medicus Novus."

LIST OF SUBSCRIBERS

TO

The Bristol Medico-Chirurgical Journal.

DECEMBER, 1899.

England.

CAMBRIDGESHIRE:

CAMBRIDGE.
G. S. Woodhead

CHESHIRE.

ALDERLEY EDGE.
J. McElfatrick

NEW BRIGHTON.
A. W. Riddell

CORNWALL.

EAST LOOE.
L. F. Houghton

LISKEARD.
S. E. Rigg

ST. AUSTELL.
W. Mason

HELSTON.
B. C. Kendall

PENZANCE.
W. S. Bennett
J. A. Fox
J. Symons

WEEK-ST -MARY.
S. H. Rentzsch

DEVONSHIRE.

BABBACOMBE.
T. Finch

CHAGFORD.
A. D. Hunt

NEWTON ABBOT.
J. Culross

BAMPTON.
A. R. Down

CULLOMPTON.
G. G. Gidley

PAIGNTON.
J. Alexander

BARNSTAPLE.
C. H. Gamble
J. Harper
M. Jackson

DARTMOUTH.
R. B. Searle

PLYMOUTH.
G. F. Aldous
R. H. Clay
Medical Society
E. B. Thomson
W. L. Woollcombe

BRIXHAM.
G. C. Searle

DEVONPORT.
F. E. Row

BROAD CLYST.
J. Somer

EXETER.
J. M. Ackland
H. Davy
R. V. Solly
E. B. Steele-Perkins
R. Thomas
L. H. Tosswill

PLYMPTON.
C. Aldridge
W. D Stamp

BUDLEIGH SALTERTON.
T. G. C. Evans

26

DEVONSHIRE *(Continued).*

TORQUAY.

SOUTH MOLTON.

H. J. Smyth

H. Humphreys
W. Odell
R. Pollard

W. Powell
C. H. Wade

WINKLEIGH.

J. H. Norman

DORSETSHIRE.

DORCHESTER.

P. W. MacDonald

STURMINSTER NEWTON.

J. C. Leach

WEYMOUTH.

J. M. Lawrie

ESSEX.

NEWPORT.

W. A. Smith

GLOUCESTERSHIRE.

ALMONDSBURY.

J. C. MacWatters

BRISTOL.

W. R. Ackland
J. Ambrose
T. R. Atkinson
W. M. Barclay
T. G. L. Baretti
B. J. Baron
A. E. Blacker
A. F. Blagg
E. C. Board
C. W. J. Brasher
H. F. Briggs
J. Broom
F. St. J. Bullen
E. F. H. Burroughs
J. P. Bush
A. Carr
T. M. Carter
W. F. Carter
T. Carwardine
R. H. Chilton
J. M. Clarke
T. V. Coker
H. Cook
F. N. Cookson
W. Cotton
R. J. Coulter
F. R. Cross
J. Dacre
D. S. Davies
N. C. Dobson
E. A. G. Dowling
E. L. W. Dunbar
E. Eberle
F. H. Edgeworth
W. Elder
C. Elliott
J. Ewens
E. Fawcett
R. G. Fendick
J. L. Firth
T. Fisher
A. L. Flemming

E. L. Fox
J. Freeman
W. J. Fyffe
E. B. Garland
T. T. Genge
W. C. Gent
D. S. Gerrish
A. N. G. Gibbs
J. S. Griffiths
L. M. Griffiths
W. B. T. Gubbin
C. D. G. Hailes
A. H. Haines
H. E. Harris
A. J. Harrison
W. H. Harsant
A. G. Hayman
C. A. Hayman
J. C. Heaven
C. K. C. Herapath
H. E. Hetling
H. Hill
T. Hill
General Hospital
G. A. Imlay
H. W. Kendall
F. P. Lansdown
R. G. P. Lansdown
A. E. A. Lawrence
E. L. Lees
R. C. Leonard
W. Ligertwood
J. J. S. Lucas
F. W. McCrea
A. B. McKee
G. Metcalfe
W. A. Milligan
H. F. Mole
A. T. Morgan
C. A. Morton
G. T. Myles
B. G. Neale

W. N. Nevill
C. Newman
W. H. C. Newnham
T. D. Nicholson
C. O'Brien
A. Ogilvy
G. S. Page
G. Parker
J. H. Parry
A. W. Peake
H. C. Pearson
W. A. Perry
C. F. Pickering
W. E. Pountney
J. J. Powell
A. W. Prichard
J. E. Prichard
A. B. Prowse
B. M. H. Rogers
F. Rose
W. B. Roué
C. K. Rudge
H. T. Rudge
J. E. Shaw
E. J. Sheppard
E. M. Skerritt
G. M. Smith
R. S. Smith
E. H. E. Stack
W. H. Steele
C. Steele
J. B. Stephenson
W. H. Stevens
F. W. Stoddart
J. Swain
J. G. Swayne
S. H. Swayne
W. C. Swayne
J. O. Symes
J. Taylor
W. J. Tivy
H. Waldo

GLOUCESTERSHIRE (Continued).

BRISTOL (continued).

C. H. Walker
C. H. Wallace
J. H. Wathen

C. J. Whitby
J. Wilding
E. C. Williams
P. W. Williams

W. R. Williams
H. W. Windsor-Aubrey
C. Wintle

CHELTENHAM.

W. J. K. Millard
G. A. Peake
E. Trevithick
L. Winterbotham

GLOUCESTER.

R. W. Batten
W. R. Hadwen
W. Hodges
J. G. Soutar

STONEHOUSE.

G. T. B. Watters

STOW-ON-THE-WOLD.

E. Dening

CHIPPING SODBURY.

F. F. Fox
A. Grace

HAMBROOK.

E. Crossman
F. W. Crossman
W. F. B. Eadon

STROUD.

A. S. Cooke

KINGSWOOD.

L. W. Powell

TETBURY.

W. Wickham

CIRENCESTER.

W. R. Cossham
O. H. Fowler
C. Mackinnon

LYDNEY.

W. P. Kennedy

THORNBURY.

E. M. Grace
L. H. Williams

COLEFORD.

L. B. Trotter

PARKEND.

W. C. Halpin

REDFIELD.

J. W. Rodgers

WESTBURY-ON-TRYM.

A. Harvey
H. L. Ormerod

DOWNEND.

H. Skelton

ST. GEORGE.

J. Young

WINTERBOURNE.

R. Eager
W. Eager

FISHPONDS.

W. Brown

STAPLETON.

H. A Benham

STOKE BISHOP.

H F Parsons.
C. E. Wedmore

WOTTON-UNDER-EDGE.

J. G. Boyce
D. H. Forty

HAMPSHIRE.

ALTON.

W. L. P. Bevan

CARISBROOKE.

J. Groves

FLEET.

H. Wilcox

SOUTHAMPTON.

W. R. Y. Ives

BOURNEMOUTH.

C. H. Ackland
J. S. Dickie
J. G. Harsant

LYMINGTON.

J. Rendall

SOUTHSEA.

J. W. Cousins

HUNTINGDONSHIRE.

ST. NEOT'S.

T. C. Grey

LANCASHIRE.

LIVERPOOL.

G. A. Hawkins-Ambler

PRESTON.

J. E. Garner

MIDDLESEX.

LONDON.

Bayer Co.
J. Berry
T. C. Fox
M. Handfield-Jones

W H. A. Jacobson
H. M. Jones
Lord Lister
E. J. Maclean
J. Macready

A. L. Marshall
F. T. Roberts
W. J. Seward
E. C. Taylor

TOTTENHAM.

W. H. Plaister

MONMOUTHSHIRE.

NEWPORT.

W. Basset
C. B. Gratte
O. E. B. Marsh
C. Matthews
A. G. Thomas
H. E. Williams

PONTYPOOL.

J. R. Essex
S. B. Mason

RHYMNEY.

T. H. Redwood

TREDEGAR.

G. A. Brown

NORFOLK

WALPOLE ST. ANDREWS.

R. Smith

NOTTINGHAMSHIRE.

NOTTINGHAM.

C. B. Taylor
W. M. Willis

OXFORDSHIRE.

OXFORD.

H. P. Symonds

SOMERSETSHIRE

BATH.

W. D. Akers
E. J. Cave
F. S. Cowan
S. Craddock
W. M. Ellis

A. E. W. Fox
T. B. Goss
P. King
F. Lace
T. P. Lowe
W. S. Melsome

R. J. H. Scott
L. H. Walsh
L. A. Weatherly
J. Wigmore
A. S. Wohlmann

BRIDGWATER.

F. J. C. Parsons
J. L. K. Pringle
R. H. F. Routh

BRISLINGTON.

B. B. Fox
W. M. Morton
C. M. Phillips

BURNHAM.

F. C. Berry

CHEDDAR.

R. W. Statham

CLEVEDON.

H. J. Capron
T. Davis
W. J. Hill
J. Martin

CREWKERNE.

W. J. Penny
W. W. Webber

CURRY RIVEL.

R. H. Vereker

FRESHFORD.

C. E. S. Flemming

FROME.

A. W. Dalby
J. M. Rattray
C. R. Wood

HAM GREEN.

F. P. Mackie

ILMINSTER.

C. Munden

KEYNSHAM.

G. G. D. Willett

SOMERSETSHIRE *(Continued).*

LANGPORT.
J. Morgan

LEIGH WOODS.
J. Harvey.

MILVERTON.
C. Randolph

PILL.
T. W. S. Morgan

PORTISHEAD.
G. Boyd
W. Monckton
C. A. Wigan

SOUTH PETHERTON.
S. W. MacIlwaine

TAUNTON.
H. T. S. Aveline
Taunton Hospital
H. T. Rutherford

TIMSBURY.
F. Woods

WEDMORE.
J. Ford
R. P. Tyley

WELLINGTON.
J. Meredith

WELLS.
W. Fairbanks
W. A. L. Smith

WESTON-SUPER-MARE.
H. T. M. Alford
H. S. Ballance
C. P. Crouch
G. B. Fraser
E. F. Martin
G. F. Rossiter
R. Roxburgh
J. W. Smith
G. H. Temple
J. Wallace

WORLE.
F. St. J. Kemm

WRINGTON.
H. C. Bristowe
H. W. Collins

YEOVIL.
W. R. M. Semple

SUFFOLK.

BECCLES.
F. H. Hudson.

SURREY.

VIRGINIA WATER.
S. R. Philipps

WARWICKSHIRE.

LEAMINGTON.
A. W. W. Hoffman

WILTSHIRE.

BRADFORD-ON-AVON.
W. J. A. Adye
J. Beddoe

CALNE.
W. S. Batten

DEVIZES.
C. Eddowes

SWINDON.
W. Howse
J. C. Maclean

FOVANT.
C. Clay

MALMESBURY.
R. Kinneir

WARMINSTER.
R. L. Willcox

WORCESTERSHIRE.

WORCESTER.
R. W. Brimacombe

Ireland.

ANTRIM.

BELFAST.

J. W. Browne   A. Jamison   J. A. Lindsay

Wales.

BRECONSHIRE.

TALGARTH.

W. Howells

CARMARTHENSHIRE.

FERRYSIDE.   LLANELLY.

P. Williams   S. J. Roderick

CARNARVONSHIRE.

ST. CLEARS.

R. Thomas

GLAMORGANSHIRE.

ABERDARE.

E. Jones

CARDIFF.

P. R. Griffiths   W. Price   J. L. Thomas
T. G. Horder   A. Sheen   H. R. Vachell
D. R. Paterson   Medical Society   J. Williams

GORSEINON.

T. Mitchell

MERTHYR TYDVIL.
W. W. Jones   PENARTH.   PORTH.
C. E. G. Simons   R. F. Nell   H. N. Davies
J. L. W. Ward
                SWANSEA.   TREHARRIS.
    R. C. Elsworth   E. Le C. Lancaster   W. W. Leigh

PEMBROKESHIRE.

HAVERFORDWEST.

E. P. Phillips

Belgium.

COURTRAI.

Dr. Lauwers

Switzerland.

DAVOS-PLATZ.

W. R. Huggard

Cape Colony.

FORT BEAUFORT.
J. Shaw
KING WILLIAM'S TOWN.
H. M. Chute

United States.

COLORADO.
S. E. Solly
CHICAGO.
Columbus Medical Library

Italy.

GENOA.

S. Biamonti

Egypt.

ALEXANDRIA.
J. Mackie

CAIRO.
M. A. Ruffer

New Zealand.

LOWER HUTT.
J. R. Purdy

India.

BHAGELPORE.
N. Muzumider

INDEX.

Aarons, Dr. S. J.—Golden rules of gynæcology (Review), 362.

Abdominal surgery, Ovariotomy and—H. Cripps (Review), 265.

Abdominal surgery, Some groups of interesting cases of—C. A. Morton, 203.

Achondroplasia—Dr. F. H. Edgeworth, 27; C. E. S. Flemming, 21.

Allbutt, Dr. T. C. [Ed.]—A system of medicine (Review), 56, 346.

American Pediatric Society, Transactions of the (Review), 75.

American Physicians, Transactions of the Association of (Review), 364.

American Surgical Association, Transactions of the (Review), 275.

American year-book of medicine and surgery (Review), 157.

Anæsthetists, The transactions of the Society of (Review), 277.

Anastomosis, Intestinal, 248.

Anatomy, Tablets of—T. Cooke and F. G. H. Cooke (Review), 54.

Anderson, Dr. T. M'C.—Contributions to clinical medicine (Review), 255.

Animal as a prime mover, The—R. H. Thurston (Review), 359.

Annual and analytical cyclopædia of practical medicine (Reviews), 157, 277.

Antrum of Highmore, Muco-purulent catarrh of the, 338.

Aphasia and other speech defects—Dr. H. C. Bastian (Review), 268.

Apoplexy, On the temperature in cases of—Dr. J. M. Clarke, 97.

Archives provinciales de médecine (Review), 159.

Army, Recollections of thirty-nine years in the—Sir C. A. Gordon (Review), 53.

Arterial disease, Ophthalmoscopic evidence of, 47.

Asthma, On so-called spasmodic—Dr. E. Kingscote (Review), 360.

Atkinson, Dr. T. R.—Aids to examinations (Review), 270.

Baby feeding (Review), 155.

Bacteria, Pathogenic—Dr. J. McFarland (Review), 272.

Bacteriology, An atlas of—Dr. C. Slater and E. J. Spitta (Review), 261.

Bacteriology, A manual of—Dr. R. T. Hewlett (Review), 353.

Bacteriology of some suppurations complicating pulmonary disease—Dr. J. O. Symes, 30.

Baldy, Dr. J. M. [Ed.]—An American text-book of gynecology (Review), 354.

Bangs and W. A. Hardaway, Drs. L. B. [Eds.]—An American text-book of genito-urinary diseases, syphilis, and diseases of the skin (Review), 64.

Bannatyne, Dr. G. A.—Rheumatoid arthritis (Review), 72.

Barclay, Dr. W. M.—Report on surgery, 331.

Baron, Dr. B. J.—Report on larngology and rhinology, 336.

Bastian, Dr. H. C.—A treatise on aphasia and other speech defects (Review), 268.

Beard, J.—On certain problems of vertebrate embryology; The span of gestation and the cause of birth (Reviews), 141.

Bell, Dr. J.—Notes on surgery for nurses (Review), 365.

Bell, Dr. R.—Chloroform: its absolutely safe administration (Review), 272.

Bergey, Dr. D. H.—An investigation on the influence upon the vital resistance of animals to the micro-organisms of disease' brought about by prolonged sojourn in an impure atmosphere (Review), 272.

Bicêtre—Recherches cliniques et thérapeutiques sur l'épilepsie, l'hystérie, et l'idiotie (Review), 156.

Birth, The span of gestation and the cause of—J. Beard (Review), 141.

Blake, Dr. E.—On the study of the hand for indications of local and general disease (Review), 359.

Blood, The—Dr. A. C. Coles (Review), 55.

Boston Society of Medical Sciences, Journal of the (Review), 77.

Bradycardia, A case of extreme—R. G. Fendick and Dr. G. Parker, 113; Notes on the eye symptoms—F. R. Cross, 113.

Breast, Cancer of the, 128.

Breast, Diseases of the—Dr. A. M. Sheild (*Review*), 266.

Breast, Extensive operations for cancer of the, 331.

Bristol in the eighteenth century, Medical—W. H. Harsant, 297.

Bristol Medico-Chirurgical Society, 79, 161, 367.

British food journal, The (*Review*), 159.

British physician, The (*Review*), 278·

Brodie, Sir Benjamin Collins—T. Holmes (*Review*), 140.

Brodie, Dr. T. G.—The essentials of experimental physiology* (*Review*), 54.

Bronchitis, On the treatment of sub-acute—Dr. F. H. Edgeworth, 197.

Burghard, Drs. W. W. Cheyne and F. F.—A manual of surgical treatment (*Review*), 350.

Burr, Dr. C. B.—A primer of psychology and mental diseases (*Review*), 357.

Bush, J. P.—Some unusual operations on lunatics and their results, 219.

Caledonian medical journal (*Review*), 278.

Cancer and tuberculosis, The ferment treatment of—Dr. H. Manders (*Review*), 262.

Cancer of the breast, 128.

Cancer of the tongue, 130.

Cardio-vascular repair, Observations on—Dr. W. B. Thorne (*Review*), 360.

Carless, W. Rose and A.—A manual of surgery (*Review*), 143.

Carpus backwards, A case of dislocation of the hand and—Dr. T. Mitchell, 121.

Carwardine, T.—Report on surgery, 244.

Case paper—Drs. J. K. Crouch and E. Le C. Lancaster (*Review*), 365.

Cataract, A treatise on "unripe"—Dr. W. A. M'Keown (*Review*), 356.

Cataract extraction, 46.

Catheterisation of the ureters, 244.

Cautley, Dr. E.—The natural and artificial methods of feeding infants and young children (*Review*), 69.

Cerebro-spinal meningitis, Epidemic—Drs. W. T. Councilman, F. B. Mallory, and J. H. Wright (*Review*), 270.

Chavasse's Advice to a mother (*Review*), 73; Advice to a wife (*Review*), 73.

Chemistry, Practical organic—S. Rideal (*Review*), 154.

Cheyne and F. F. Burghard, Drs. W. W.—A manual of surgical treatment (*Review*), 350.

Childhood, Medical diseases of infancy and—Dr. D. Williams (*Review*), 151.

Children, An American text-book of the diseases of—Dr. L. Starr [Ed.] (*Review*), 355.

Children, Clinical examination and treatment of sick—Dr. J. Thomson (*Review*), 151.

Children, Dementia in, 330.

Children, General paresis in, 329.

Children, Lumbar puncture in, 326.

Children, Nervous diseases following acute specific fevers in, 328.

Children, Pocket formulary for the treatment of disease in—Dr. L. Freyberger (*Review*), 363.

Children, The study of—Dr. F. Warner (*Review*), 69.

Children's teeth, The diseases of—R. D. Pedley (*Review*), 74.

Chirurgie, Association Française de. 11° Congrès. Procès-verbaux (*Review*), 156.

Chloroform—Dr. R. Bell (*Review*), 272.

Chreiman, M. A.—Health loss and gain (*Review*), 155.

Clarke, Dr. J. M.—On the temperature in cases of apoplexy, and on the occurrence (1) of œdema and (2) loss of the knee-jerk in the paralysed limbs in hemiplegia, 97; Report on medicine, 326.

Climatology, Medical—Dr. S. E. Solly (*Review*), 145.

Clinical investigation, Atlas of methods of—Dr. C. Jakob (*Review*), 142.

Clinical Society of London, Transactions of the (*Review*), 274.

Clouston, Dr. T. S.—Clinical lectures on mental diseases (*Review*), 258.

Coles, Dr. A. C.—The blood : how to examine and diagnose its diseases (*Review*), 55.

Consumptive sanatorium for the people, The erection of a—Dr. Nahm (*Review*), 362.

Consumptives, Sanatoria for—Dr. F. R. Walters (*Review*), 348.

Cooke, T. and F. G. H.—Tablets of anatomy (*Review*), 54.

Corfield, Dr. W. H. — Dwelling houses: their sanitary construction and arrangement (*Review*), 155.

Cory, Dr. R. — Lectures on the theory and practice of vaccination (*Review*), 153.

Cotton, Dr. W.—A simple form of influence machine for X-ray work, 222.

Councilman, F. B. Mallory, and J. H. Wright, Drs. W. T.— Epidemic cerebro-spinal meningitis and its relation to other forms of meningitis (*Review*), 270.

Crile, Dr. G. W.—An experimental research into surgical shock (*Review*), 352.

Cripps, H.—Ovariotomy and abdominal surgery (*Review*), 265.

Cross, F. R.—Notes on the eye-symptoms of a case of extreme bradycardia, 113.

DaCosta, Dr. J. C.—A manual of modern surgery (*Review*), 259.

Darwin and the theory of natural selection, Charles—E. B. Poulton (*Review*), 254.

Dementia in the young, 330.

Dermatitis, 249.

Dermatological Society of Great Britain and Ireland, Transactions of the (*Review*), 76.

Dermatology, Report on—Dr. H. Waldo, 249.

Devon and Exeter Medico-Chirurgical Society, 175.

Diabetes mellitus and its treatment —Dr. R. T. Williamson (*Review*), 60.

(Diabetes mellitus), Wesen, ursache und behandlung der zuckerkrankheit—Dr. A. Lenné (*Review*), 61.

Diagnosis, A clinical text-book of medical—Dr. O. Vierordt (*Review*), 344.

Diarrhœa, Treatment of summer— Irrigation of the large intestine, 339; Lavage of the stomach, 340.

Dictionary, Lippincott's medical (*Review*), 138.

Dictionary of medical terms (English -French)—H. de Méric (*Review*), 342.

Diet and food—Dr. A. Haig (*Review*), 269.

Diet in chronic kidney disease, 244.

Diphtheria, Epidemic—Dr. A. Newsholme (*Review*), 70.

Diphtheria, Vomiting and cardiac failure in connection with, 339.

Directory of booksellers and bibliophile's manual, The international (*Review*), 366.

Dislocation of the hand and carpus backwards, A case of—Dr. T. Mitchell, 121.

Dispensing for nurses, Notes on pharmacy and—C. J. S. Thompson (*Review*), 155.

Dowse, Dr. T. S.—The treatment of disease by physical methods (*Review*), 361.

Dwelling houses—Dr. W. H. Corfield (*Review*), 155.

Ear, Diseases of the—Dr. E. B. Gleason (*Review*), 273.

Edgeworth, Dr. F. H.—Achondroplasia, 27; On the treatment of subacute bronchitis, 197.

Edinburgh medical journal (*Reviews*), 158, 278.

Edinburgh Obstetrical Society, Transactions of the (*Reviews*), 276, 365.

Edkins, Drs. E. Klein and J. S.— Elements of histology (*Review*), 154.

Electro-therapeutics, Conservative gynecology and—Dr. G. B Massey (*Review*), 150.

Embolism of the mesenteric vessels, 41.

Embryology, On certain problems of vertebrate—J. Beard (*Review*), 141.

Encyclopædia medica—Dr. C. Watson [Ed.] (*Review*), 344.

Endocarditis, A case of acute ulcerative—Dr. H. L. Ormerod, 15.

English sanitary institutions—Sir J. Simon (*Review*), 138.

Épilepsie, l'hystérie et l'idiotie, Recherches cliniques et thérapeutiques sur l' (*Review*), 156.

Epiphyses, Traumatic separation of the—J. Poland (*Review*), 260.

Examinations, Aids to—Dr. T. R. Atkinson (*Review*), 270.

Eyeball, Excision of the, 48.

Eyeball, Use of electro-magnet in extracting foreign bodies in the, 45.

Eye-reflexes in infants, Condition of the pupils and, 327.

Eye, System of diseases of the— Drs. W. F. Norris and C. A. Oliver [Eds.] (*Review*), 267.

Fayrer, Sir J.—Inspector-General Sir James Ranald Martin (*Review*), 50.

Feeding infants and young children, The natural and artificial methods of—Dr. E. Cautley (*Review*), 69.

Fendick and Dr. G. Parker, R. G.—A case of extreme bradycardia, 113.

Fenwick, E. H.—Golden rules of surgical practice (*Review*), 361.

Ferment treatment of cancer and tuberculosis, The—Dr. H. Manders (*Review*), 262.

Filters, An inquiry into the relative efficiency of water—Drs. G. S. Woodhead and G. E. C. Wood (*Review*), 71.

Firth, J. L.—Report on surgery, 41.

Fisher, Dr. T.—Report on medicine, 36.

Flemming, C. E. S. — Achondroplasia, 21.

Forensic medicine and toxicology—Dr. J. D. Mann (*Review*), 70.

Formulæ, Physicians' book for private (*Review*), 280.

Freyberger, Dr. L. — The pocket formulary for the treatment of disease in children (*Review*), 363.

From our dead selves to higher things—F. J. Gant (*Review*), 72.

Frontal sinus, Chronic empyema of the, 337.

Fürbringer, Dr. P.—Text-book of diseases of the kidneys and genitourinary organs (*Review*), 65.

Fürstner, Dr. C. — Wie ist die fürsorge für gemüthskranke von aerzten und laien zu fördern? (*Review*), 270.

Gadd, H. W.—A synopsis of the British Pharmacopœia, 1898 (*Review*), 272.

Gant, F. J.—From our dead selves to higher things (*Review*), 72.

Gastric ulcer, 238.

Gemüthskranke von aerzten und laien zu fördern, Wie ist die fürsorge für—Dr. C. Fürstner (*Review*), 270.

General paresis in the young, 329.

Genito-urinary diseases, syphilis, and diseases of the skin, An American text-book of—Drs. L. B. Bangs and W. A. Hardaway [Eds.] (*Review*), 64.

Genito-urinary surgery and venereal diseases—Drs. J. W. White and E. Martin (*Review*), 144.

Gestation and the cause of birth, The span of—J. Beard (*Review*), 141.

Gibson, Dr. G. A.—Diseases of the heart and aorta (*Review*), 257.

Glands, The surgical anatomy of the lymphatic—Dr. C. H. Leaf (*Review*), 349.

Glasses for prevention of eye injuries, Protective, 46.

Gleason, Dr. E. B.—Essentials of the diseases of the ear (*Review*), 273.

Glycerin, The properties and uses of pure—M.D. (*Review*), 362.

Gordon, Sir C. A.—Recollections of thirty-nine years in the army (*Review*), 53.

Gowers, Sir W. R.—A manual of diseases of the nervous system (*Review*), 347.

Grant College Medical Society Transactions of the (*Review*), 274.

Grèce médicale, La (*Review*), 158.

Greene, R.—The Schott treatment for chronic heart diseases (*Review*), 271.

Grünwald, Dr. L.—Atlas and abstract of the diseases of the larynx (*Review*), 357.

Gynæcology, Golden rules of—Dr. S. J. Aarons (*Review*), 362.

Gynæcology, Report on—Dr. W. C. Swayne, 131.

Gynecology, An American text-book of—Dr. J. M. Baldy [Ed.] (*Review*), 354.

Gynecology and electro-therapeutics, Conservative—Dr. G. B. Massey (*Review*), 150.

Gynecology, Operative—Dr. H. A. Kelly (*Review*), 263.

Haig, Dr. A.—Diet and food, considered in relation to strength and power of endurance, training and athletics (*Review*), 269.

Halliburton, Dr. W. D.—Kirkes' hand-book of physiology (*Review*), 343.

Hallucinations and illusions — E. Parish (*Review*), 55.

Hand and carpus backwards, A case of dislocation of the—Dr. T. Mitchell, 121.

Hand for indications of local and general disease, On the study of the—Dr. E. Blake (*Review*), 359.

Hardaway, Drs. L. B. Bangs and W. A. [Eds.]—An American text-book of genito-urinary diseases, syphilis, and diseases of the skin (*Review*), 64.

Hare, Dr. F. E.—The cold-bath treatment of typhoid fever (*Review*), 258.

Hare, Dr. H. A.—A text-book of practical therapeutics (*Review*), 62.

Harley, George—Mrs. A. Tweedie [Ed.] (*Review*), 342.

Harsant, W. H.—Medical Bristol in the eighteenth century, 297.

Headache, Nasal and aural disease as a cause of, 336.

Health loss and gain.—M. A. Chreiman (*Review*), 155.

Health resorts of Europe, The mineral waters and—Dr. H. and F. P. Weber (*Review*), 146.

Heart and aorta, Diseases of the —Dr. G. A. Gibson (*Review*), 257.

Heart diseases, The Schott treatment for chronic—R. Greene (*Review*), 271.

Hemiplegia, On the occurrence (1) of œdema, and (2) of loss of the knee-jerk in the paralysed limbs in—Dr. J. M. Clarke, 97.

Hemorrhage, Post-partum, 131.

Herz, Dr. H.—Die störungen des verdauungsapparates als ursache und folge anderer erkrankungen (*Review*), 255.

Hewlett, Dr. R. T.—A manual of bacteriology (*Review*), 353.

Histology, Elements of—Drs. E. Klein and J. S. Edkins (*Review*), 154.

Hofmann, Dr. E. von—Atlas of legal medicine (*Review*), 358.

Holmes, T.—Sir Benjamin Collins Brodie (*Review*), 140.

Hospitals and charities, Burdett's (*Review*), 365.

Hurst, Drs. A. M. Marshall and C. H.—A junior course of practical zoology (*Review*), 343.

Hysterectomy for fibroid tumour of uterus —Dr. W. H. C. Newnham, 8.

Ἰατρικὴ Πρόοδος (*Review*), 158.

Illusions, Hallucinations and—E. Parish (*Review*), 55.

Index-catalogue of the library of the Surgeon-General's Office, United States Army (*Review*), 76.

Index medicus, The, 189.

Infancy and childhood, Medical diseases of—Dr. D. Williams (*Review*), 151.

Infancy and childhood, Therapeutics of—Dr. A. Jacobi (*Review*), 68.

Infants and young children, The natural and artificial methods of feeding—Dr. E. Cautley (*Review*), 69.

Infants, Condition of the pupils and eye-reflexes in, 327.

Influence machine for X-ray work, A simple form of—Dr. W. Cotton, 222.

Intestinal anastomosis, 248.

Intussusception, On irreducible— Dr. G. L. K. Pringle, 322.

Iowa State Medical Society, Transactions of the (*Review*), 274.

Ireland, Transactions of the Royal Academy of Medicine in (*Review*), 274.

Irrigation of the large intestine in summer diarrhœa, 339.

Jacobi, Dr. A. — Therapeutics of infancy and childhood (*Review*), 68.

Jakob, Dr. C.—Atlas of methods of clinical investigation, with an epitome of clinical diagnosis and of special pathology and treatment of internal diseases (*Review*), 142.

Jellett, Dr. H.—A short practice of midwifery (*Review*), 149.

Johns Hopkins hospital reports (*Review*), 74.

Journal of the Boston Society of Medical Sciences (*Review*), 77.

Journal of tropical medicine, The (*Review*), 77.

Keen, Dr. W. W.—The surgical complications and sequels of typhoid fever (*Review*), 351.

Kelly, Dr. H. A.—Operative gynecology (*Review*), 263.

Kelynack, Dr. T. N.—Renal growths (*Review*), 145.

Kidney disease, Diet in chronic, 244.

Kidney, Rupture of the, 44.

Kidneys and genito-urinary organs, Diseases of the—Dr. P. Fürbringer (*Review*), 65.

King's College hospital reports (*Review*), 156.

Kingscote, Dr. E. — On so-called spasmodic asthma (*Review*), 360.

Kirkes' hand-book of physiology— Dr. W. D. Halliburton (*Review*), 343.

Klein and J. S. Edkins, Drs. E.— Elements of histology (*Review*), 154.

Knee-jerk in the paralysed limbs in hemiplegia, Loss of—Dr. J. M. Clarke, 97.

Knowledge (*Review*), 279.

Laryngology, Report on—Dr. B. J. Baron, 336.

Larynx, Atlas and abstract of the diseases of the—Dr. L. Grünwald (*Review*), 357.

Lazarus - Barlow, Dr. W. S.—A manual of general pathology (*Review*), 147.

Leaf, Dr. C. H.—The surgical anatomy of the lymphatic glands (*Review*), 349.

Legal medicine, Atlas of—Dr. E. von Hofmann (*Review*), 358.

Lenné, Dr. A.—Wesen, ursache und behandlung der zuckerkrankheit (Diabetes mellitus) (*Review*), 61.

Library of the Bristol Medico-Chirurgical Society, 89, 177, 282, 370.

Liebig, Justus von—W. A. Shenstone (*Review*), 140.

Lippincott's medical dictionary (*Review*), 138.

Liver, Operative treatment of cirrhosis of the, 247.

Local medical notes, 92, 181, 287, 374.

London, Transactions of the Clinical Society of (*Review*), 274.

Loomis and W. G. Thompson, Drs. A. L. [Eds.] — A system of practical medicine by American authors (*Review*), 58.

Lumbar puncture in children, 326.

Lunatics, Some unusual operations on—J. P. Bush, 219.

McFarland, Dr. J.—A text-book upon the pathogenic bacteria (*Review*), 272.

M'Keown, Dr. W. A.—A treatise on "unripe" cataract (*Review*), 356.

Maddox, Dr. E. E.—Tests and studies of the ocular muscles (*Review*), 152.

Malaria, 236.

Malaria, Notes on—Surgeon-Major E. M. Wilson (*Review*), 154.

Malarial fevers, Lectures on the— Dr. W. S. Thayer (*Review*), 59.

Mallory, and J. H. Wright, Drs. W. T. Councilman, F. B.—Epidemic cerebro-spinal meningitis and its relation to other forms of meningitis (*Review*), 270.

Manders, Dr. H. — The ferment treatment of cancer and tuberculosis (*Review*), 262.

Mann, Dr. J. D.—Forensic medicine and toxicology (*Review*), 70.

Manson, Dr. P.—Tropical diseases (*Review*), 260.

Marshall and C. H. Hurst, Drs. A. M.—A junior course of practical zoology (*Review*), 343.

Martin, Drs. J. W. White and E.— Genito-urinary surgery and venereal diseases (*Review*), 144.

Martin, Inspector-General Sir James. Ranald—Sir J. Fayrer (*Review*), 50.

Martindale, W.—Drs. Harvey and Davidson's syllabus of materia medica (*Review*), 361.

Martindale and Dr. W. W. Westcott, W.—The extra pharmacopœia (*Review*), 73.

Massey, Dr. G. B.—Conservative gynecology and electro-therapeutics (*Review*), 150.

Materia medica, Drs. Harvey and Davidson's syllabus of—W. Martindale (*Review*), 361.

Materia medica, pharmacy, pharmacology, and therapeutics — Dr. W. H. White (*Review*), 155.

Medical annual (*Review*), 158.

Medical Council, Minutes of the General (*Review*), 270.

Medical defence, A year's work in (*Review*), 278.

Medical Society of London, Transactions of the (*Review*), 364.

Medicine, A system of—Dr. T. C. Allbutt [Ed.] (*Reviews*), 56, 346.

Medicine, A system of practical, by American authors — Drs. A. L. Loomis and W. G. Thompson [Eds.] (*Review*), 58.

Medicine, Contributions to clinical —Dr. T. M'C. Anderson (*Review*). 255.

Medicine, History of—Dr. R. Park (*Review*), 50.

Medicine, Practice of—Dr. F. Taylor (*Review*), 255.

Medicine, Reports on—Dr. J. M. Clarke, 326; Dr. T. Fisher, 36; Dr. G. Parker, 236; Dr. R. S. Smith, 121.

Medico - chirurgical transactions (*Review*), 363.

Mental diseases—Dr. T. S. Clouston (*Review*), 258.

Merck's annual report (*Review*), 277.

Méric, H. de—Dictionary of medical terms (English–French) (*Review*). 342.

Mesenteric vessels, Thrombosis and embolism of the, 41.

Mexico—Informes rendidos por los inspectores sanitarios de cuartel y por los de los distritos al consejo superior de salubridad (*Review*). 363.

Michigan State Medical Society, Transactions of the (*Review*), 364.

Microbes, The war with the—E. A. de Schweinitz (*Review*), 362.

Middlesex hospital reports (*Review*), 74.

Midwifery—Dr. H. Jellett (*Review*), 149; Dr. W. S. Playfair (*Review*), 354; Dr. D.,L. Roberts (*Review*), 67.

Mineral waters and health resorts of Europe—Drs. H. and F. P. Weber (*Review*), 146.

Mitchell, Dr. T.—A case of dislocation of the hand and carpus backwards, 121.

Moore, Dr. J. E.—Orthopedic surgery (*Review*), 67.

Morris, H.—On the origin and progress of renal surgery (*Review*), 259.

Morris, M.—Diseases of the skin (*Review*), 273.

Morton, C. A.—Report on surgery, 126; Some groups of interesting cases of abdominal surgery, 203.

Mother, Chavasse's Advice to a (*Review*), 73.

Muscular atrophy, A case of neuritic —Dr. J. E. Shaw, 319.

Myoma of the uterus, The surgical treatment of—W. R. Williams, 1.

Nahm, Dr.—The erection of a consumptive sanatorium for the people (*Review*), 362.

Nasal obstruction—W. J. Walsham (*Review*), 152.

Nervensystems, Pathologie und pathologischen anatomie des central-—Dr. A. Pick (*Review*),148.

Nervous diseases following acute specific fevers in children, 328.

Nervous system, A manual of diseases of the—Sir W. R. Gowers (*Review*), 347.

Newnham, Dr. W.H. C.—A case of hysterectomy for fibroid tumour of the uterus, with intra-abdominal treatment of pedicle, 8.

Newsholme, Dr. A.—Epidemic diphtheria; a research on the origin and spread of the disease from an international standpoint (*Review*), 70.

New York, Transactions of the Medical Society of the State of (*Review*), 275.

Norris and C. A. Oliver, Drs. W. F. [Eds.]—System of diseases of the eye (*Review*), 267.

Nurses, Notes on pharmacy and dispensing for—C. J. S. Thompson (*Review*), 155.

Nursing directory, Burdett's official (*Review*), 279.

Obstetrics, Report on—Dr. W. C. Swayne, 131.

Ocular muscles, The—Dr. E. E. Maddox (*Review*), 152.

O'Dwyer, Memorial to Dr. Joseph, 189.

Œdema in the paralysed limbs in hemiplegia—Dr. J. M. Clarke, 97.

Ohio State Medical Society, Transactions of the (*Review*), 275.

Oliver, Drs. W. F. Norris and C. A. [Eds.] — System of diseases of the eye (*Review*), 267.

Ophthalmia neonatorum, 49.

Ophthalmological Society of the United Kingdom, Transactions of the (*Review*), 276.

Ophthalmology, Report on—C. H. Walker, 45.

Ormerod, Dr. H. L.—A case of acute ulcerative endocarditis, 15.

Orthopedic surgery—Dr. J. E. Moore (*Review*), 67; Dr. W. M. Shaffer (*Review*), 74.

Ovariotomy and abdominal surgery —H. Cripps (*Review*), 265.

Paresis in the young, General, 329.

Parish, E.—Hallucinations and illusions (*Review*), 55.

Park, Dr. R.—An epitome of the history of medicine (*Review*), 50.

Parker, Dr. G.—Report on medicine, 236.

Parker and R. G. Fendick, Dr. G.— A case of extreme bradycardia, 113.

Patella, Fracture of the—A. W. Prichard, 104.

Pathology, General — Dr. W. S. Lazarus-Barlow (*Review*), 147.

Pedley, R. D.—The diseases of children's teeth (*Review*), 74.

Penrose, Dr. C. B.—A text-book of diseases of women (*Review*), 150.

Peritoneum after severe injuries, Tolerance of the, 248.

Pharmacopœia, 1898, A synopsis of the British—H. W. Gadd (*Review*), 272.

Pharmacopœia, The extra — W. Martindale and Dr. W. W. Westcott (*Review*), 73.

Pharmacy and dispensing for nurses, Notes on—C. J. S. Thompson (*Review*), 155.

Philadelphia monthly medical journal, The (*Review*), 159.

Philadelphia, The College of Physicians of, 381.

Philadelphia, Transactions of the College of Physicians of (*Review*), 75.

Physiology, Kirkes' handbook of— Dr. W. D. Halliburton (*Review*), 343.

Physiology, The essentials of experimental—Dr. T. G. Brodie (*Review*), 54.

Pick, Dr. A.—Beiträge zur pathologie und pathologischen anatomie des central nervensystems (*Review*), 148

Pityriasis rosea, 251.

Pityriasis rubra, 249.

Playfair, Dr. W. S.—A treatise on the science and practice of midwifery (*Review*), 354.

Poland J.—Traumatic separation of the epiphyses (*Review*), 260.

Poliomyelitis, Causes of acute, 329.

Polyclinic, The (*Review*), 160.

Poulton, E. B.—Charles Darwin and the theory of natural selection (*Review*), 254.

Prichard, A. W.—Fracture of the patella, 104.

Pringle, Dr. G. L. K.—Irreducible intussusception : with notes on a fatal case, 322.

Psilosis or "sprue"—Dr. G. Thin (*Review*), 143.

Psychology and mental disease, A primer of—Dr. C. B. Burr (*Review*), 357.

Pterygium, Etiology of, 47.

Purdy, Dr. C. W.—Practical uranalysis and urinary diagnosis (*Review*), 359.

Renal growths—Dr. T. N. Kelynack (*Review*), 145.

Renal surgery—H. Morris (*Review*), 259.

Renal tuberculosis, 239.

Respiratory tract, Diseases of the upper—Dr. P. W. Williams (*Review*), 74.

Retinitis proliferans, 48.

Rheumatoid arthritis — Dr. G. A. Bannatyne (*Review*), 72.

Rhinology, Report on—Dr. B. J. Baron, 336.

Rideal, S.—Practical organic chemistry (*Review*), 154.

Roberts, Dr. D. L.—The practice of midwifery (*Review*), 67.

Roentgen ray, Archives of the (*Review*), 278 ; A simple form of influence machine for X-ray work —Dr. W. Cotton, 222 ; X-rays in ophthalmology, 46.

Rogers, Dr. B. M. H.—Idiopathic thrombosis of the portal and contributory veins, 107 ; Report on therapeutics, 339.

Rose and A. Carless, W.—A manual of surgery (*Review*), 143.

Rotunda hospitals, Clinical report of the (*Review*), 75.

Saint Bartholomew's hospital reports (*Review*), 157.

Saint Thomas's hospital reports (*Review*), 365.

Sanatoria for consumptives — Dr. F. R. Walters (*Review*), 348.

Sanatorium for the people, The erection of a consumptive—Dr. Nahm (*Review*), 362.

Sanitary institutions, English—Sir J. Simon (*Review*), 138.

Schenk, Dr. L.—The determination of sex (*Review*), 72.

Schott treatment for chronic heart diseases, The—R. Greene (*Review*), 271.

Schweinitz, E. A. de—The war with the microbes (*Review*), 362.

Scraps, 93, 190, 295, 381.

Sex, The determination of—Dr. L. Schenk (*Review*), 72.

Shaffer, Dr. N. M.—Brief essays on orthopædic surgery (*Review*), 74.

Shaw, Dr. J. E.—A case of neuritic muscular atrophy ("peroneal" type), 319.

Sheild, Dr. A. M.—A clinical treatise on diseases of the breast (*Review*), 266.

Shenstone, W. A.—Justus von Liebig : his life and work (*Review*), 140.

Shock, An experimental research into surgical—Dr. G. W. Crile (*Review*), 352.

Sick, Preparations for the, 77, 160, 280, 366.

Simon, Sir J.—English sanitary institutions (*Review*), 138.

Skene, Dr. A. J. C.—Treatise on the diseases of women (*Review*), 68.

Skin, An American text-book of genito-urinary diseases, syphilis, and diseases of the—Drs. L. B. Bangs and W. A. Hardaway [Eds.] (*Review*), 64.

Skin, Diseases of the—M. Morris (*Review*), 273.

Slater and E. J. Spitta, Dr. C.— An atlas of bacteriology (*Review*), 261.

Smith, Dr. R. S.—Report on medicine, 121.

Soap, The antiseptic and disinfectant properties of—Dr. J. O. Symes, 193.

Societies : Bristol Medico-Chirurgical, 79, 161, 367 ; Devon and Exeter Medico-Chirurgical, 175.

Solly, Dr. S. E.—A handbook of medical climatology (*Review*), 145.

South Carolina Medical Association, Transactions of the (*Reviews*), 275, 364.

Spencer, W. G.—Outlines of practical surgery (*Review*), 62.

Spitta, Dr. C. Slater and E. J.—An atlas of bacteriology (*Review*), 261.

Starr, Dr. L. [Ed.]—An American text-book of the diseases of children (*Review*), 355.

Stevenson, Surgeon-Colonel W. F.— Wounds in war (*Review*), 63.

Stewart, Dr. R. W.—The diseases of the male urethra (*Review*), 66.

Stroebe, Dr. H.—Ueber die wirkung des neuen tuberkulins TR auf gewebe und tuberkelbacillen (*Review*), 261.

Suppurations complicating pulmonary disease, The bacteriology of some—Dr. J. O. Symes, 30.

Surgery, Atlas and epitome of operative—Dr. O. Zuckerkandl (*Review*), 351.

Surgery—Dr. J. C. DaCosta (*Review*), 259 ; W. Rose and A. Carless (*Review*), 143 ; R. F. Tobin (*Review*), 272.

Surgery for nurses, Notes on—Dr. J. Bell (*Review*), 365.

Surgery, Practical—W. G. Spencer (*Review*), 62.

Surgery, Reports on—W. M. Barclay, 331 ; T. Carwardine, 244 ; J. L. Firth, 41 ; C. A. Morton, 126.

Surgical practice, Golden rules of— E. H. Fenwick (*Review*), 361.

Surgical treatment, A manual of— Drs. W. W. Cheyne and F. F. Burghard (*Review*), 350.

Swayne, Dr. W. C. — Report on obstetrics and gynæcology, 131 ; Symphysiotomy, 11.

Symes, Dr. J. O.—The antiseptic and disinfectant properties of soap, 193 ; The bacteriology of some suppurations complicating pulmonary disease, 30.

Symphysiotomy—Dr. W. C. Swayne, 11.

Syphilis and diseases of the skin, An American text-book of genitourinary diseases — Drs. L. B. Bangs and W. A. Hardaway [Eds.] (*Review*), 64.

Taylor, Dr. F —A manual of the practice of medicine (*Review*), 255.

Teeth, The diseases of children's— R. D. Pedley (*Review*), 74.

Temperature in cases of apoplexy, On the—Dr. J. M. Clarke, 97.

Thayer, Dr. W. S.—Lectures on the malarial fevers (*Review*), 59.

Therapeutic notes (*Review*), 278.

Therapeutics of infancy and childhood — Dr. A. Jacobi (*Review*), 68.

Therapeutics, Practical—Dr. H. A. Hare (*Review*), 62.

Therapeutics, Report on—Dr. B. M. H. Rogers, 339.

Thin, Dr. G.—Psilosis or " sprue " (*Review*), 143.

Thompson, C. J. S.—Notes on pharmacy and dispensing for nurses (*Review*), 155.

Thompson, Drs. A. L. Loomis and W. G. [Eds] — A system of practical medicine by American authors (*Review*), 58.

Thomson, Dr. J. — Guide to the clinical examination and treatment of sick children (*Review*), 151.

Thorne, Dr. W. B.—Observations on cardio-vascular repair (*Review*), 360.

Thrombosis of the mesenteric vessels, 41.

Thrombosis of the portal and contributory veins, Idiopathic—Dr. B. M. H. Rogers, 107.

Thurston, R. H.—The animal as a prime mover (*Review*), 359.

Tobin, R. F.—A synopsis of surgery (*Review*), 272.

Tongue, Cancer of the, 130.

Tonsillitis, Acute, 339.

Toxicology, Forensic medicine and —Dr. J. D. Mann (*Review*), 70.

Treatment of disease by physical methods—Dr. T. S. Dowse (*Review*), 361.

Tropical diseases—Dr. P. Manson (*Review*), 260.

Tropical medicine, The journal of (*Review*), 76.

Tubercle, How to avoid—Dr. A. T. Wise (*Review*), 271.

Tuberculosis, 121.

Tuberculosis (*Review*), 365

Tuberculosis, The ferment treatment of cancer and — Dr. H. Manders (*Review*), 262.

Tuberculosis, The treatment and prevention of, 36.

Tuberkulins TR, Ueber die wirkung des neuen—Dr. H. Stroebe (*Review*), 261.

Tweedie, Mrs. A. [Ed.]—George Harley (*Review*), 342.

Typhoid fever, The cold-bath treatment of—Dr. F. E. Hare (*Review*), 258.

Typhoid fever, The surgical complications of—Dr. W. W. Keen (*Review*), 351.

Ulcerative endocarditis, A case of acute—Dr. H. L. Ormerod, 15.

Uræmia, 243.

Uranalysis, Practical—Dr. C. W. Purdy (*Review*), 359.

Ureters, Catheterisation of the, 244.

Urethra, The diseases of the male—Dr. R. W. Stewart (*Review*), 66.

Uterine fibroids, Treatment of the pedicle after the removal of, 126.

Uterine neoplasms, The varieties of —W. R. Williams, 314.

Uterus, Malignant disease of the, 133.

Uterus, The surgical treatment of myoma of the—W. R. Williams, 1.

Vaccination, The theory and practice of—Dr. R. Cory (*Review*), 153.

Venereal diseases, Genito-urinary surgery and—Drs. J. W. White and E. Martin (*Review*), 144.

Verdauungsapparates, Diestörungen des—Dr. H. Herz (*Review*), 255.

Vierordt, Dr. O.—A clinical text-book of medical diagnosis (*Review*), 344.

Viscera, Air-inflation of the hollow, 246.

Vital resistance of animals to the micro-organisms of disease brought about by prolonged sojourn in an impure atmosphere, An investigation on the influence upon the—Dr. D. H. Bergey (*Review*) 272.

Waldo, Dr. H.—Report on dermatology, 249.

Walker, C. H.—Report on ophthalmology, 45.

Walsham, W. J.—Nasal obstruction (*Review*), 152.

Walters, Dr. F. R.—Sanatoria for consumptives (*Review*), 348.

War, Wounds in—Surgeon-Colonel W. F. Stevenson (*Review*), 63.

Warner, Dr. F.—The study of children, and their school training (*Review*), 69.

Watson, Dr. C. [Ed.]—Encyclopædia medica (*Review*), 344.

Weber, Drs. H. and F. P.—The mineral waters and health resorts of Europe (*Review*), 146.

Wellcome club and institute, Programme of the inauguration of the (*Review*), 280.

Westcott, W. Martindale and Dr. W. W.—The extra pharmacopœia (*Review*), 73.

White and E. Martin, Drs. J. W. — Genito-urinary surgery and venereal diseases (*Review*), 144.

White, Dr. W. H.—Materia medica, pharmacy, pharmacology and therapeutics (*Review*), 155.

Wife, Chavasse's Advice to a (*Review*), 73.

Williams, Dr. D.—Medical diseases of infancy and childhood (*Review*), 151.

Williams, Dr. P. W.—Diseases of the upper respiratory tract (*Review*), 74.

Williams, W. R.—The surgical treatment of myoma of the uterus, 1; The varieties of uterine neoplasms and their relative frequency, 314.

Williamson, Dr. R. T.—Diabetes mellitus and its treatment (*Review*), 60.

Wilson, Surgeon-Major E. M.—Notes on malaria, in connection with meteorological conditions at Sierra Leone (*Review*), 154.

Wise, Dr. A. T.—How to avoid tubercle (*Review*), 271.

Women, Diseases of—Dr. C. B. Penrose (*Review*), 150; Dr. A. J. C. Skene (*Review*), 68.

Wood, Drs. G. S. Woodhead and G. E. C.—An inquiry into the relative efficiency of water filters in the prevention of infective disease (*Review*), 71.

Woodhead and G. E. C. Wood, Dr. G. S.—An inquiry into the relative efficiency of water filters in the prevention of infective disease (*Review*), 71.

Wright, Drs. W. T. Councilman, F. B. Mallory, and J. H.—Epidemic cerebro-spinal meningitis and its relation to other forms of meningitis (*Review*), 270.

X-rays, *see* Roentgen ray.

Year-book of scientific and learned societies (*Review*), 279.

Year-book of treatment (*Review*), 76.

Zoology, Practical—Drs. A. M. Marshall and C. H. Hurst (*Review*), 343.

Zuckerkandl, Dr. O.—Atlas and epitome of operative surgery (*Review*), 351.

Lightning Source UK Ltd.
Milton Keynes UK
UKHW021347110219
337100UK00009B/652/P